Catholic Theology of Marriage in the Era of HIV and AIDS

Catholic Theology of Marriage in the Era of HIV and AIDS

Marriage for Life

Emily Reimer-Barry

LEXINGTON BOOKS
Lanham • Boulder • New York • London

Published by Lexington Books
An imprint of The Rowman & Littlefield Publishing Group, Inc.
4501 Forbes Boulevard, Suite 200, Lanham, Maryland 20706
www.rowman.com

Unit A, Whitacre Mews, 26-34 Stannary Street, London SE11 4AB

British Library Cataloguing in Publication Information Available

Library of Congress Cataloging-in-Publication Data

Reimer-Barry, Emily.
Catholic theology of marriage in the era of HIV and AIDS : marriage for life / Emily Reimer-Barry.
p. cm.
Includes bibliographical references and index.
ISBN 978-0-7391-9628-1 (cloth : alk. paper) -- ISBN 978-0-7391-9629-8 (electronic)
1. Marriage--Religious aspects--Catholic Church. 2. Marriage--United States. 3. Catholic Church--United States. 4. AIDS (Disease)--Religious aspects--Catholic Church. 5. HIV infections--Religious aspects--Catholic Church. I. Title.
BX2250.R435 2015
261.8'3581088282--dc23
2015002507

™ The paper used in this publication meets the minimum requirements of American National Standard for Information Sciences Permanence of Paper for Printed Library Materials, ANSI/NISO Z39.48-1992.

Printed in the United States of America

Contents

Acknowledgments

I am deeply grateful for the support I received from family members, friends, mentors, and most especially the women whose stories are told in this book. My husband, Jay, has given me encouragement through the research and writing of this book and I feel very blessed to have him as my partner in life. My parents have given me unwavering support throughout my life and have modeled what *marriage for life* is all about. I'm grateful to those mentors and colleagues who have inspired and challenged me as they've shaped my thinking over the years, and especially to those who read portions of the manuscript and gave me valuable feedback: Rev. Nicholas Ayo, C. S. C., Rev. James F. Keenan, S. J., Rev. Edward C. Vacek, S. J., Patricia Beattie Jung, Susan A. Ross, Aana Marie Vigen, A. Denise Starkey, Melissa Browning, Elisabeth Vasko, Jeanine Viau, Dan Olsen, Meghan Clark, Kathryn Lilla Cox, Jennifer Beste, and Judith Liu. I would also like to thank my students at Loyola University Chicago and the University of San Diego. Their insightful questions keep me on my toes, and their enthusiasm for social justice inspires me and renews my hope. In particular, a huge thank you to Laceé Pappas for her editorial assistance and for completing the book's index and bibliography.

Many other persons helped to make this book possible. I am indebted to the case managers and community leaders who assisted in recruitment of study participants, especially Daniel T. Lunney of the National Catholic AIDS Network, Dr. Lawrence Ouellet of the University of Illinois at Chicago School of Public Health Community Outreach Intervention Project, Louise McKissick and Armando Smith of Vital Bridges, and the staff of Better Existence with HIV. I wish to thank Susana Mate for her assistance as my Spanish-English interpreter, Alissa Parra for her editorial assistance, and the blind reviewer for the helpful suggestions on revising the manuscript. A faculty research grant from the University of San Diego College of Arts and Sciences enabled me to complete the final manuscript. Thanks also to Bloomsbury Continuum, an imprint of Bloomsbury Publishing Plc., for permission to use "Church Communities and HIV-Affected Persons: Toward Abundant Life" [in *Calling for Justice throughout the World: Catholic Women Theologians on the HIV/AIDS Pandemic*, ed. Mary Jo Iozzio with Mary M. Doyle Roche and Elsie M. Miranda (Continuum, 2008), 140–146] and "The Listening Church: How Ethnography Can Transform Catholic Ethics" [in *Ethnography as Christian Theology and Ethics*, ed. Christian Scharen and Aana Marie Vigen (Continuum, 2011), 97–117] as the basis for chapters 2, 4, and 5. The original artwork on the front cover is entitled "Positive Couples," by Lucy Hunnicut. Thank you, Lucy, for giving your permission to use your artwork in this manner. I believe it captures the opennesss and the courage of the women whose stories are told in this book.

Finally, I wish to thank the courageous women who shared their stories with me. Their resilience and hope remind me that we can experience God in the daily struggles of life, and especially in the struggle to make the world more just and loving. I hope this research contributes, at least in some small way, to their flourishing and to the flourishing of other women who are living with HIV. I dedicate this book to Sue, Cheryl, Keesha, Carmen, Diva, Lettie, Crystal, and Grace, with gratitude.

Chapter One

Introduction

> Why do you see the speck in your neighbor's eye, but do not notice the log in your own eye? Or how can you say to your neighbor, "Let me take the speck out of your eye," while the log is in your own eye? You hypocrite, first take the log out of your own eye, and then you will see clearly to take the speck out of your neighbor's eye.
> Mt 7: 3–5

The first time I remember learning about Acquired Immunodeficiency Syndrome (AIDS) was in middle school. The lesson I remember went something like this: "Don't have sex before marriage because you could get sick with something terrible like AIDS." AIDS was presented as a normal, predictable consequence of a sinful action. A few years later, when celebrity basketball player Earvin "Magic" Johnson publicly disclosed that he was living with the Human Immunodeficiency Virus (HIV), which causes AIDS, my teachers relied on the same kind of logic: "He was promiscuous." I interpreted this to mean that "he broke the rules," so he got AIDS. In my early teens, I had the impression that people with AIDS must have done something wrong to deserve this disease. But if I remained pure and chaste, I would be safe. The moral message I absorbed emphasized personal responsibility: Be good, and you won't become a victim. These messages—by teachers who cared deeply about me and my classmates—still had the effect of making us judgmental and of perpetuating stigma instead of nurturing compassion. But it took me a long time to recognize the log in my eye.

When I was in my mid-twenties, I began to volunteer at an AIDS outreach agency on the north side of Chicago. This organization, which had twelve staff members and over fifty regular volunteers, provided free HIV testing, case management, housing placement, educational outreach, medical education seminars, art therapy, massage therapy, support groups, free condoms, and needle exchange. My job was to answer the phones, welcome walk-in clients, and do whatever organizational task needed to be accomplished that day. After the volunteer orientation, I felt equipped and ready to do my part. But then clients started to ask me questions.

- If my doctor prescribed a drug that isn't on the ADAP[1] approved list, how do I get it?
- Do I have to tell my boss that I'm positive?
- How do I get on the waiting list for residential drug treatment?
- Can my landlord evict me because I'm HIV-positive?
- ¿Me puede recomendar un grupo de apoyo para habla español?
- My doctor wants me to participate in a drug trial but I don't understand the medicines he wants to give me, so can you help me?

I learned very quickly that I had a lot to learn. My conversations with clients and staff members at that agency helped me to understand the gravity and complexity of the epidemic in Chicago at the time. I began to understand the social dimensions of individual behaviors and some of the barriers to behavior change. Hearing their stories, and learning about the brokenness of the health care delivery system in the United States, led me to experience a range of emotions, from anger and cynicism to empathy and concern. After some time, I began to think of my work as a part of their struggle, and eventually, I began to recognize our common struggle against the virus and the complex forces that feed it. It was through a gradual immersion into the world of the AIDS epidemic that I came to better understand my own limitations and gaps of knowledge but also the people hurt by this disease. They had names and faces; they were no longer simply statistics. And they were not evil people. Sure, they were imperfect (as we all are), but most of the people I met were kind, friendly, even funny. It became a running joke that in the lobby of this organization, we always started talking about the weather but two minutes later we would be talking about politics or religion. Through relationships with these women and men affected by HIV and AIDS I became more involved in fundraising and educational outreach initiatives. I volunteered to staff the information booth at summer music festivals and craft fairs, I walked in the AIDS walk, and I began to teach a course on HIV and AIDS at my university. Gradually, my new friends helped me to recognize the log in my eye.

In Matthew's gospel, Jesus tells his followers to stop focusing on the speck in our neighbor's eye when our own vision is obstructed by a log. But sometimes we don't notice the log in our eye. We think our answers are compassionate. We assume that women in abusive relationships can *just leave* their partners. We think that gay Christians *should be happy* living the celibate single life. We think people with addictions can *just decide to stop* using drugs. But what happens when we start to uncover the falsity of so many of our assumptions? How do we work to correct our vision, to ask for help in removing the log in our eye?

While the agency where I began to learn about AIDS is not affiliated with any religious group, many of the clients are people of faith, and I too found myself thinking about my faith when I encountered their stories. During one particular lunch table conversation, shortly after the election of Pope Benedict XVI, one of the social workers complained about how difficult it was to help clients who were in denial about their HIV-positive status. From her perspective, the Catholic Church was part of the problem. She explained that some of the devout Christians in her caseload were overcome by debilitating guilt, thought of themselves exclusively as sinners, had not fully accepted their HIV-positive status, and thought that their sickness was somehow part of God's plan, or that they would be healed by God if they only had enough faith. She called this "warped moral formation." I asked her if she thought the Catholic Church could be part of the solution, but even in my mind I did not yet know what that might mean.

As that lunch-table conversation wrapped up, I had more questions than answers. Was it fair, I wondered, to describe the Catholic Church as part of the problem? I felt some ambivalence about the question. On the one hand, Catholic teachings on disciplined sexual loving offer a beautiful description of self-gift in mutual, loving, marital relationships, and affirm the goodness and stability of family life. Catholic magisterial teaching forbids both nonmarital sex and direct contraception. The US bishops have also condemned needle exchange (clean syringe) programs. Yet in my work as a volunteer I had encountered many Chicagoans who had engaged in risky behaviors, some of whom came to this particular agency to attend support groups or to access free condoms or acquire clean needles. While I saw only a glimpse of their struggles, I heard some of their stories of homelessness, violence, and unemployment. My perception was that many were doing their best in a difficult situation, and that any attempt to help them reduce harmful consequences of risky behaviors, and to seek help for addictive lifestyles, was at least in some ways positive. Nevertheless I remained conflicted, wondering about the status of the church's more ideal position in light of these real stories of human struggle. I did not believe that my co-worker's description of "warped moral formation" described my own experience of faith formation within the church. I wondered if I was out of touch with the experiences of other Catholics in the area. As I reflected on this, more questions arose. What does compassion require? Is church teaching *good news* for people living with HIV? What did Jesus mean when he said that he wanted people to have abundant life (Jn 10:10)? What does abundant life look like for someone living with HIV?

Around the same time, I became aware of a report that named marriage as a risk factor for HIV for women across the world because of cultural expectations for women in the institution of marriage.[2] These include the expectation that women will have children, the imbalance of power between partners, which prevents some women from demanding abstinence or from negotiating barrier methods of birth control, and violence against women. This report ignited my interest in the plight of Catholic married women. Since the Catholic Church names marriage as a sacrament (that is, as a vocation that enables a graced encounter with God), how do these data from the public health community challenge our understanding of the sanctity of marriage? If a marriage is unhealthy because it exposes a spouse to a deadly virus, is it still a sacrament? Has my church been complicit in harm to married women? I began to see that in addition to my commitment to volunteer at this agency, I might make an additional contribution by proposing a theology of marriage that would be both realistic and life-affirming for women and men living with HIV and AIDS.

In conceiving of this research project I could not envision a book about the church and HIV that does not start with the stories of real people living with HIV. While I was aware of the severe impact that AIDS has had in other parts of the world—from Haiti to Zimbabwe to China—I was concerned that the experiences of persons living with HIV in my city had been overlooked. Moreover, little attention had been paid to the struggles of married women in the US context. Thus, I decided to interview Catholic married women in Chicago who are living with HIV in order to learn how the church might better support them.[3]

THEOLOGY "IN THE MIDDLE": THE ETHNOGRAPHIC TURN IN CHRISTIAN ETHICS

It is worth reflecting, at the outset, on the epistemological and theo-ethical assumptions underlying the methodology of this project. When I say epistemological assumptions, I mean that we need to ask the question: How do I know what I know? How is my knowledge conditioned by my experiences and social location? And is it possible that someone else has different knowledge precisely because of different experiences? Theology is always written from a particular context, by human beings embedded in particular historical, linguistic, and geographical spaces. These contexts shape the worldview of the theologian, although sometimes theologians do not admit to this. As a white, well-educated, healthy, and economically privileged lifelong Catholic, my life experiences are different than the life experiences of the women who are my collaborators in this book. But that, of course, is precisely why I knew that I needed their input in order to think about the church's teachings on

HIV, AIDS, and marriage. Still, I am the author of this book, and their voices are filtered through my own research. This is somewhat problematic, in that the reader experiences their stories through mine. But still it is their stories that are told. I will engage in critical self-reflection throughout as a reminder to the reader that I am interpreting their contributions and shaping my response in reaction to their stories, but I also invite readers to engage in critical self-reflection as you read, think, and react to this text. My book is not the final word but rather a modest contribution to communal ecclesial discernment about a better construction of marriage in light of the experiences described within these pages.

Some might consider this book more sociological than theological. But increasingly, theologians and ethicists have come to the conclusion that our theology and ethics cannot be written from research silos detached from reflection on the ordinary experiences of human persons in community; thus the work of sociology, economics, politics, and other forms of critical engagement, are all properly considered resources for theo-ethical reflection. Liberation theologian Gustavo Gutierrez explains the task of theology in this way:

> Theology is utterly practical, a reflection not merely on theories and concepts but on life as it really is and as it really can be. The various challenges to human life—economic, political, environmental, and medical—may seem disconnected from theology, but they are not. Theology is a reflection about life in light of the reality of God. And this means that theology is very historical. It develops in the history of the church as we try to announce the gospel within a concrete situation and in a way relevant for daily life. Thus theology is "in the middle," between the living faith of believers and the task of announcing that faith in the world.[4]

Seen from the perspective of Gutierrez, then, this book is an example of doing theology "in the middle"—in the middle of the lives of women living with HIV. This method engages women in the midst of thinking about the reality of God in their lives and about how their experiences of marriage have shaped their understanding of God's loving care for them.

Pope Francis echoes this call when he writes, in *Evangelii Gaudium*, that theology should be "in dialogue with other sciences and human experiences" and that theologians "must always remember that the Church and theology exist to evangelize, and not be content with a desk-bound theology."[5] In that same exhortation, the pope tells readers that an evangelizing community is a community that shows mercy and that gets involved in people's lives.

> An evangelizing community gets involved by word and deed in people's daily lives; it bridges distances, it is willing to abase itself if necessary, and it embraces human life, touching the suffering flesh of Christ in others. Evangel-

> izers thus take on the "smell of the sheep" and the sheep are willing to hear their voice. An evangelizing community is also supportive, standing by people at every step of the way, no matter how difficult or lengthy this may prove to be.[6]

I have found reassurance in the pope's message here because it reframes the ethical task, insisting that theologians encounter Christ not only in the sacraments mediated by the church but also, and perhaps especially, through lived encounters with people who are suffering. Theology cannot be "desk-bound" if it is to witness to the good news of God's love in the messiness of our daily lives. This is why the pope emphasizes the theology of accompaniment, which means walking alongside one another and privileging compassion and encouragement.[7] This theology of accompaniment informs the methodology of this project.

My primary theological commitments, as will be seen in the unfolding argument of this book, are two-fold: fidelity to the gospel and fidelity to lived experience. With regard to the first commitment—fidelity to the gospel—I identify as a Christian theological ethicist, and my work is animated by my faith in Jesus as the Christ. I believe that in the encounter with Jesus we experience the abundance of God's love and that salvation, experienced through the community of believers, makes demands on the body of Christ. As Catholic ethicist Lisa Sowle Cahill explains: "Salvation transforms individual persons and social relationships, but it is also always a corporate reality, with social and political dimensions."[8] Jesus privileged the needs of the poor, welcomed the outcast, healed the sick, challenged the use of the law to enslave instead of to liberate, and Jesus suffered death as a witness to the transformative power of living in right relationship with God.[9] A goal of this project is thus to craft a theology of marriage that will be *good news* to women today. The church must embody the inclusive, salvific love of Christ in our broken world. As we make meaning in our lives, Christians have the opportunity to evangelize in words and actions by demonstrating to those we encounter "God loves you and desires your full flourishing." This is both a personal and a corporate mission. Thus preaching the good news of God's love is part of the task of this book.

The second theological commitment of this book is fidelity to lived experience. I mean this in two different ways. First, this research is my attempt to make sense of my own life experience. My social location and life experiences have shaped my theology of God, my understanding of the human person, and my approach to theological ethics. I grew up in a loving and stable family in Mobile, Alabama, and had a happy childhood. I grew up in a predominantly white affluent neighborhood and went to private Catholic schools. Both of my parents are college graduates and both earned graduate degrees as well: my father is a physician, and my mother is a stay-at-home mother who also works part-time as a spiritual director. Only recently have I begun to understand how my experiences of privilege shaped my vision of the world, my values, and my identity. As I have become more aware of the literature on social determinants of health, for example, I realize how my family's socioeconomic status insulated me from the harsh realities of poverty and lack of health care access that threaten the lives of so many others. As I learn more about social psychology and the formation of children in early childhood, I realize that my basic sense of trust in the goodness of the human person may be rooted not only in the theological claim that God created each person with inherent dignity, but also rooted in my own experience of being loved and of learning to trust others in intimate relationships. Today I write as a married woman and feel grateful every day for the love and support of my spouse. I know from personal experience that marriage can be an empowering, affirming, mutual, and deeply fulfilling vocation for women. But a second way that I am faithful to lived experience as a component of my theological method is that I realize that my own experiences may differ from yours. The reality of our broken world is that far too many children today experience home as a place of violence and abuse.[10] In 2012, more than forty-six million people living in the United States were living in poverty,[11] and forty-nine million Americans live in food insecure households, including over fifteen million children.[12] This is the world in which I live, and yet this is not my experience. Thus, it remains critical for theologians and ethicists to probe carefully the limits of our own experiences even as we draw on our experiences in constructing our theological approaches.

This project incorporates an ethnographic method together with Christian feminist analysis. Ethnography is "a process of attentive study of, and learning from, people—their words, practices, traditions, experiences, memories, insights—in particular times and places in order to understand how they make meaning (cultural, religious, ethical) and what they can teach us."[13] In the Catholic tradition, moral theology has been understood as reflection on the implications of faith for the way Christians live their lives. Too often moral theology has been framed as a rule book, and this is especially true in the realm of sexual ethics. But increasingly theologians are recovering the understanding of moral theology as reflection on the encounter with Christ in the everyday moments of our lives.[14] And to better understand how Christians actually experience Christ in their everyday lives, theologians are turning to methods like ethnography. The task of moral theology must be "in the middle" so that theologians can both learn from people's experiences and announce the gospel in the real world in a way that it can be heard, understood, and lived.

My approach is also deeply rooted in a Christian feminist method. Christian feminists have argued for decades that women's diverse experiences are both a source and norm for Christian ethics.[15] Feminism advocates for the full flourishing of all human persons in relationships of radical interdependence. Theologically speaking, feminism functions as a normative criterion in my theological method in the classic sense articulated by Rosemary Radford Ruether: "Whatever denies, diminishes, or distorts the full humanity of women is, therefore, appraised as not redemptive. Theologically speaking, whatever diminishes or denies the full humanity of women must be presumed not to reflect the authentic nature of things, or to be the message or work of an authentic redeemer or community of redemption."[16] Feminist analysis is not anti-male; women and men must be partners in re-shaping the world to be more just, loving, and holy. But feminist theologians do pay special attention to the ways in which women's experiences are interpreted, and to the power dynamics that underlie male and female relationships. This is especially true in feminist research on marriage traditions.

THE BIBLE AND CHRISTIAN MARRIAGE: A CAUTIONARY TALE

Grounding one's theology of Christian marriage in the Bible is both necessary and potentially problematic. It is necessary because it is what makes Christian marriage *Christian*. Christians rely on the Bible as an indispensable source of moral wisdom. But this approach is also potentially problematic because the Bible was written by men in places and times very different than today. For feminist theologians this presents a difficult problem: how can theologians rely on a text that is both "the word of God" and "the words of men"?

The Bible is called God's Word because Christians believe that in the Bible God reveals or communicates God's very self. In the Catholic tradition, the Bible is considered to be *inerrant*. The bishops of the Second Vatican Council explained, in *Dei Verbum*, that "the books of scripture, firmly, faithfully, and without error, teach that truth which God, for the sake of our salvation, wished to see confided to the sacred scriptures."[17] The church thus believes that the Bible is a reliable faith text that reveals the truths of salvation for believers. Yet one still must proceed with some caution because the meaning of the Bible is not self-evident. The Bible is better thought of as a collection of books, not a single text. The books of the Bible were written by many different authors in different historical periods with various (sometimes conflicting) religious and political motivations. The bishops of the Second Vatican Council explain: "In sacred scripture, God speaks through human beings in human fashion."[18] The books of the Bible contain different genres of writing; they are not journalistic accounts of historical events but rather reflections on and interpretations of people's experiences. So the Bible must be interpreted, and the task of interpretation is a complex communal task. It involves asking questions such as: Why was this text written? When was it written, and by whom? What are some of the assumptions of the author? In what language was the text written, and why was it translated in this way? To these questions, feminist scholars will add others, such as: How does the sex and social location of the author influence the text's account of human relations? Are women in the text objects or subjects?

In *Dei Verbum*, the bishops of the Second Vatican Council recognized that "there is growth in insight into the realities and words that are being passed on" because of the contemplation and study of the biblical canon.[19] In that document, the Council fathers explained that it is the task of biblical scholars "to work towards a better understanding and explanation of the meaning of sacred scripture in order that their research may help the church's judgment to mature."[20] The faith of the church is that through the sacred scriptures "we may come to know the ineffable loving-kindness of God."[21] And yet Christians today come to know God through the writings of human beings that were limited by their own cultures, times, and places. This is especially true when one begins to consider the biblical texts that offer resources for teachings on sexuality and marriage.

Biblical scholar Luke Timothy Johnson demonstrates that the dominant motifs for Christian marriage today have biblical roots: heterosexual coupling (Gn 1–2), procreation (Gn 1:28), covenant relationship (Hosea, Jeremiah, Isaiah, Proverbs), indissolubility (Mk 10:2–12, Lk 16:18), and mutual submission (Eph 5). But Johnson also finds in these texts "complexity and ambiguity."[22] In analyzing the Old Testament (Hebrew Scriptures), Johnson writes:

> The Old Testament pays relatively little attention to the sexual or affective aspects of marriage as such, focusing instead on the command given the first couple to "be fruitful and multiply and fill the earth and subdue it" (Gen 1:28). Especially after God declares to Abraham the intention of making one family (Abraham's seed) the means by which all humans would be blessed (12:1–3), the biblical story is preoccupied with issues of fertility and descent (see, for example, Gen 15:1–6; 16:1–6; 17:1–8; 21:1-14; 25:19–34; 27:18–29). The laws written for the people's observance in the land of Israel likewise concentrated on issues of descent through the male seed and the preservation of the chosen people through marriage and childbearing within the proper boundaries (Num 25:6–15; Deut 7:3). Adultery and the coveting of another's wife is forbidden (Exod 20:17; Deut 22:22), as is the marrying of foreign women. The male perspective in all of this is dominant. Thus, the man can divorce a woman who displeases him (Deut 24:1–4). And while Proverbs describes the ideal wife (Prov 31:10–31), it does not mention the ideal husband.[23]

As Johnson points out, one cannot escape the fact that these texts—texts revered as sacred scripture by Christians—are written from a male perspective. Pamela Dickey Young explains that in the Bible, women were often cast in the "male-defined roles" of wife, mother, virgin, temptress, and whore."[24]

Can texts that describe women as property or as dangerous seductresses be "good news" for contemporary women?[25] It is no exaggeration to claim that the biblical view of marriage is heavily influenced by *patriarchy*: "a social system based on the *patria potestas*, in other words, the absolute and unaccountable power over wives and concubines, children, servants, slaves, animals, and real property enjoyed by the *paterfamilias*, in other words, the father who is head of the family, tribe, or clan."[26] The New Testament does not offer a simple corrective to the problem of patriarchy; our attempt to construct a biblical account of Christian marriage must proceed with caution. As theologian Julie Hanlon Rubio explains, family is not a central idea in the New Testament.

> In fact, it hardly mentions family at all. Moreover, in those few passages in which the New Testament writers do take up the subject of marriage, their words are often more disabling than affirming. Followers of Jesus are told to hate their families, leave them behind, put service to the kingdom first. The earliest Christian sources point away from the primacy of family duty. Jesus, the model for all humans who call themselves Christian, was an itinerant celibate preacher for whom family ties were unimportant. Discipleship with this Jesus, according to the Gospel writers, asks people to decentralize family, not focus on it.[27]

Consider the following passages:

- Who are my mother and brothers? And looking at those who sat around him, he said, "Here are my mother and my brothers! Whoever does the will of God is my brother and sister and mother. (Mk 3:33–35)
- Let the dead bury their own dead. But as for you, go and proclaim the kingdom of God. (Lk 9:60, Mt 8:21–22)
- While he was saying this, a woman in the crowd raised her voice and said to him, "Blessed is the womb that bore you and the breasts that nursed you!" But he said, "Blessed rather are those who hear the word of God and obey it!" (Lk 11:27–28)
- Jesus said, "Truly I tell you, there is no one who has left house or brothers or sisters or mother or father or children or fields, for my sake and for the sake of the good news who will not receive a hundredfold now in this age—houses, brothers and sisters, mothers and children, and fields, with persecutions—and in the age to come eternal life." (Mk 10:29–30)
- And call no one your father on earth, for you have one Father—the one in heaven. (Mt 23:9)
- Now large crowds were traveling with him; and he turned and said to them, "Whoever comes to me and does not hate father and mother, wife and children, brothers and sisters, yes, and even life itself, cannot be my disciple. Whoever does not carry the cross and follow me cannot be my

disciple. For which of you, intending to build a tower, does not first sit down and estimate the cost, to see whether he has enough to complete it?" (Lk 14: 25–28)

As Rubio interprets this pattern within the New Testament, she finds evidence that Jesus preached the importance of a "new family" that would have challenged his listeners' assumptions about family life. Drawing on biblical scholars Richard Horsley and Elisabeth Schüssler Fiorenza, Rubio claims that Jesus rejected the patriarchal family of his own culture and promises a new family based on the community of disciples who follow Jesus, a community of equals.[28] Similarly, Lisa Sowle Cahill argues that the Christian family is "domestic church" because "the primary values defining the Christian family are the same values that define the "new family in Christ": other concern and compassionate love that overlooks socially normative boundaries and is willing to sacrifice to meet the needs of others."[29] But Rubio offers caution: "patriarchy does not end overnight."[30] While scholars point out the radical nature of Jesus's preaching of egalitarian relationships, some early Christian texts perpetuated a patriarchal understanding of marriage and placed limits on the participation of women in church communities, indicating the persistence of patriarchy even in the New Testament (1 Cor. 11:7–12, Col 3:18, 1 Tim. 2:12–15).

Thus, our contemporary theology of marriage, which must be grounded in sacred scripture, must also be keenly sensitive to the reality of patriarchy in the Bible and in the Christian tradition of biblical interpretation. Texts must be scrutinized, challenged, and evaluated according to the criterion set out by the bishops in *Dei Verbum*: Does this interpretation disclose the ineffable loving-kindness of God? In other words, is it *good news*? Elisabeth Schüssler Fiorenza calls this the task of "critical dialectical mode of biblical interpretation," which insists that "the litmus test for invoking Scripture as the Word of God must be whether or not biblical texts and traditions seek to end relations of domination and exploitation."[31]

A liberationist reading of the Bible, such as the one proposed by Schüssler Fiorenza, coheres with this book's attempt to propose a *life-affirming* theology of marriage for contemporary women living with HIV. For many in our world today, everyday life is marked by struggle and suffering. If theology is "in the middle"—learning from people's experiences and announcing the good news in everyday life—then theologians must understand better the world in which we live. It is a world in flux, a world in which vast inequalities are exposed by the devastation caused by HIV and AIDS, and a world in which marriage laws and marriage traditions seem to be changing dramatically. Attention to these "signs of our times" will provide an introduction to some of the challenges reported by the women in this study.

READING THE SIGNS OF THE TIMES, PART ONE: HIV AND AIDS IN THE UNITED STATES

One of the major themes of the Second Vatican Council was the importance of "reading the signs of the times and of interpreting them in the light of the Gospel."[32] Sadly, one of the signs of our times is the HIV pandemic, an unfolding catastrophe that continues to reveal the "fractures, stresses, and strains" of human society.[33] The root causes of HIV infection are complex, especially when one takes into account the impact of culture and social context on behavior and attitudes.

HIV is the virus that causes AIDS.[34] HIV was discovered in 1981 and since then has become a major worldwide pandemic.[35] HIV causes AIDS by attacking the body's immune system, compromising the body's ability to defend itself against illness and infection.[36] Persons with AIDS are at risk for developing opportunistic infections such as cancer or pneumonia; these opportunistic infections become the cause of death for persons with late-stage AIDS. The stages of HIV and AIDS are marked by CD4-counts, which indicate the number of T-cells per cubic millimeter of blood.[37] HIV is spread through unprotected sex with an infected partner, contact with infected blood, sharing of contaminated needles, use of contaminated medical equipment, prenatal transmission from mother to child, and transmission from mother to child through breast milk. HIV has a long asymptomatic latency period—as long as ten years for some patients. The only way to know that someone is infected when he or she is asymptomatic is to have a blood test performed that shows the presence of the HIV virus or antibodies to the virus.[38] While drug therapies are improving and becoming more widely available,[39] these drug treatment regimens do not cure the disease and they are very expensive.[40]

The Joint United Nations Programme on HIV/AIDS (UNAIDS) estimates that over thirty-five million people across the globe are living with human immunodeficiency virus (HIV); almost half are women.[41] While Sub-Saharan Africa continues to bear the heaviest burden of HIV and AIDS, no country or region is unaffected.[42] In order to contextualize the stories of the women in this study, it is important to have greater clarity about the impact of HIV in the United States.

More than one million people in the United States are living with HIV infection, many of whom do not know that they are infected.[43] Over the past decade, the number of people living with HIV in the United States has increased, while the annual number of new HIV infections has remained relatively stable. In the United States, men who have sex with men remain most seriously affected by the disease; nearly two thirds of new infections in 2012 occurred among this population.[44] In 2012 women accounted for 20 percent of new HIV infections;[45] 24 percent of those living with HIV infection in the United States are women.[46] New HIV infections among women are primarily attributed to unprotected heterosexual sex; the second highest mode of transmission for women is through intravenous drug use.[47] Access to treatment for HIV infection remains a critical problem for women in the United States; the CDC reports that only about half of women who are diagnosed with HIV receive regular medical care and only 40 percent have the virus under control.[48]

Racial and ethnic minorities continue to be disproportionately affected by the HIV epidemic in the United States. Although African-Americans represent about 12 percent of the population, they accounted for 44 percent of new HIV infections in 2010. Unless the course of the epidemic changes, at some point in their lifetime, an estimated one in sixteen black men and one in thirty-two black women will be diagnosed with HIV infection. Hispanics/Latinos are also disproportionately affected by HIV. Hispanics/Latinos represented 16 percent of the population but accounted for 21 percent of new HIV infections in 2010. The incidence rates are especially jarring when compared to the impact among white Americans: African American men and women have an HIV incidence rate *eight times higher* than the incidence rate among whites.[49] The rate of new HIV infections for Latino males is *almost three times* that for white males, and the rate of new infections for Latinas was *four times* that for white females.[50]

Seven of the eight women interviewed for this study live in Chicago, Illinois; one lives in a nearby rural area but travels to Chicago regularly to access medical care and to attend support group meetings. In the United States, HIV prevalence remains highest in large metropolitan cities.[51] Chicago is the highest population center in the Midwest, and is the epicenter for the AIDS epidemic in the state. Approximately 87 percent of Illinois residents with HIV diagnoses reside in the Chicago metro area.[52] An estimated 22,346 Chicagoans are living with HIV or AIDS. Male-to-male sexual contact is the leading mode of transmission (75 percent), followed by heterosexual contact (16 percent) and injection drug use (3 percent). Unprotected heterosexual sex is the leading mode of transmission among women (86 percent), while the second highest mode of HIV transmission for women in Chicago is injection drug use.[53] Minority communities bear a disproportionate burden of HIV infection in Chicago.[54] In 2013, 81 percent of new female HIV infections were among non-Hispanic Black women.[55]

Womanist theologian Emilie Townes encourages readers to understand the US AIDS epidemic through the prism of systemic racism and structural injustices.[56] While Townes is writing particularly for the African American community to discourage apathy with regard to sexual education, her analysis is compelling for a wider group of Christians. HIV and AIDS flourish because of social injustices, including poverty, gender inequality, racism, social stigma, and disparities in health care access. Persons who are marginalized by these social injustices are more vulnerable to HIV and are less able to get the care they need. A good first step is to have a more open conversation about the devastation caused by HIV and AIDS, and Townes argues that the churches should initiate this conversation. "Injecting drugs, unprotected sex, and sex among unmarried heterosexuals—all high-risk behaviors that make people vulnerable to HIV and AIDS—are also subjects that are often shunned. Meaningful discussions about these behaviors have not taken place within many African American communities. Therefore, it is extremely difficult to have substantive conversations about HIV/AIDS."[57] Townes explains that we face a "deadly dynamic that makes it difficult to sort through the massive issues, stereotypes, phobias, and outright bigotry and hatred that accompany any discussion of AIDS in the Black community."[58] To fully understand the AIDS pandemic, then, we will have to talk about sex, drugs, poverty, racism, and many other difficult topics; this is precisely what "reading the signs of the times" in our day requires.

READING THE SIGNS OF THE TIMES, PART TWO: MARRIAGE IN THE UNITED STATES

Catholic bishops in the United States are concerned about marriage,[59] and rightly so. Official church teachings on marriage assert that marriage is the cornerstone of a healthy society,[60] so Catholic leaders are right to focus their attention on any troubling signs of the deterioration of society rooted in a rejection of the goods of the family. A healthy marriage benefits the spouses and children of married households by providing emotional attachments, support of kinship networks, economic stability, and a safe space for identity formation and value education. Yet marriage, as a social institution, is changing rapidly. Attitudes and beliefs about marriage are also undergoing a major shift in the United States.[61] More couples are choosing not to marry.[62] More are waiting until later in life to marry.[63] More challenge traditional gender roles.[64] And there is growing support for same-sex partnerships.[65] In a Pew Research survey, 39 percent of survey respondents said they agree that marriage is becoming "obsolete."[66]

It is into this context that the US Conference of Catholic Bishops wrote their pastoral letter, *Marriage: Love and Life in the Divine Plan.*[67] The bishops rightly point out that "conditions in contemporary society do not always support marriage."[68] They note the troubling elements of "lustful, self-centered pleasures of our culture" and affirm the value of intimate relationships grounded in "trust instead of shame."[69] The bishops argue that four dominant challenges in our culture "are directed at the very meaning and purpose of marriage."[70] They are: contraception, same-sex unions, divorce, and cohabitation.[71] The bishops restate what they consider to be the most important components of a Catholic theology of marriage and then address these four challenges.

The bishops define marriage as "a lifelong partnership of the whole of life, of mutual and exclusive fidelity, established by mutual consent between a man and a woman, and ordered towards the good of the spouses and the procreation of offspring."[72] Since "God is the author of marriage," Catholic theology of marriage is presented as wisdom received by God and passed on to the wider culture through the church, not as something constructed by human agents in history.[73] The document explains that male-female complementarity is essential to marriage, drawing on the story of creation in Genesis 1–2 to argue that "man and woman have been made to come together in the union of marriage."[74] The bishops focus especially on physical complementarity of male and female partners: "The roots of marriage can be seen in the biological fact that a man and a woman can come together as male and female in a union that has the potential for bringing forth another human person. This kind of union fills the need for the continuation of the human race."[75] In addition to these biological goods, sexual intercourse in marriage has "personal and spiritual dimensions" which enable the couple to "form a communion of persons."[76] The document then explains that the two purposes of marriage are the good of the spouses and the procreation of children, and that these two ends are "inseparable."[77]

According to the bishops, contraception threatens marriage because it separates the unitive and procreative meanings of the marital act and is thus a "refusal to give oneself entirely" to one's spouse.[78] The bishops find it deeply problematic that so many couples "readily treat, as separate choices, the decisions to get married and to have children."[79] They diagnose this as a "mentality in which children are seen not as integral to a marriage but as optional," arguing that this leads to "damaging consequences."[80] The bishops describe the act of sexual intercourse as "the act most symbolic and expressive of the marriage as a whole" because the spouses give of themselves completely and are thus united as a communion of persons.[81]

The bishops explain that same-sex unions are a threat to marriage because marriage "is the permanent bond between one man and one woman whose two-in-one-flesh communion of persons is an indispensable good at the heart of every family and every society" and same-sex unions "are incapable of realizing this specific communion of persons."[82] The document further argues that it would be gravely unjust to "*intentionally* deprive children of the right to a mother and a father" by redefining marriage.[83]

A third major threat to marriage today, according to the bishops, is divorce, which "claims to break the contract, to which the spouses freely consented, to live with each other until death."[84] The bishops note that conflict, quarrels, and misunderstandings are found in all marriages, yet "God's plan for marriage persists, and he [sic] continues to offer mercy and healing grace."[85] The bishops recognize, however, that "divorce may be the only solution to a morally unacceptable situation," as is the case when a spouse is abusive.[86] In these cases, the bishops encourage readers to make frequent use of the sacraments and to consider seeking a declaration of nullity.[87]

The fourth major threat to marriage today, according to the bishops, is the practice of living together without marriage (cohabitation). "Only the public and legal commitment of marriage expresses the complete gift of self that is the basis of marriage," argue the bishops.[88] In their view, the unions of cohabiting couples lack "unconditional trust" and "complete self-giving."[89] Citing concerns for the welfare of children, the bishops argue that cohabitation puts children at risk, and that "the most human and humanizing context for welcoming children" is a stable marriage.[90]

An overarching theme of the marriage pastoral is the importance of self-sacrificial love in Christian marriage. In fact the bishops go so far as to say that marital love, a love of "complete self-giving," "is most completely expressed by Jesus's death on the cross."[91] The image of the cross is used repeatedly and without qualification throughout the pastoral letter.[92]

Is the marriage pastoral *good news* for married women living with HIV? There are certainly some affirming messages within the document, especially the call to fidelity and mutual love between spouses and the bishops' concern for the welfare of children. Women deserve to be treated with respect, to be cherished and loved by a sexual partner. This is good news for women. Families do not exist in a vacuum but rather are embedded in particular social contexts; families require social support and assistance. The promise of this support is good news for families. And the promise of God's mercy and the church's ongoing support is undoubtedly good news for married persons—people living the messiness of everyday marital life.

But when we further consider the complexities of life with HIV and AIDS, the plot thickens. Why is the church's teaching on the obligation to follow one's conscience absent from this document? How would a sexually transmitted infection necessarily alter the church's reflection on the "symbolism" of the marital act? When we begin to apply the marital norms within this document in ministry with HIV-positive persons in pastoral settings, we face new dilemmas that merit further consideration. The bishops argue that a married Christian couple has a "responsibility to serve life by being open to children."[93] But does this necessarily apply to all married couples, even those couples in which one or both spouses is living with HIV? For example, is procreation a purpose of marriage for couples in which one or both partners is living with HIV infection? Should women consider the decision to marry as distinct from the decision to have sexual relations that could lead to pregnancy? With regard to divorce, from the perspective of the bishops divorce is a tragedy, but from the perspective of a battered woman, could divorce instead be seen as a symbol of freedom and the possibility of reclaiming one's human dignity? And finally, is marital love best symbolized by the death of Jesus on the cross? Such descriptions seem to imply that marital love is primarily characterized by renunciation of self and even uncritical acceptance of suffering. This portrait of marriage can be dangerous for women if it fails to affirm a woman's proper care for self. If spouses are not counseled to consider their own needs, desires, or vocations at all, but rather are instructed to focus *all* of their love and attention on their partner and children—*totally and completely*—this hardly affirms a vision of marriage rooted in an understanding of one's own dignity and worth.[94] It would be very troubling if the bishops' portrait of Christian marriage is heard by women as a call to self-neglect without care for their own well-being. It is clear, then, that more work needs to be done in this area so that couples who are trying to discern God's will in difficult circumstances may have more resources for thinking about their obligations as Christians in marriage.

PERSONS OVER PAPERWORK: IN SEARCH OF A LIFE-AFFIRMING THEOLOGY OF MARRIAGE

The aim of this book is to listen to and learn from the life experiences of married women living with HIV, and to recommend a theology of Christian marriage that would be life-affirming for people living with HIV and AIDS. I call this a pro-life approach to marriage and HIV and AIDS; this is not a reductionistic method that looks only to the physical health of a married couple, but rather in a holistic way this method seeks the full human flourishing of both spouses in body, mind, and spirit. In much of Christian history and theology women have been silenced, spoken for, and sexually subordinate to men. Unfortunately these patterns persist, and the task of contemporary feminist scholarship is to affirm the equal dignity of women, enable women to speak for themselves about their life experiences, and empower them to be treated as equal partners in sexual relationships.

Employing the criterion of human flourishing is not a new method of moral argument in Christian ethics.[95] Todd Salzman and Michael Lawler find evidence that the bishops of the Second Vatican Council employed "the principle of the human person adequately considered" as a foundational principle for judging all human activity, including sexual activity.[96] My approach is situated in the personalist strand of natural law ethics, which requires reflection on human experiences in order to draw moral norms about what is right and wrong.[97]

The women interviewed for this study did not consistently hear empowering messages in their faith communities. Lettie, for example, explained that in her experience "sometimes the church just seems more concerned with the paperwork than with helping." Lettie's experience was shared by other collaborators who felt that church leaders cared more about lifting up marital ideals than dealing with everyday realities. It is no longer tenable to treat the institution of marriage with more respect than we treat the persons who are married. With theologian Kevin Kelly, then, I affirm that "marriage is made for persons, not persons for marriage."[98] The approach of this book is to ask what constructions of Christian marriage affirm women as fully human, and to propose HIV interventions and a revised theology of Christian marriage that promote the full flourishing of married persons.

The next two chapters focus on my collaborators' experiences of marriage and HIV and AIDS. Each woman told me of her HIV diagnosis, her coping strategies, and her experiences of marriage, family life, and church involvement. In these stories of messy, ordinary struggles, the women reflect on what practices have been life-affirming and what messages have been death-dealing. I analyze the themes that emerged from their stories and how the church has been both a place of comfort as well as a source of stigma and shame. Surely some of these women's struggles and needs will be very different from the struggles and needs of women in other parts of the world. When I address the implications of this research I note those areas that are more universal in scope and those areas that are particular to the contexts in which these women's stories are embedded. My hope is that Christians will be both challenged and enriched by listening to these women's stories.[99]

In the second half of the book, I build on the descriptive analysis from my fieldwork and move to consider in greater detail the implications of my collaborators' experiences for the church. Since the women in my study reported challenges to self-care both before and after their HIV diagnosis, I explore the theological foundations for affirming self-concern in Christian discipleship. Further, I discerned two important dimensions of their experiences that were equally significant and yet intertwined: each woman recounted how HIV affected her marriage, and likewise how her marriage shaped her experience of HIV. And yet both of these areas—the experience of being HIV-positive and their experiences of marriage—yielded specific implications for church teachings. In the fifth chapter I build on the women's descriptive experiences to develop a more adequate Catholic response to HIV and AIDS, one that affirms self-concern and enables women to control their sexual decision making. I also argue that church communities should promote comprehensive sexual education, should defend harm reduction strategies of HIV prevention, and should actively work to reduce stigmatizing behaviors within church communities. In the sixth chapter, I begin to construct a life-affirming theology of Christian marriage that is rooted in what Vatican II called "the good of the spouses": A marriage must affirm the inherent dignity of each spouse so that in marriage one is safe from physical and emotional abuse and can care for oneself while simultaneously loving one's partner. In this way, Christian marriage holds together the personal and social dimensions of the love commandment, balancing appropriate self-concern with self-giving love. In the seventh chapter I describe implications of the argument for liturgical practice, marriage preparation programs, sexual education programs, and family ministries including pastoral ministries with HIV-affected families. Since the purpose of an ethnographic methodology within Christian feminist ethics is not only to describe the experiences of particular women, but also to advocate for social justice,[100] I suggest how the church can better respond to these women's needs, and to the needs of other similarly situated women whose stories have yet to be heard.

NOTES

1. ADAP stands for AIDS Drug Assistance Program. See US Department of Health and Human Services (HHS) Health Resources and Services Administration (HRSA), "Part B: AIDS Drug Assistance Program," http://hab.hrsa.gov/abouthab/partbdrug.html (Accessed August 3, 2014).
2. UNAIDS, *Women and HIV/AIDS: Confronting the Crisis* (New York: United Nations Publications, 2004).
3. While my research does not focus on the experiences of married men, of persons who identify as gay or lesbian, of single persons, or of children, these groups of persons should not be neglected in the theological examination of issues related to HIV and AIDS. But by limiting my study to the experiences of married women I am able to focus more attention on an analysis of the unique factors that prevent their full flourishing. Sustained attention to the experiences of men and children affected by HIV and AIDS, while necessary, is beyond the scope of this project.
4. Gustavo Gutierrez, "Saying and Showing to the Poor: God Loves You," in *In the Company of the Poor: Conversations with Dr. Paul Farmer and Fr. Gustavo Gutierrez,* ed. Michael Griffin and Jennie Weiss Block (Maryknoll: Orbis, 2013), 28.
5. Pope Francis, Apostolic Exhortation *Evangelii Gaudium*: The Joy of the Gospel (Washington, DC: United States Conference of Catholic Bishops, 2013), no. 133.
6. Ibid., 24.
7. Ibid., 169.
8. Lisa Sowle Cahill, *Global Justice, Christology and Christian Ethics* (New York: Cambridge University Press, 2013), 76.
9. An in-depth exploration of Christology is beyond the scope of this book. Still, it is important to note that Jesus was embedded in the Judaism of his time. It is important to remember that the gospels are not eye witness accounts but rather texts written after the death of Jesus by communities who endeavored to explain the significance of Jesus; in other words, they are "faith texts" and should be interpreted as such.
10. See US Department of Health and Human Services, *Child Maltreatment 2012* (Washington DC, 2013). Available online: http://www.acf.hhs.gov/sites/default/files/cb/cm2012.pdf and National Coalition against Domestic Violence, "Domestic Violence Fact Sheet." Available online: http://www.ncadv.org/files/DomesticViolenceFactSheet%28National%29.pdf (Accessed June 23, 2014).
11. United States Census, Current Population Survey (CPS), 2013 Annual Social and Economic Supplement (ASEC): https://www.census.gov/hhes/www/poverty/about/overview/ (Accessed June 23, 2014).
12. "Food Insecurity Statistics," Website of Feeding America: http://feedingamerica.org/hunger-in-america/hunger-facts/hunger-and-poverty-statistics.aspx# (Accessed June 23, 2014).
13. Christian Scharen and Aana Marie Vigen, *Ethnography as Christian Theology and Ethics* (New York: Continuum, 2011), 16. See also Christopher P. Vogt, "Locating the Church

in the World: Ethnography, Christian Ethics, and the Global Church" *Journal of Moral Theology* 2:2 (2013): 158–172.

14. Contextual theologies have led the way on this. Stephanie Y. Mitchem argues that "in black theology, the everyday realities of black people's lives become an important basis for construction. This approach requires a willingness to utilize a variety of sources as well as to listen to stories of past and present." See Stephanie Y. Mitchem, *Introducing Womanist Theology* (Maryknoll: Orbis, 2002), 44. Ada Maria Isasi-Diaz is one of the most well-known Cuban-American mujerista theologians, and *lo cotidiano* was a central theme of her reflections, valuing the importance of reflection on the everyday realities of the poor. See her *En La Lucha: A Hispanic Women's Liberation Theology* (Minneapolis: Fortress, 1993) and *Mujerista Theology: A Theology for the Twenty-First Century* (Maryknoll: Orbis, 1996).

15. See Pamela Dickey Young, *Feminist Theology, Christian Theology: In Search of Method* (Eugene, Oregon: Wipf and Stock, 2000), Stephanie Y. Mitchem, *Introducing Womanist Theology* (Maryknoll: Orbis, 2002), and *Readings in Moral Theology, No. 9: Feminist Ethics and the Catholic Moral Tradition*, eds. Charles E. Curran, Margaret A. Farley, and Richard A. McCormick, S.J. (New York: Paulist, 1996).

16. Rosemary Radford Ruether, *Sexism and God Talk* (Boston: Beacon Press, 1983), 19.

17. Second Vatican Council, *Dogmatic Constitution on Divine Revelation (Dei Verbum)*, (November 18, 1965), no. 11.

18. Ibid., no. 12.

19. Ibid., no. 8.

20. Ibid., no. 12.

21. Ibid., no. 13.

22. Luke Timothy Johnson, "The Biblical Foundations of Matrimony." In *Readings in Moral Theology, No. 5: Marriage*, eds. Charles E. Curran and Julie Hanlon Rubio (Mahwah, NJ: Paulist Press, 2009), 3–7, at 6–7. See also Michael G. Lawler, "Marriage in the Bible," and Theodore Mackin, S.J., "The Primitive Christian Understanding of Marriage," in Kieran Scott and Michael Warren, eds., *Perspectives on Marriage: A Reader* (New York: Oxford University Press, 2001), 7–21, 22–28.

23. Ibid., 4.

24. Pamela Dickey Young, *Feminist Theology*, 13.

25. Classic feminist texts on this issue include Mary Daly, *The Church and the Second Sex* (New York: Harper and Row, 1975); Rosemary Radford Ruether, ed., *Religion and Sexism: Images of Women in the Jewish and Christian Traditions* (New York: Simon and Schuster, 1974); Letty Russell, ed., *The Liberating Word: A Guide to Nonsexist Interpretation of the Bible* (Philadelphia: Westminster, 1976); and Sandra M. Schneiders, *Women and the Word* (New York: Paulist, 1986).

26. Schneiders, *Women and the Word*, 11.

27. Julie Hanlon Rubio, *A Christian Theology of Marriage and Family* (New York: Paulist, 2003), 46.

28. Rubio, *A Christian Theology of Marriage and Family*, 50-64. Rubio cites Richard Horsley, *Sociology of the Jesus Movement* (New York: Crossroad, 1989) and Elisabeth Schüssler Fiorenza, *In Memory of Her: A Feminist Theological Reconstruction of Christian Origins* (New York: Crossroad, 1989).

29. Lisa Sowle Cahill, *Family: A Christian Social Perspective* (Minneapolis: Fortress Press, 2000), 134.

30. Rubio, *A Christian Theology of Marriage and Family*, 57.

31. Elisabeth Schüssler Fiorenza, *Bread Not Stone: The Challenge of Feminist Biblical Interpretation* (Boston: Beacon, 1984), xiii.

32. Second Vatican Council, *Gaudium et Spes*: Pastoral Constitution on the Church in the Modern World (December 7, 1965), no. 4. Available online: http://www.vatican.va/archive/hist_councils/ii_vatican_council/documents/vat-ii_const_19651207_gaudium-et-spes_en.html (Accessed June 20, 2014).

33. Alan Whiteside, *HIV/AIDS: A Very Short Introduction* (New York: Oxford University Press, 2008), 39.

34. The claim that HIV causes AIDS has been challenged by some notable public figures, including President Mbeki of South Africa, but the scientific community has come to a firm consensus on this causal relationship. See "Evidence that HIV is the Cause of AIDS," in Darrell E. Ward, *The AmFAR AIDS Handbook: The Complete Guide to Understanding HIV and AIDS* (New York: W. W. Norton, 1999), 386–390. See also NIAID, "How HIV Causes AIDS," available online at http://www.niaid.nih.gov/factsheets/howhiv.htm (Accessed 3/11/2008) and NIAID, "The Evidence that HIV Causes AIDS," available online at http://www.niaid.nih.gov/factsheets/evidhiv.htm (Accessed 3/11/2008).

35. See Darrell E. Ward, "The Emergence and Early Years of the HIV/AIDS Epidemic," *AmFar AIDS Handbook*, 1999, 366–385. See also R. Bayer, *Private Acts, Social Consequences: AIDS and the Politics of Public Health* (New York: Free Press, 1989).

36. National Institutes of Allergy and Infectious Diseases (NIAID), "HIV Infection and AIDS: An Overview," (October 2007) Available online at http://www.niaid.nih.gov/factsheets/hivinf.htm (Accessed 3/11/2008). HIV-infected pregnant women will pass the virus to their babies during pregnancy and delivery in about 15 to 20 percent of cases and an additional 5 to 20 percent of infants will become infected post-natally through breastfeeding, for an overall risk of 30 to 45 percent transmission from mother to child. The World Health Organization (WHO) recommends that HIV-positive women breastfeed their infants exclusively for the first six months of life unless replacement feeding is acceptable, affordable, feasible, sustainable, and safe for them and for their infants. When these conditions are met, WHO recommends avoidance of all breastfeeding for HIV+ women. Mixed feeding has been associated with higher rates of mother to child transmission (MTCT) of HIV and is not recommended. See WHO, *HIV Transmission Through Breastfeeding: A Review of Available Evidence* (Geneva, Switzerland: World Health Organization Publications, 2004).

37. See Michael DiSpezio, *The Science of HIV*, 2nd ed. (Arlington, VA: NSTA Press, 2000); see also Ward, 1999).

38. CDC guidelines recommend routine voluntary HIV testing, sometimes called the "opt-out" plan. See CDC, "Revised Recommendations for HIV Testing of Adults, Adolescents, and Pregnant Women in Health-Care Settings," *Morbidity and Mortality Weekly Report* 55:14 (2006): 1–17.

39. UNAIDS reports that there has been a forty-fold increase in access to anti-retroviral therapy between 2002 and 2012; in 2012 9.7 million people in low and middle income countries had access to anti-retroviral therapies. UNAIDS, AIDS by the Numbers 2013 (Geneva, UNAIDS, 2013). Available online: http://www.unaids.org/en/media/unaids/contentassets/documents/unaidspublication/2013/JC2571_AIDS_by_the_numbers_en.pdf (Accessed June 24, 2014).

40. Access to anti-retroviral therapy was given significant attention in the 2012 World AIDS Day Report (Geneva: UNAIDS, 2012). Available online: http://www.unaids.org/en/media/unaids/contentassets/documents/epidemiology/2012/gr2012/jc2434_worldaidsday_results_en.pdf (Accessed June 24, 2014).

41. Joint United Nations Program on HIV/AIDS (UNAIDS), "AIDS Info." http://www.unaids.org/en/dataanalysis/datatools/aidsinfo/ (Accessed June 11, 2014).

42. In 2012 more than twenty-five million people in Sub-Saharan African were living with HIV. Joint United Nations Program on HIV/AIDS (UNAIDS), "Fact Sheet." http://www.unaids.org/en/resources/campaigns/globalreport2013/factsheet/ (Accessed June 24, 2014). For an excellent treatment of the dangers of Christian marriage for women in Sub-Saharan Africa, see Melissa Browning, *Risky Marriage: HIV and Intimate Relationships in Tanzania* (Lanham, MD: Lexington, 2014).

43. The CDC reports that an estimated 15.8 percent of people living with HIV in the United States are unaware of their infection. Centers for Disease Control and Prevention, "HIV in the United States: At A Glance." Available online: http://www.cdc.gov/hiv/statistics/basics/ataglance.html (Accessed June 23, 2014).

44. As this book went to press, the latest surveillance data available from the Centers for Disease Control and Prevention was the *HIV Surveillance Report*, vol 24 (November 2014), available online at http://www.cdc.gov/hiv/pdf/statistics_2012_HIV_Surveillance_Report_vol_24.pdf (Accessed December 10, 2014). Even though the report was published in 2014, it

analyzes data through 2012. In 2012, male-to-male sexual contact accounted for 67 percent of new HIV infections (CDC, HIV Surveillance Report, 7). The Centers for Disease Control and Prevention track infections by behavior not sexual orientation, so MSM (men who have sex with men) includes gay, bisexual, and men who have sex with men but do not self-identify as gay or bisexual.

45. Centers for Disease Control and Prevention, *HIV Surveillance Report, 2012*. vol. 24 (US Department of Health and Human Services: Atlanta, Georgia, 2014), 6.

46. According to the CDC, women accounted for 25 percent (7,949) of the estimated 32,052 AIDS diagnoses (including children) in 2011 and represent 20 percent (232,902) of the 1,155,792 cumulative AIDS diagnoses (including children) in the United States from the beginning of the epidemic through the end of 2011. Centers for Disease Control and Prevention, "HIV Among Women" Fact Sheet. http://www.cdc.gov/hiv/risk/gender/women/facts/index.html (Accessed December 26, 2014).

47. New HIV infections among women are primarily attributed to heterosexual contact (84 percent) or injection drug use (16 percent). Injection drug users represented 8 percent of new HIV infections and 16 percent of those living with HIV. Centers for Disease Control and Prevention, "HIV in the United States: At A Glance." Available online: http://www.cdc.gov/hiv/statistics/basics/ataglance.html (Accessed June 23, 2014).

48. Centers for Disease Control and Prevention, "HIV Among Women." Available online: http://www.cdc.gov/hiv/risk/gender/women/facts/index.html (Accessed June 24, 2014).

49. Centers for Disease Control and Prevention, "HIV Among African Americans." Rev. December 10, 2014. http://www.cdc.gov/hiv/risk/racialethnic/aa/facts/index.html (Accessed December 26, 2014).

50. Centers for Disease Control and Prevention, "HIV Statistics: Basics." Rev. October 15, 2014. http://www.cdc.gov/hiv/statistics/basics/ (Accessed December 26, 2014).

51. These data do not discount the growing epidemic in the rural South. A 1998 *Morbidity and Mortality Weekly Report* reported that the Southern region of the United States accounted for the largest proportion (34 percent) of new AIDS cases and over half (54 percent) of AIDS cases among residents of rural areas. *MMWR* 47:45 (11/20/1998): 974–9798. According to the CDC, from 2001 to 2005, the estimated number of AIDS cases increased 24 percent in the Midwest, 9 percent in the South, and 2 percent in the Northeast, and decreased 3 percent in the West. During the same time period, the estimated number of AIDS deaths decreased in the Northeast, Midwest, and West, and increased in the South. For more information about HIV/AIDS in rural areas of the United States, see the website of the National Rural Health Association at http://www.nrharural.org/opporty/sub/rural_HIV.html (Accessed 3/11/2008).

52. AIDS Foundation of Chicago, "HIV/AIDS in Chicago 2010." http://aidschicago.org/pdf/chicago_factsheet_2010.pdf (Accessed June 24, 2014).

53. Chicago Department of Public Health, *HIV/STI Surveillance Report, December 2014*. (Chicago, IL: Chicago Department of Public Health, 2014), 6.

54. African Americans account for a disproportionately large share of the HIV/AIDS epidemic in Chicago. While representing 36.8 percent of the Chicago population, they represent 59 percent of Chicagoans reported as living with HIV. Caucasians represented 42 percent of the population and 23 percent of 2009 HIV cases, and Latinos represent 26 percent of the population but 16 percent of new HIV cases. See AIDS Foundation of Chicago "HIV/AIDS in Chicago 2010." Available online: http://aidschicago.org/pdf/chicago_factsheet_2010.pdf (Accessed June 24, 2014).

55. Chicago Department of Public Health, *HIV/STI Surveillance Report, December 2014*. (Chicago, IL: Chicago Department of Public Health, 2014), 6

56. Emilie M. Townes, *Breaking the Fine Rain of Death: African American Health Issues and a Womanist Ethic of Care* (New York: Continuum, 2001), 121–144. Many African American women theologians self-identify as *womanist* in order to note the particularity of their experiences as different from, but complementary to, *white feminist* theology. See also Emilie M. Townes, *Womanist Ethics and the Cultural Production of Evil* (New York: Palgrave Macmillan, 2006) and *In a Blaze of Glory: Womanist Spirituality As Social Witness* (Nashville: Abington, 1995).

57. Townes, *Breaking the Fine Rain of Death,* 131.

58. Townes, *Breaking the Fine Rain of Death,* 125.

59. In June 2014, marriage was one of the top concerns of the United States bishops at their Assembly in New Orleans. The USCCB press release contains more information: http://www.usccb.org/news/2014/14-074.cfm (Accessed June 23, 2014). The bishops encouraged the faithful to support and attend the March for Marriage: http://www.usccb.org/issues-and-action/marriage-and-family/marriage/promotion-and-defense-of-marriage/upload/Ltr-re-2014-March-for-Marriage.pdf (Accessed June 23, 2014).

60. The bishops of the Second Vatican Council summarize it this way: "The well-being of the individual person and of human and Christian society is intimately linked with the healthy condition of that community produced by marriage and family." Second Vatican Council, *Gaudium et spes,* no. 47. Full text available online: http://www.vatican.va/archive/hist_councils/ii_vatican_council/documents/vat-ii_const_19651207_gaudium-et-spes_en.html (Accessed June 23, 2014).

61. Ibid., 10.

62. The Pew Research Center reports that there have been significant changes in the past fifty years in the United States. In a comparison of marriage rates between 1960 and 2010, the Pew Research Center reports that in 2010, 51 percent of adults ages 18 or over were married, compared to 72 percent in 1960. This decline is especially notable for young adults: 20 percent of 18- to 29-year-olds were married in 2010, compared with almost 60 percent in 1960. See Pew Research Center: Social and Demographic Trends, "Barely Half of U.S. Adults are Married—A Record Low." (December 14, 2011), 1. Full text available online: http://www.pewsocialtrends.org/files/2011/12/Marriage-Decline.pdf (Accessed June 23, 2014).

63. In 2011, the median age at first marriage was an estimated 28.7 for men and 26.5 for women. That means half of men don't marry until at least about age 29, and half of women don't marry until at least about age 27. In 1960, the median age at first marriage for both men and women was in the early 20s. Ibid., 2, 9. For international statistics, see United Nations, Department of Economic and Social Affairs, Population Division, World Fertility Report 2012 (Geneva: United Nations Publication, 2013) .

64. Pew Research Center, "Breadwinner Moms," (May 29, 2013): http://www.pewresearch.org/key-data-points/gay-marriage-key-data-points-from-pew-research/ (Accessed June 23, 2014). This study reports that mothers are the sole or primary provider for 40 percent of households with children in the United States. Women make up half the labor force in the United States and 79 percent of survey respondents reject the claim "women should return to their traditional roles in society."

65. The rise in support for same-sex marriage from 2003 to 2013 is among the largest changes in opinion on any policy issue over this time period. In 2013, 51 percent of those surveyed approved of same-sex marriage. The reason most cited for changing views on same-sex marriage was having a gay family member, friend, or acquaintance. The Millenial generation is far more open to gay rights than previous generations; thus many see this as a growing trend in the US context. See Pew Research Center, "Gay Marriage: Key Data Points from Pew Research." (June 11, 2013). Available online: http://www.pewresearch.org/key-data-points/gay-marriage-key-data-points-from-pew-research/ (Accessed June 23, 2014).

66. Ibid. Although it is interesting to note that within that same study, most people who have never married say they would like to marry someday (including many who agree that marriage is becoming obsolete).

67. United States Conference of Catholic Bishops (hereafter USCCB), *Marriage: Love and Life in the Divine Plan* (Washington, DC: USCCB Publishing, 2009), available online at: http://www.usccb.org/issues-and-action/marriage-and-family/marriage/love-and-life/upload/pastoral-letter-marriage-love-and-life-in-the-divine-plan.pdf(Accessed June 25, 2014). Page numbers of subsequent references are taken from this online version.

68. Ibid., 17.

69. Ibid., 47.

70. Ibid., 17.

71. Ibid., 17.

72. Ibid., 7. The documents cites USCCB, *Catechism of the Catholic Church*, 2ed. (Washington, DC: USCCB, 2000), no. 1601.

73. Ibid., 7. The document cites Second Vatican Council, *Constitution on the Church in the Modern World (Gaudium et spes)*, no. 48.

74. Ibid., 9.

75. Ibid., 10.

76. Ibid., 10.

77. Ibid., 11–17, citing *Gaudium et spes*, no. 48, *Catechism* nos. 1604, 1652, and 2363, and *Humanae vitae*, no. 9.

78. Ibid., 18–19.

79. Ibid.,, 4.

80. Ibid., 4.

81. Ibid., 17.

82. Ibid., 22–23. An extended critique of this argument is beyond the scope of this book, but Lisa Fullam makes a compelling argument when she notes that the bishops seem to collapse the two distinct ends (unitive love and procreative love) of *Gaudium et Spes*. Fullam writes: "According to the bishops, the 'communion of persons' of *Gaudium et Spes* is revealed in the procreative capacity of couples: while the Council taught that non-procreative marriages are still marriages, the USCCB roots the unitive end of marriage in the procreative possibility of heterosexual marriage." See Lisa Fullam, "Same Sex Marriage: A Catholic Affirmation." Bondings 2.0: The Blog of New Ways Ministry, http://newwaysministryblog.wordpress.com/civil-same-sex-marriage-a-catholic-affirmation/ (Accessed June 30, 2014). See also Stephen J. Pope, "The Magisterium's Arguments against Same-Sex Marriage: An Ethical Analysis and Critique," in *Readings in Moral Theology, No. 15: Marriage*, eds. Charles E. Curran and Julie Hanlon Rubio (New York: Paulist, 2009), 300–329.

83. USCCB, *Marriage,* 23.

84. Ibid., 24, citing *Catechism*, no. 2384.

85. Ibid., 25.

86. Ibid., 25.

87. Ibid., 25–26.

88. Ibid., 27, citing Pontifical Council for the Family, "Family, Marriage, and De Facto Unions." (Washington, DC: USCCB, 2001), no. 25.

89. Ibid., 27.

90. Ibid., 27.

91. Ibid., 32.

92. References to the cross can be found in nos. 18, 21, 31–33, and 47–48. The word "self-giving" appears twenty-one times, while "self-gift" appears twelve times. "Gift of self" and "sacrifice" appear eight and five times, respectively.

93. USCCB, *Marriage,* 4.

94. "Conjugal love, the love proper to marriage, is present in the commitment to the complete and total gift of self between husband and wife." USCCB, *Marriage*, 8. In a later section, the bishops argue that contraception "makes the act of intercourse signify, or speak, something less than the unreserved self-gift intended in the marriage promises." USCCB, *Marriage*, 18. On page 46, the grace of the sacrament should make one feel gratitude for "the always undeserved gift of love," which seems to imply that one does not deserve to be loved, a strange claim indeed.

95. Kevin Kelly explains that the basic criterion is the principle of "respect for the human person." Kevin T. Kelly, *New Directions in Sexual Ethics: Moral Theology and the Challenge of AIDS* (London: Geoffrey Chapman, 1998), 140.

96. Todd A. Salzman and Michael G. Lawler, *Sexual Ethics: A Theological Introduction* (Washington DC: Georgetown University Press, 2012), 47. See also Kelly, *New Directions*, 140.

97. See Richard M. Gula, S.S., *Reason Informed by Faith: Foundations of Catholic Morality* (New York: Paulist, 1989), 63–73, 220–249; Charles E. Curran, "Natural Law" in *The Development of Moral Theology: Five Strands* (Washington DC: Georgetown University Press, 2013), 73–147.

98. Kelly, *New Directions*, 9–10.

99. Other important works on Christian ethics and HIV/AIDS include: James Olaitan Ajayi, *The HIV/AIDS Epidemic in Nigeria: Some Ethical Considerations* (Rome, Italy: Gregorian University Press, 2003), Elias K. Bongmba, *Facing a Pandemic: The African Church and the Crisis of AIDS* (Waco: Baylor, 2007), Melissa Browning, *Risky Marriage: HIV and Intimate Relationships in Tanzania* (Lanham: Lexington, 2014), Maria Cimperman, *When God's People Have AIDS: An Approach to Ethics* (Maryknoll, New York: Orbis, 2005), Musa W. Dube, ed., *HIV/AIDS and the Curriculum* (Geneva: World Council of Churches, 2003), Musa W. Dube and M. Kanyoro, eds., *Grant Me Justice! HIV/AIDS and Gender Readings of the Bible* (Maryknoll: Orbis, 2004), Robin Gill, ed., *Reflecting Theologically on AIDS: A Global Challenge* (London: SCM Press, 2007), T. M. Hinga, A. N. Kubai, P. Mwaura, H. Ayanga, Eds., *Women, Religion, and HIV/AIDS in Africa: Responding to Ethical and Theological Challenges* (Pietermaritzburg, South Africa: Cluster, 2008), Robert H. Iles, ed., *The Gospel Imperative in the Midst of AIDS* (Wilton, Conn.: Morehouse, 1989), James F. Keenan, S. J., ed., *Catholic Ethicists and HIV/AIDS Prevention* (New York: Continuum, 2000), Kenneth R. Overberg, S. J., *Ethics and AIDS: Compassion and Justice in Global Crisis* (Lanham, MD: Rowman & Littlefield, 2006), Gillian Paterson, *Women in the Time of AIDS* (Maryknoll, New York: Orbis, 1996), Timothy Radcliffe, Lytta Basset, and Eric Fassin, *Christians and Sexuality in the Time of AIDS* (New York: Continuum, 2007), and Cassie J. E. H. Trentaz, *Theology in the Age of Global AIDS and HIV: Complicity and Possibility* (New York: Palgrave Macmillan, 2012). The 2007/3 edition of *Concilium: The International Journal of Theology* was edited by Regina Ammicht-Quinn and Hille Hacker and focused on AIDS (London: SCM, 2007).

100. Beverley Haddad, for example, describes herself as an "activist-intellectual." Beverley Haddad, "Living It Out: Faith Resources and Sites as Critical to Participatory Learning with Rural South African Women," *Journal of Feminist Studies in Religion* 22:1 (2006): 135–154. Ada Maria Isasi-Diaz, identifies herself as an "activist theologian" in *Mujerista Theology* (Maryknoll, NY: Orbis, 1996). For these theologians, the goal of their research is advocacy for social justice. Liberationist methodologies typically entail the goal of personal conversion and social transformation.

Chapter Two

Learning by Listening: The Life Experiences of Eight Catholic Women

> He left that place and entered their synagogue; a man was there with a withered hand, and they asked him, "Is it lawful to cure on the sabbath?" so that they might accuse him. He said to them, "Suppose one of you has only one sheep and it falls into a pit on the sabbath; will you not lay hold of it and lift it out? How much more valuable is a human being than a sheep! So it is lawful to do good on the sabbath." Then he said to the man, "Stretch out your hand." He stretched it out, and it was restored, as sound as the other.
> Mt 12: 9–13

If your sheep fell into a pit, you would want to grab on to it and lift it out, Jesus tells the people. But how much more valuable is a human being than a sheep? When we witness the struggles of our fellow human beings, we are sometimes moved with compassion. Stories can stir in us a desire to help, to look into the pit and offer a helping hand. Perhaps hearing the stories of these eight women will have a similar impact. These eight women, all Catholic and HIV-positive, shared intimate details of their lives for this study.[1] All are women of extraordinary courage, resilience, and faith, who are also vulnerable, fragile, imperfect, and not without their share of fears. Only two had disclosed their HIV-status within their parish, so for most this was the first time they had been invited to share their personal story of faith for the benefit of the wider church community.

Listening to the experiences of others can be deeply moving, unsettling, and de-centering. The process of listening creates a collaboration between the listener and the speaker. In my experience of listening I came to appreciate my collaborators' struggles, perceptions, and worldviews and began to examine privileges in my own life, all the while sharing a profound solidarity with these women.[2]

The church, too, can benefit from listening to these women's experiences. But this process of listening might also be unsettling and de-centering for the church; listening to and honoring these women's stories may challenge some previously held assumptions underlying church teachings. Even knowing this, Christians must cultivate the practice of listening. When Jesus encountered the man with the withered hand, he recognized his value as a human person and wanted to restore his health. Jesus challenged his followers to prioritize love and concern over the letter of the law. As a church called to continue the mission of Jesus—to preach God's transformative love and to work in solidarity against the injustices of our world—the process of listening should precede any action. We need to listen before we speak, preach, and advocate for changes in public policy. Pope Francis repeatedly calls the church to listening as a way to demonstrate openness to the other and ministry of presence.

> We need to practice the art of listening, which is more than simply hearing. Listening, in communication, is an openness of heart which makes possible that closeness without which genuine spiritual encounter cannot occur. Listening helps us to find the right gesture and word which shows that we are more than simply bystanders. Only through such respectful and compassionate listening can we enter on the paths of true growth and awaken a yearning for the Christian ideal: the desire to respond fully to God's love and to bring to fruition what he has sown in our lives.[3]

It is interesting that the pope calls listening an art, for certainly listening requires a kind of attunement and sensitivity often associated with creativity of expression. But all of us can learn to be better attuned to the needs and concerns of others, even if we do not consider ourselves artists. Compassionate listening communicates to the speaker that her voice *matters*, that she *counts*. It communicates: *I'm here. You are not alone. We are in this together.* Pope Francis and his predecessors have continually emphasized the priority of love.[4] And it is this call, "to see God in others and to go forth from ourselves to seek the good of others"[5] that grounds this demand to listen to the voices of people living with HIV before we begin to construct a church response to the moral crisis of HIV and AIDS. Towards that end, the stories in this chapter introduce my collaborators and offer a glimpse into the complicated, messy, confusing situation in which each woman finds herself so that we may begin to understand her stresses and anxieties, and the way that she sees her world.[6]

When this project began in 2006, the women were between the ages of thirty-seven and fifty-nine years old; seven lived in Chicago, and one lived in a rural Midwest town but traveled to Chicago for support-group meetings. All described themselves as Catholic. Six were married, one was widowed, and one was married but separated from her husband. Of these eight women, four are African-American/Black, two are Hispanic/Latina, and two are Caucasian/White. Six of the eight had children. Three had sero-discordant marriages; that is, their partners were not HIV-positive. Five had HIV-positive partners. Each spoke to the ways that HIV forever changed her marriage, her relationships with family members, and her sense of financial stability and social dependence on others and on the government. Each found solace in prayer and found strength in her personal faith; all had suggestions to the church for how to address AIDS more adequately.

SUE MELTON[7]

Sue Melton does not fit any AIDS stereotype. When we met in 2006, Sue was fifty years old and had been married for thirty-three years. She has two grown children and one grandchild. Sue lives in a rural Midwest town but traveled to Chicago for support-group meetings. Sue described herself as a cradle Catholic and Caucasian/White. She was exposed to HIV during a surgery in 1981, but was only diagnosed in 1993. "So I had been living with HIV for twelve years, and it went undiagnosed, but I was living in a rural area so the doctors always had other reasons for thinking I was sick. Now I've been living with HIV for twenty-five years. That's a long time." Sue was eager to tell me her story, and while she was soft-spoken and gently led me through a description of her personal journey at the beginning of our discussion, she also became exasperated in telling me about the people who make her angry.

Sue encountered a great deal of ignorance, stigma, and fear from people in her town and in her church community. Her husband helped her to stay strong. Especially frustrating was the ignorance of AIDS from her local church, and once she was asked to leave a Catholic bookstore because she was putting up a poster advertising an AIDS family camp on their public bulletin board. Fellow parishioners avoided her, and her pastor refused to break the silence. This went on for fourteen years.

> It's kind of like, they know I'm sick, but let's not really talk about it, that's kind of how it's been. There's nobody else in my church that's AIDS-affected. I tried to get them to do AIDS Compassion Sunday. That's a service for those who are infected and affected. But after the bookstore incident last year, that was dropped. And I really felt that there was a lack of leadership in our church. So this last year has been extremely difficult for me. I don't feel close to my church.

And yet Sue's relationship with God remains strong. "It's during those times that I hurt the most that I feel closest to God. If I didn't have my faith, I know I'd be dead by now." Sue's faith grounds her and gives her hope, even though she does not always feel comforted by her participation in her local parish.

Sue and her husband endured many difficult years of financial stress, anxiety, and, for Sue, complications with medications. They were frequently unable to pay all of their bills, and her insurance coverage was very limited. Despite so many hardships, she has a deep faith and remains committed to educational outreach, especially to family members of the newly diagnosed. Since Sue has lived so long with HIV infection—and continues to live a happy, busy life—her story can give them hope and help them to see that one can live a stable, happy life with HIV. Sue's goals for the rest of her life are simple: take care of herself as much as possible, love her family, see her granddaughter grow up, support her husband emotionally, and work to change the church in any small way she can by helping people in her own community understand HIV and AIDS more deeply. Sue told me that these simple goals are often complicated in real life, but they help keep her focused on what is most important. She refuses to be silent, even though people resist change and her story makes them uncomfortable.

CHERYL KING[8]

When we first met in 2006, Cheryl King was fifty-three years old and full of energy and self-confidence. Cheryl is African-American/Black and has six grown children. Her husband of three years was also HIV-positive. They speculate that they were infected through intravenous drug use. Cheryl converted to Catholicism as an adult, and Cheryl's childhood experiences in the Missionary Baptist church also form her spirituality in significant ways. Cheryl first discovered she was HIV-positive in 1999 when she had flu symptoms that would not go away. She did not believe the nurse who gave her the results, and went through a long period of denial. Looking back, Cheryl says she should have known that she was in trouble, because she was using drugs at the time and her life was in a downward spiral, but it was not until she hit "rock bottom" that she accepted her status. She has since completed a drug and alcohol rehabilitation program and attends Alcoholics Anonymous (hereafter AA) meetings regularly. Cheryl was proud that she has been "clean" since 2003. Cheryl is a person of deep faith and explained that she often prays to God.

> At night, I just thank God for that day. It helps me rest, helps me drift to sleep, because I'm in a state of gratitude. I forget my burdens. I've learned to slow down a little bit now too. When I leave the house, I just ask God to watch over me, carry me through this day. Sometimes in the morning if I'm in a sour mood, I'll say to God, "God I don't know what is wrong with me today but

> whatever hardness I have in my heart, remove it. Help me feel better. Don't let me walk around like this all day."

Her husband remains a source of strength for Cheryl in dealing with the burdens of being HIV-positive.

> He's my honey. He does everything he can for me. See after my last surgery, he had to go to work, but it was cute how worried he was for me. He laid everything out on the counter, all my meds and things for me to eat, and, see, my daughter pretended she had something better to do, so I was all alone that day, but I was okay. But he was so worried. He called and checked up on me. And that means a lot, you know.

Their lives were filled with struggles to pay their bills, and they both had frequent appointments with doctors, therapists, case managers, and support groups. But Cheryl was quick to count her blessings: her children, her husband, his job, their apartment, their church, and their network of support. Cheryl remained realistic about her illness and how it affected her marriage.

> It's the little bitty things that you really need to appreciate. If I don't feel like cooking, he'll go out and get some fried chicken, and we'll eat it right from the bucket in the middle of our bed watching a movie. We're casual like that. But every day is a challenge, you know. We aren't perfect, nobody is perfect. You have your good days and your bad days, but we are in this thing together, me and him. And we support each other. This is a big process, a big struggle, HIV. So I think being married helps you deal with it.

Cheryl tried to remain positive, despite all of her struggles. She and her husband depend on each other and support each other in big and small ways alike. She also depends on governmental assistance programs and networks of support through her health-care provider and social-service agencies. These have all been tremendously helpful as she copes with her illness.

KEESHA WALKER[9]

When we met in 2006, Keesha was thirty-seven years old, and had been living with HIV for twenty years. Thin and tall with bright eyes, Keesha described herself as African-American/Black. On the day of our first interview she arrived late, her hair pulled back, complaining of feeling ill from her medications. She felt drowsy, she said, and looked forward to going back home to bed. She told me that even though she felt ill, she wanted to tell me her story. She *needed* to tell me her story.

As a rape survivor who was infected by a sexual partner at age seventeen, Keesha still had a hard time accepting her status. Substance abuse helped

Keesha escape from her pain, for a time, but addictions caused her even more problems. "Truthfully, I think I still can't accept it. Because that's some rotten sh—. Excuse me, I was going to say something else. That's some rotten stuff. And finding out what you got, and that it's going to kill you, that can make you crazy." Keesha told me that she still feels dirty and used.

In twenty years of living with HIV, Keesha had a variety of doctors and medications. She struggled with understanding her drug regimens and taking her medicines, but as the regimens improved[10] she became better at taking her medications.[11]

Her nine-year marriage to Shawn, who worked for the Park District, provided many happy memories. When we spoke in 2006 they were separated, but Keesha was emphatic that they were *not* divorced. She told me "we *will* work out our problems."[12] Keesha told me that she was motivated to attend her Alcoholics Anonymous (AA) meetings regularly and meet with her sponsor, and to take good care of herself, since failing to do so contributed to their marital separation. Keesha said Shawn lost trust in her, and did not want to be with her anymore. She admitted that it was probably very difficult for him to be married to her because she continued to struggle with drug and alcohol addictions. Keesha told me she was trying to turn her life around because she missed Shawn daily.

> But now, you know, sometimes you don't really think about a person until they're really gone. I think about him every single day. Every day of my life. I'm always going to love him. But I was just scared. You know, it still hurts me. If I just think about him being with somebody else, ah. I will never get that through my head, you know. Because that's my husband, you know. And I was thinking today, I think once you get married one time you can't get married again.

Keesha confided about her broken marriage to her support group that she attended regularly, and she developed many strong friendships with the HIV-positive members of that group. She told me that she prayed to God every day to keep her safe and give her strength, but she did not attend church regularly anymore. "It's hot and cold for me. They always ask for money. I don't like that. God doesn't need my money. God ain't asking for nothing but us. That's what I think."

Although Keesha was tired and feeling sick, and I wondered whether it would be best to cut our interview short, she was determined to answer my questions and kept saying that it felt good to tell someone about what she has endured. Despite the layers of tragedy in her story, from sexual violence to drug abuse to a broken marriage, she was doing her best to cope day by day and was grateful that she had found networks of support (though not within her church). Her greatest fear was to be alone, so she was determined to continue to reach out to these networks and to seek reconciliation with her husband.

CARMEN RAMIREZ[13]

My interview with Carmen Ramirez was conducted with the help of an interpreter, as Carmen is not fluent in English and I am not fluent in Spanish. Carmen graciously welcomed Susana (our interpreter) and myself into her home on a hot August afternoon. Carmen lived in a predominantly Latino/a neighborhood peppered with bustling neighborhood markets and street vendors selling merchandise from the sidewalk. We sat on her oversized couch in the living room, decorated in pale pastel colors and family pictures. Her neighbors outside greeted us with smiles and music as we made our way to the house.

On that hot summer day in 2006, Carmen described herself as forty-four and Hispanic.[14] She has three daughters and had been HIV-positive for ten years. She complained about her figure and her daily fatigue, but was eager to share her story. Carmen was convinced that she acquired HIV while hospitalized for a tubal-ligation surgery[15] after her third pregnancy in 1995. The physicians and social workers at that hospital insist that this is highly unlikely, and they contend she most likely contracted the virus through sexual contact.[16] Carmen is animated and furious when talking about these hospital employees.

Carmen first discovered she was HIV-positive in December of 1996 when she was hospitalized for pneumonia and the doctor asked if she would consent to an HIV test.

> And the day they told me, I'm telling you, I felt sick. My feet were numb because with this illness, you get your feet numb, because of the weakness, my hands too. The only thing I remember is that my daughters were first, and when they told me, I screamed, screamed and cried that it could not be possible that I had this illness. "It can't be," I said, and "no." And then they told me: "And why can't it be?" "It's that, it can't be," I told them. "Because the father of my daughters, I don't know, He is not sick," I told them. "And can it be," they told me, "that he had passed the illness to me?" And I even started to suspect him. But what I was telling them is that it can't be because he never fell ill.

She is motivated to survive now so that she can care for her daughters, and that helps her to live and to avoid despair, but Carmen says that she will never accept her disease.

Carmen's first marriage took place in Honduras before she came to the United States. She has one daughter from that marriage. Her first husband is still in Honduras, and their marriage ended when she came to the United

States looking for a better life. After a difficult period of separation, she and her first husband divorced. Carmen's eldest daughter is in Honduras with Carmen's first husband. She proudly showed me her eldest daughter's picture in her living room.

Carmen's second marriage took place in the United States, and she has two daughters from that marriage. This husband was tested for HIV after Carmen was diagnosed HIV-positive, but his tests came back negative. Overall her second husband was supportive and helped to cheer her up and helped her focus on her family and the good things in her life. But that marriage ended in 1998 when he was deported after being arrested for drug possession. So Carmen cared for her two daughters here in the United States for five years by herself. During that time she was close to despair on many occasions and even contemplated suicide. She says, "If I hadn't had my daughters, I would have taken my own life a long time ago."

At the suggestion of her case manager, Carmen began to attend support group meetings, and she has found an important nonjudgmental community there. They call her "the Crying Woman."

> Crying woman, you know, there comes the crying woman. Because I cry. Because of the disease, I always cry. And before that I never spoke about my disease, and now I speak up in the groups and I explain then the steps I had to take. I was close to taking my own life, and that life is beautiful, and that they mustn't take their lives. Now I am one of the advisors, you know?

It was through that support group that Carmen met her third husband. They married in 2003, and she said they were companions more than anything else. They are both HIV-positive and taking medicines. She tells me that "sex is not the same anymore." They show their love in other ways, by taking care of each other. She says they are good for each other because neither wants to be alone. But Carmen and her husband are in therapy because they still have some problems. He sometimes becomes bitter about being HIV-positive, and he has expectations for Carmen that she does not always agree with, so they often argue.

Carmen has never told her pastor that she is HIV-positive but she continues to attend Mass regularly. She also prays to God directly and has devotions to Mary and to particular saints.

DIVA JACKSON[17]

When I first interviewed Diva Jackson in 2006 she was fifty-two years old and proudly showed me pictures of her six grown children and five grandchildren. On the day we met she was feeling strong, healthy, and ready to share her story so that other women could hear what she had been through.

Diva described herself as African-American/Black; she converted to Catholicism as an adult.

When she was first diagnosed with HIV in 1999, Diva went through a two-year period of denial. She said she did not feel sick, and could not understand how she could have the virus. She had used drugs in the past and had a history of alcohol abuse, and when she was informed about being HIV-positive, she continued to use alcohol as an escape. This was part of her denial, but with the help of her priest, Diva enrolled in a residential drug-treatment program; when we first talked Diva had been drug- and alcohol-free for two years.

> I was going to the Catholic Church. I found out you could talk to the priest more openly. That's actually when I first started realizing that I had HIV. I was staying sick all the time. And my priest told me, he said, "Why don't you go ahead and stop being in denial? And just face facts. But God forgives all sinners. And just do what you have to do to survive."

While Diva had accepted her illness, she remained afraid to tell her children. She told her children that she had cancer, which was true, but was not the whole truth.[18] Her youngest children lived with her eldest daughter, so Diva was not the primary caretaker for any of her children anymore. She continued to pray about this dilemma and asked God to help her disclose her status to her children at the "right time."

Even though Diva faithfully took her medications, she did not like the idea of being dependent on them and hated to think that she needed medicines to survive.

> See, each day I wake up in the morning, and I know I got a life-threatening disease, and I look at all those twenty-eight pills sitting on my dresser, and sometimes I just want to take each and every bottle and throw them out the back door. But I know that if I don't take my medicine, I can't thrive. I can't be there for my grandchildren. I can't go to the mall, I can't get my hair done, can't get my nails done, I can't move around. And I love to shop, know what I mean? But the faith that I have in God helps me keep going every day. And I have to keep that faith. And I just take my pills, put a smile on my face, and drink a lot of water, and say okay, and just go on. But some days, you just want to say, "I'm tired. I'm fed up! I'm tired of taking medicine."

Diva had an active prayer life and was quick to describe her reliance on God. I asked her whether her struggles to take her medications ever make her angry with God. She explained:

> Yes, it makes me angry at everybody, including God. But then, you're not supposed to get angry at God. God don't put nothing too much on you that you cannot bear. He gave me something to live with and I know I can bear it. But

> the thing is, I know I can live a productive life and be a productive member of society. I can go anywhere, and no one has to know that I am HIV-positive unless I tell them. So that's the way that I look at it.

Even though Diva admitted that her situation angered her, she trusted that God would give her the strength to bear her burdens. Her faith in God renewed her energy and enabled her to face her illness and the frustrations that come with it, including fatigue and depression.

> Cause when that depression sets in, nothing will help until it passes over. You know, it's like a film that comes over, a bubble, and it has a lock on it, and not until that lock is unlocked do you feel like getting up and doing something. Sometimes it takes a day, sometimes a week, or whatever. But me, I pray. I say, "Lord, whatever it is that I'm going through, help me."

In addition to relying on her relationship with God, Diva relied on her husband, Lamar. Diva and Lamar had been married for almost two years when we met in 2006, although they had known each other for six years. Lamar was already AIDS-diagnosed. Diva explained that their marriage is built on trust and companionship. They took care of each other and expected that since they were both living with HIV, they would have to take care of each other a lot in the future. Diva was confident that when the time came to care for Lamar she would be able to do it, but she told me that she tried not to think about that too much.

LETTIE MENDOZA[19]

My interview with Lettie Mendoza took place in her home on a hot July afternoon in 2006. Lettie is bilingual, so the interview was conducted in English. At the time, Lettie was fifty-nine years old; she described herself as Hispanic and a cradle Catholic.[20] Although born in Mexico, Lettie came to Chicago when she was fifteen years old. She has three children and five grandchildren.

Lettie's first husband was abusive, and when she felt her children were old enough to cope with the inevitable disruption in their lives, she left her first husband.

> And that's when my life began, actually, because I was never really happy with my husband. Then I dated, started going out and dating. I dated one guy for three years. And then I dated another guy for three years, and I think that is the one that had the HIV. Because he got really sick with pneumonia. And at that time I didn't know anything about HIV or AIDS or anything like that. I was always home, you know? I was always with my grandmother or my

> children. I was home. See I was always either at work or at home. I was never on the street. So I didn't know much about what was going on, or AIDS.

Lettie's second husband, Cesar, was not HIV-positive. When we met in 2006, Lettie and Cesar had been together for twelve years. When they first met, Lettie did not know of her own status. When she got sick in 1998 and was tested for HIV, she was shocked to find out she was HIV-positive. Her family has been extremely supportive of her, especially Cesar.

Lettie had still not told her friends or coworkers of her HIV-positive status, and feared that if her employer knew she could be discriminated against at work. This caused her a lot of anxiety. She also explained that her medications were expensive, but she had insurance through her employer, so she did not have to worry as much as other HIV-positive people.

Lettie attended church every week, and she knew her parish priest, but she said that there was no support for her at her church, and so she remained involved in the support groups recommended by her case manager.

Lettie explained that HIV was part of her whole life now. Sometimes it was difficult for her to remember to take her medication, and sometimes she resisted taking it, but Cesar always helped to remind her and encouraged her when she resisted.

> There are moments when I don't think about it, but it is still there, you know. Sometimes I try to turn the switch off and enjoy my day, and it all depends on what I'm trying to do. And I still have to take my medication. That's very hard for me. Sometimes I leave the house without bringing my medication with me, and then I get back and I take it later than I'm supposed to. When I get home, he always reminds me, "Did you take your medication?" It is amazing how many times I still forget. That's the hardest thing, taking medication.

Lettie constantly felt overwhelmed, as if she could not catch up with her life. She juggled doctor appointments, therapy and support-group meetings, and family obligations, but still worked full-time and could not afford to retire. She hoped that in the next six years her health would remain stable and healthy so that she could retire at age sixty-five. She was thankful every day for the love and support of her husband.

CRYSTAL SMITH[21]

Crystal Smith is a thin, petite, and energetic woman who is a rapid-fire conversationalist. When we first met in 2006 she was forty-seven years old and described herself as African-American/Black. She was raised Catholic, but said that she attended Mass irregularly. She made a special effort to attend Mass during Lent and Easter, which are her favorite liturgical seasons.

Crystal discovered her HIV-positive status during a time in her life when she was addicted to drugs and alcohol and living on the streets. Her mother raised her two sons when Crystal was living on the streets. Crystal does not remember why she was in the emergency room in the first place, but that is where she was tested for HIV/AIDS.

> When I first found out that I was HIV positive I was stuck. I'm like, "I'm hearing it, but I don't want to hear what you're saying." That was fifteen years ago. I didn't even go in to be tested for that, but they asked if I would consent to the HIV test. When I found out I had it, I just couldn't believe it.

Since that first experience of shock, Crystal found ways of coping with her illness. She said that she never blamed God, but took responsibility for her own actions.

> But throughout it all, I mean I know I did some things. So I would never say, "Poor me, why me?" To God, I mean. I say instead, "Well why not me?" I still am blessed. I'm living. It hasn't stopped me from doing anything yet. Stuff comes up, I catch stuff quicker than others, but if I do what I'm supposed to then I can get right back on track.

Crystal tried to avoid feelings of self-pity and was determined to live a healthy lifestyle. She had taken responsibility for her past actions but still tried to see the blessings in her life.

Crystal is dependent on governmental assistance programs, but expressed frustration about long waiting periods and slow response times. She learned to be her own self-advocate, but this is often exhausting.

Crystal has two adult sons. When we met in 2006, one son was serving in the US military and the other lived with his grandmother, Crystal's mother. Crystal had been married since 2004. She met her husband in 2001 at an AA meeting; they are each recovering drug addicts and alcoholics. They were together for three years before they married. Crystal admitted that it had been a difficult relationship because "he has a bit of an anger problem" and because Crystal carries the trauma of being a rape survivor.

Crystal explained that although she and her husband were both HIV-positive, they were still asymptomatic, thus they had not had to work very hard to take care of each other. But they accompanied each other to their doctor appointments and supported one another in their daily living.

> He goes to my doctor appointments with me, and I go to his appointments with him, so we both know that we need to take care of each other. Sometimes we use condoms. We know about the risk of not using it, because he's not on meds, and he's undetected, but I'm on meds, even though my count is high. I'm confused about that, but sometimes you know in the heat of the moment, I

> go, like, "No, we better back it up. We've got to use a condom." And his faith is not as strong as mine. So occasionally he'll just get pissed off at the world.

Crystal described the need for mutual care-giving in her marriage, including condom use as part of that call. She also described her husband's willingness to accompany her at the doctor's office as a sign of his commitment to her. Further, Crystal explains that her husband continued to struggle with his addictions, and she tried to be a positive influence in his life.

> He thinks it's a death sentence. I know that we're going to die from this. But I got hit by a car last year; I could've died then. So, uh, we don't too much approach the subject. We don't too much talk about it. He gets angry though. It upsets him, it disturbs him. As a matter of fact, he's pretty healthy himself. You know, he can walk from here to kingdom come, but he says things like, "I want to get drunk, I might as well, I'm dying anyway." And when he gets in that sour mood, can't nobody get him out. So sometimes I just say, "Go ahead, but just be back here to pick me up when I get out of this meeting."

While her husband struggled with anger, depression, and alcoholism, Crystal tried to see how she could help him and support him. While Crystal anticipated that she might become more of a caregiver to her husband if he were to become ill, they had not encountered that yet in their relationship.

> No, we're not at that stage. See he's pretty healthy. And I don't really get sick that often. Now one time when he did have the flu—he was real messed up—and we're pretty good at waiting on each other. When he's like that, he doesn't have to get out of the bed. I bring him anything he wants, and vice versa. Naturally I'm more nurturing, that's what women do. You know, men are big babies. He brings me two cups of soup and he's tired. But anything that he wants or needs I get him through it. That's pretty much all we dealt with though, just a simple cold. We haven't been sick sick sick.

While a "simple cold" is all they've had to encounter so far, Crystal's view of herself and her role in their marriage can be detected here. She saw herself as a strong and courageous woman, and her role was to help and take care of her husband. She offered few descriptions of her own self-care.

While Crystal was active in support groups, she had also confided in her primary-care doctor that her husband had a history of abusive behavior. She said that at every appointment her doctor checks her out for signs of abuse, which made Crystal feel better. Also, her husband had begun therapy for anger management, and planned to begin couple's therapy soon. Crystal had a strong network of support including her doctors, case manager, social worker, and support groups, but she was still a recovering addict and alcoholic, and a survivor of sexual violence. Her marriage was threatened by poverty, violence, and the potential instability caused by ill health.

GRACE CEKIK[22]

Grace Cekik had just turned thirty-nine years old when we met in 2006. She was warm and friendly and she began to tell me about her life. She describes herself as Caucasian/White, and was raised Catholic in a middle-class Italian-Catholic family. Grace's husband, Sam, died of AIDS-related complications in 1993. They had been married for less than two years. Her story challenges many stereotypes about persons living with HIV/AIDS, and yet a growing number of young women like Grace are being exposed to HIV through heterosexual sex.

Grace met Sam in the summer of 1990, after she had just graduated from college. She was excited about her new job, and felt confident about her future. She met Sam at a concert that summer. Sam introduced her to gourmet food, travel, romance, and culture. They really loved each other, and even talked about marriage. Then, when coming back from a vacation, everything changed. Grace explains:

> Well, we went on vacation, and there was something weird going on with him. He felt very distant from me, and I had a yeast infection for a year, and when I treated it, it wouldn't go away, and when we were on vacation he insisted we use condoms, and I was like, hmm, but he said, "Well, it's the yeast infection." So then when we were driving back from the airport at the end of our vacation, he said his ex-girlfriend called and said she was positive; and he said: "I got tested and I'm positive." He didn't say HIV but I knew what he was talking about. And my first thought was, "Oh my God, I don't want to lose you."
> That was my first thought. I finally had this wonderful beautiful man in my life, who is everything your mother says you should have, and I didn't want to lose him. So that was a hard day. And I was tested. And I knew I was positive. I was educated. I was already working in the social-work field, and by then I saw the signs. I knew I was positive because of the yeast infection and when I thought about the window period, I remembered I had gone through flu-like symptoms, and I knew I was positive. But actually my first test was negative. And then three months later it was positive.

Grace and Sam first went to a priest friend, Father Karl, who offered them comfort and support during this difficult time. Father Karl presided at their wedding, and then not long after, at Sam's funeral. Grace admitted that her spiritual life was greatly challenged by her relationship with Sam and the struggle of watching him die. "All the time, I asked, 'Why me, God?' I thought I had lived a pretty good life, you know, so I just wondered why me. I had given a lot of myself in my career, helping others. You know, I was angry. I was angry with God and with my situation."

Grace and Sam became involved in educational outreach and advocacy when they found out about their HIV-positive status, and Grace continued to do this work after Sam's death. Because Grace struggled with the way that people treated Sam, she wanted to raise awareness about HIV and AIDS.

> Like going to the hospital with Sam, and these medical professionals would ask him, "How'd you get it?" After they had already asked about drug use and risks and then they would look at me and say, "Do you have it too?" And there was just a fear. They couldn't even say "AIDS." And people would be afraid to touch us. One time we were in the hospital, and the nurse was afraid to clean up after him. Just regular garbage! Another time a nurse was afraid to help him to the bathroom. And a few times people didn't want to give him his medicine. And that always made me sad, to see the fear people had. I told myself, "I don't want other people to go through this." So I became an activist, and I started teaching people about AIDS and prevention.

Her presentations have been well received because she's "just a normal person who was in a loving relationship and it can happen to anyone." She encourages all sexually active persons to get tested, and all engaged couples to talk openly about their sexual past with their partners. Grace hopes that other people can learn from her story.

Grace admitted that for many years after Sam's death, she struggled with her grief and anger, and often felt bitter. She did not think she could ever meet anyone she loved as much as Sam and she missed him. She worried that her own HIV-positive status would prevent her from ever loving again, and she was actually looking forward to death. But after a while, and with the encouragement of friends, she began to dabble in the positive/positive Internet dating scene.[23] That is how she met Paul, the man she was living with in 2006. They had begun to talk about marriage and were preparing to buy their first home together, but Grace said that it was important that they take it slowly.

> He's not Catholic, so that's different. It was hard for my family at first, because he is Buddhist, and that is quite a change for my Italian relatives. But we are real open in talking about all that. We've talked about marriage, and we're getting ready to buy our first home together, and we've talked about children, so, it's good. It's not the same. I think I spent a long time looking for what I had with Sam. And this is not the same. But I finally realized, you never have the same love twice. It is always going to be different. It can be wonderful, but it won't be the same.

I asked Grace how she would describe this difference. She explained:

> Well, I think with Sam, I grew up with him. I was just a kid. And with Paul I already had a lot of who I was. So I think that you, well that's difficult too, because I had been alone for so long in between, from 1993 to 1999. And I had anticipated just being alone. So being in another relationship was a big adjustment for me. And, he's also HIV-positive. And he was very sick when we first

> met. And I purposely did not want anything serious with him because I knew what death is like, and I said I would never do that again. But, at the same time, I knew that I loved him. So for two years I tried really hard to only be friends. But finally in 2001 we started having a serious long-distance relationship. And he got healthier. And sometimes I think, "He better never get sick." I think I could handle it if it happened, I just hope it never does.

Although Grace's journey has been difficult, she was quick to say that she believed she was a stronger and better person because of HIV. Thirteen years after her husband's death, she realized that her life could go on, and she believed that Sam would be happy knowing that she is in love again. Grace had learned that living with HIV brings its own unique struggles, and caring for a dying spouse is a particularly draining and difficult challenge. But she said that she was blessed because of the people she had met during her journey with HIV, and that, while it is possible to love again, each love will be different.

A COMPLEX PICTURE

In telling their stories of HIV, most women began not with a telling of how they became infected, but rather a description of their diagnosis. Of course, even though they were living with the virus prior to their diagnosis, most women were unaware of that fact. Instead, the date of their diagnosis, and the context—the room, the person who told them the news, their initial reactions—are memories full of fresh wounds. This was a day of awakening, a day of shock, fear, anger, doubt, devastation, and despair. After this point, nothing would be the same. Whether they were told by a doctor, nurse, or sexual partner, this day became the beginning of their personal medical journeys (some would say, nightmares): new infectious-disease (ID) consults, new medicines, a fresh awareness of their bodies, awareness of their limitations, and—perhaps most upsetting—awareness of the reality of their own mortality.[24]

Their personal struggles include their medical struggles and how their medical condition shapes their view of themselves. They are *infected*. They have a virus in their bodies. On the day of their diagnosis they were told that there is no cure. This new knowledge transformed each woman's sense of herself. Sometimes that self was divided, as when Keesha tried to escape, or Diva lived in denial, or Lettie tries to "turn off the switch" and ignore the HIV. Most disclosed their status exclusively within their families and safe spaces like support groups for people living with HIV/AIDS.[25] In doing so they force themselves to withhold this information about their identity in public places, including work and church, further complicating the divided sense of self, since they were not open with all acquaintances. This lack of full disclosure is understandable in light of their experiences of stigma and their awareness of the ignorance of colleagues and acquaintances.[26] But it also meant that they lived a divided life, sometimes fearing that something would slip and they would have to explain this personal information to someone who might reject them.

After that life-changing day, their relationships were profoundly altered. This new reality of being *infected* radically changed their marriages, their relationships with their children, their friendships, their relationships with coworkers. For some, their HIV-status also opened up a new circle of friendships, especially through support groups and collaborations for political advocacy. Lettie, Carmen, and Sue explained that their support groups were like family, but this time it was a family who understood them and their most intimate fears and struggles. Lettie laughed when she told me about the gay men in her support group who became dear friends in the eight years they had been meeting weekly. She was certain they would have never met otherwise.

As people of faith, these women have asked difficult questions of their God.[27] Why would you let this happen to me? Why do people of my church avoid talking to me? What did I do to deserve this? What am I supposed to do? Despite not finding complete answers to these profound spiritual questions, they have found comfort, joy, and peace in their relationship with God. Some have been especially consoled in the stories of Jesus healing the sick, extending forgiveness to sinners, and accepting the suffering of the cross. As Diva tells me, "God won't give you burdens too heavy to bear." Keesha, perhaps the most sinned-against,[28] tells me that she prays to God to give her strength and protect her. The women's stories were often layered with details of their medical journey and of acceptance of HIV, as well as stories of intimate relationships and feelings about God and the church. The next chapter explores four emergent themes: survival, intimacy, faith, and self-care.

NOTES

1. I refer to these women as research participants, collaborators, interviewees, and, more generically, "the women of my study." All of these descriptors are meant to convey the research partnership as a mutual collaboration, though I take full responsibility for the written report and for my own analysis.

2. On "unearned privilege," see Peggy McIntosh, "Unpacking the Invisible Backpack," *Independent School* 49:2 (Winter 1990): 31–36. See also Laurie M. Cassidy and Alex Mikulich, eds., *Interrupting White Privilege: Catholic Theologians Break the Silence* (Maryknoll, NY: Orbis Books, 2007).

3. Pope Francis, Apostolic Exhortation *Evangelii Gaudium: The Joy of the Gospel* (Washington DC: United States Conference of Catholic Bishops, 2013), no. 171.

4. Ibid., no. 39.

5. Ibid.

6. The women were first interviewed in 2006 in Chicago, Illinois. The study was approved by the Institutional Review Board of Loyola University Chicago. No real names are given for

my collaborators, their family members, case managers, priests, hospitals, or any other persons or institutions named in the in-person interviews. Each woman selected a pseudonym for the book. I interviewed two women at their homes, one at her office, one at her case manager's office, and four in my office. In each case I accommodated the collaborator's preference and schedule. I had follow-up conversations with each woman by telephone after the initial in-person interview. In the Afterword I give an update on each collaborator.

7. Melton, Sue [pseud.]. Interviewed by the author, July 18, 2006, Chicago, IL.

8. King, Cheryl [pseud.]. Interviewed by the author, October 18, 2006, Chicago, IL.

9. Walker, Keesha [pseud.]. Interviewed by the author, August 4, 2006, Chicago, IL.

10. The first Highly Active Anti-Retroviral Therapy (HAART) cocktails required that patients take twenty to thirty pills a day on a strict schedule. Some of the advantages of current dosing regimens include fewer side effects and fewer pills. Information about available medications, including the HIV Drug Chart, can be found at the webpage of Test Positive Awareness Network: http://positivelyaware.com/2014/14-03/drugguide.shtml (Accessed June 20, 2014).

11. For an analysis of social factors that impede patient compliance, see Paul Farmer, Margaret Connors, Janie Simmons, eds., *Women, Poverty, and AIDS: Sex, Drugs, and Structural Violence* (Monroe, ME: Common Courage Press, 1996).

12. Italics represent her emphasis in conversation.

13. Ramirez, Carmen [pseud.]. Interviewed by the author, August 13, 2006, Chicago, IL.

14. Carmen was born in Honduras. She tells me that she calls herself Hispanic.

15. This surgical procedure is a female sterilization.

16. I have no evidence that Carmen is lying. She clearly believes that she was exposed to HIV during this surgical procedure. She says that she tested negative for HIV during her third pregnancy. Her first symptoms of HIV infection occurred in December 1996. To her knowledge, neither her first nor second husband has become ill. It is possible that her sexual partners were HIV-positive but asymptomatic. I did not request access to any of Carmen's medical records, nor did I interview the heath care workers she describes.

17. Jackson, Diva [pseud.]. Interviewed by the author, March 16, 2006, Chicago, IL.

18. Diva's cancer is an opportunistic infection to which she is susceptible because of her underlying HIV infection. To tell her children the "whole truth" would involve that she disclose her HIV status.

19. Mendoza, Lettie [pseud.]. Interviewed by the author, July 14, 2006, Chicago, IL.

20. Lettie was born in Mexico and describes herself as Hispanic.

21. Smith, Crystal [pseud.]. Interviewed by the author, August 3, 2006, Chicago, IL

22. Cekik, Grace [pseud.]. Interviewed by the author, October 11, 2006, Chicago, IL.

23. The "positive/positive" dating scene refers to persons who are HIV-positive who are seeking dating or long-term relationships with partners who are also HIV-positive.

24. I do not intend to imply that these experiences are unique to women who have just discovered an HIV-diagnosis. Someone with a cancer diagnosis, for example, might also feel angry, shocked, afraid, and aware of one's mortality.

25. Sue and Grace are exceptions here. Both have publicly disclosed their HIV-status and are involved in education and outreach in their communities.

26. To say that this privacy is "understandable" is not to approve of it. To withhold information from persons who have a right to know would clearly be problematic. Diva, for example, who has kept her children in the dark, continues to feel conflicted and afraid to fully disclose her status with them. If her secrecy prevents her children from getting tested themselves, then she could be endangering them further.

27. I do not intend to imply that these questions are unique of HIV-positive women.

28. I describe Keesha as "sinned-against" because she is a rape survivor. I am grateful to Denise Starkey for encouraging me to think critically about sin-talk from the perspective of survivors of violence. See A. Denise Starkey, *The Shame That Lingers: A Survivor-Centered Critique of Catholic Sin-Talk* (New York: Peter Lang, 2009).

Chapter Three

"Everything Has Changed": Themes of Survival, Sex, Faith, and Self-Care in the Women's Stories

> One of them, a lawyer, asked him a question to test him. "Teacher, which commandment in the law is the greatest?" He said to him, "'You shall love the Lord your God with all your heart, and with all your soul, and with all your mind.' This is the greatest and the first commandment. And a second is like it: 'You shall love your neighbor as yourself.' On these two commandments hang all the law and the prophets."
> Mt 22:36–40

The three-fold love commandment is arguably one of the central ethical motifs of the synoptic gospels. In this teaching, Jesus draws on Jewish law, explaining the priority of love for God, as well as the importance of love for neighbor and love of self. The love commandment presents an ongoing challenge for people of faith. How are we, in every action, to love God, neighbor, and self? Do these loves ever compete in the messiness of everyday life? These are questions without easy answers, but they are especially important for the stories told here. The three-fold love commandment attends to both the personal and social dimensions of Christian love. But what does it mean for the women of this study to "love your neighbor as yourself"? Must one first recognize one's own dignity and inherent worth before one can give of oneself in marriage or another form of neighbor love? Is it ever appropriate to express anger at God when one faces suffering? These and other difficult questions must be considered if we are to craft an understanding of Christian discipleship through the lens of the three-fold love commandment.

In further unpacking the life stories of the women in this study, four related themes surfaced: survival, sex, faith, and self-care. These themes share interlocking ethical concerns. The first theme uniting the women's stories is the challenge of everyday living with HIV. Their day-to-day lives were complicated by their infections, and to get through each day they had to muster the determination and willpower to survive. The second theme is the threat to intimacy in their relationships with their spouses and children, captured in the single statement: "Everything has changed." The third theme involves the challenges they wrestled with as women of faith. A fourth theme is the realization of the need for self-love and the difficulties of self-care. Some women have had to recognize acts of self-neglect in their past, and all have had to accept, forgive, and begin to take care of themselves.

"I WISH I DIDN'T HAVE TO WORRY ABOUT IT ALL": SURVIVAL IN A LIFE COMPLICATED BY HIV

The most basic theme that emerges from the stories of these HIV-positive women is the sheer willpower they must exert to survive given the threats they face on a daily basis. Some women have been socialized to always consider the needs of others before the needs of themselves, but the failure to care for oneself can be deadly. Recall that in the United States only half of HIV-positive women receive regular medical care and only 40 percent have the virus under control. In this context, advocating for oneself and prioritizing self-care is essential for physical health.

The women in this study have faced their difficulties with courage. On a good day—that is, a day when one is feeling strong and stable—time can be consumed not only by typical activities like work, grocery shopping, and paying bills, but also by attending support groups, taking one's medicines, picking up prescriptions, or going to a routine doctor appointment.[1] On a bad day, nothing is simple. Fatigue, depression, opportunistic infections, and side effects from medications turn a day topsy-turvy. Over and over again the women told me that there is no such thing as a typical day with HIV since one must daily confront bureaucratic health care systems, inefficient social-work agencies, communities fraught with stigma and ignorance, and the financial burdens of just being sick. For these women, HIV replaced dreams with nightmares.

Healthy people might not be conscious of this difference. Healthy people rarely have to convince themselves to get out of bed in the morning. Healthy people do not depend on pills for survival, or schedule their eating throughout the day according to a schedule of doses of medicines, some of which require food and some of which require an empty stomach. For healthy people, a common cold is just a cold. For someone with a compromised immune system, a common cold is never just a cold. Instead, a cold can last weeks or longer and can further weaken one's immune system. Cheryl explained that she worries whenever she or her husband gets a cold because she knows that a cold can be "the beginning of the end." Cheryl explained that for someone living with HIV, nothing can be taken for granted. To surmount these obstacles one needs to make daily choices, and each day offers fresh opportunities to affirm one's determination to survive. Each day one must actively resist any temptations to give up.

The stresses that come with HIV often involve an interrelated pattern of medical, emotional, psychological, and financial stress, as Sue, Lettie, and Crystal describe. For Sue, a specific challenge she has faced is how to pay for her medications:

> It has been very difficult. I couldn't be covered by my husband's insurance because it was considered a preexisting condition. And I didn't have my own coverage at that time. And nobody would take me on an insurance program because I was AIDS-diagnosed. But then, we didn't qualify for state assistance because of my husband's income. See, because we are married, the state counts both of our incomes, not like a gay couple where only one income is counted. I was told to get a divorce, and then the state would help me. So, financially, it has been very difficult. I don't qualify for a lot of programs. I don't qualify for anything that is Medicare Part D because of my husband's income. So, there have been a lot of times where we had to choose between medicines or food. Or medicines or paying our electric bill. Um, it's not easy to be married and have this.

Sue's descriptions expose the flawed systems of medical coverage in the United States. The implementation of the Patient Protection and Affordable Care Act has since begun to rectify some of these flaws, although many issues remain.[2] In Sue's case, the fact that she and her husband worked still did not ensure that she would have the protection of basic medical benefits because her HIV diagnosis was classified as a "pre-existent condition" that excluded her from receiving medical benefits. Even though Sue worked part-time and her husband had full time employment, they could not afford to pay both their food and their medical bills. I asked Sue to describe one of those times when she and her husband tried to decide whether to buy food or prescriptions. She explained:

> Well, in January of 2006. See, we used to have a program that helped us with our medicines. And when the Medicare Part D program went into effect, it basically said, everybody would qualify. But I got a call from my pharmacist saying that none of my medicines were covered. So I had to discuss with my family whether I should go off the medicines and die, because we couldn't afford them, and that's hard. And we are just living month to month right now.
> *ERB: How did you and your husband decide what to do?*

> Sue: [Starts to cry] Uh, we just decided that we would be there for each other, no matter what. Um, he'd just work harder. He didn't want to lose me. We just had each other.

In a year in which the United States spent $6,100 per capita on health care,[3] a working-class family in rural America still had to decide between food or medication. Sue experienced daily anxieties as a result of her inability to access stable, affordable medical care.[4] And Sue is not alone.

Lettie also told me that she felt "stressed out all the time" because of the way her HIV status impacted her health, her emotional well-being, and her financial status. In particular, she juggled a very busy schedule in order to get by. Lettie learned soon after her diagnosis that in order to cope she would need to have a great deal of personal determination. Through trial and error she learned how to ask for help and how to advocate for herself to get the care she needed. Taking the initiative to access the care available, Lettie explained how she navigated the network of support in Chicago:

> So then they assigned me a doctor. I was still sick, and the doctor said, "You know, you need to get help." And she gave me the number of an agency that has support groups, and she told me to keep calling them until they assigned me to a group. So I did. I went in right away, and they assigned me a case manager. I got a lot of support from them. It has been eight years and I still go there. I only miss [going to] support groups when I'm sick but other than that I am faithfully there.

Personal persistence led Lettie to first access medical care and then to join a support group. Fearing dismissal, Lettie did not disclose her HIV-status to her employer so that she could remain insured. Also hesitant to confide her fears and stresses with her family because she did not want to burden them, her HIV-positive support group provided her the safe space to process her questions, fears, and new experiences, while obtaining valuable information and making deep friendships. At these support-group meetings Lettie could talk about the changes in her body as well as the stresses in her family relationships.

> My experience is that after I started the treatment it was bad. I started getting side effects. That's when it was really, really—well, my real life [with HIV] began. I cried all the time. And I said all the time, "Why me?" Only in the last year did I stop crying when I talk about my situation. Besides then, I just cried and cried and cried. I guess the support groups helped me a lot.

For Lettie, her support group listened to her as she described her angers and fears, gave her the opportunity to ask difficult questions, and gave her the safe space to grieve about her situation and to accept her HIV infection.

While these support groups were a very valuable resource for Lettie, sometimes it became difficult for her to squeeze sessions into her busy schedule. She worked full-time, and needed to work, but even having a full-time job did not prevent her from experiencing financial stresses. Thankful that her job provided health insurance, Lettie counted this as a huge blessing in her life. Under her insurance plan, many of her medications were covered. But the co-payments increased significantly over the years, creating a financial burden.

> It is getting harder because not everything is covered now. See, some of the side effects cause these other problems like high cholesterol, which require other drugs that are also expensive. My insurance went up, and I have seven drugs each month, and that is twenty-five dollars per drug each month. So $175 per month just for drugs. For me, that's a lot. That's a lot. When I started, it was only ten dollars a month. Now they are twenty-five dollars *each* [her emphasis]. So that is a jump.

Taking her medication remained a difficult part of Lettie's daily routine. Her husband often had to remind her.

> My HIV cocktail is twelve pills a day. That's just my cocktail, not the other drugs, for my cholesterol and stuff. Every time I get home, he says, "Did you take your medication?" Very seldom do I miss it because of him! But if it were up to me, I don't know. I guess I depend on him, to remind me. And when I first started, oh my God, it was awful. It was like, your life depends on this medication, but you don't want to take it. So you're battling with yourself and the medication, oh, it is so hard. It is the worst feeling.

While some of her drug combinations changed over the years, Lettie had been on some form of a drug cocktail since her diagnosis. Lettie struggled to adjust to being dependent on medications, and remained frustrated by the medications' side effects and prohibitive cost.

Lettie also had a dilemma: should she begin phased retirement for the sake of her health, or should she continue to work full-time to maintain health-insurance benefits? Lettie concluded then that she should keep working full-time, even as her stressful schedule was filled with meetings and appointments.

In our first conversation, Lettie explained that she worked forty-five hours a week, commuted forty minutes each way and had four evening meetings each week (two support-group meetings, therapy, and alternative medicine), attended church services on Sundays, and on top of all of that still tried to spend time with her husband, children, and grandchildren. When she was sick or has routine doctor appointments, her schedule was further complicated. Taking it one day at a time and slowing down when possible was Lettie's survival strategy. Like Sue, Lettie relied on her family for love and support, but it was her own self-reliance and personal determination that she emphasized. Lettie found inner strength to cope with the challenges that resulted from her sickness.

> Well, it is definitely more stressful. I just want to enjoy life, and enjoy my grandkids, but I have to stay on top of all this, and get my medications. And I work, so I can't apply for all the government money, and I have insurance, so everybody thinks they should pay, but they don't cover everything. So it is complicated. I wish I didn't have to worry about it all. It is not easy at all. I have a lot of support, so I try not to think about it, and I'm in therapy. I've been in therapy since I started. I don't know what I'd do without my therapy. I go once a week. Yeah. And they are real good to me. Plus I take care of my grandchildren, and they give me help, my kids. Yeah. So, but it's not easy. It's hard. Very hard.

Lettie wished she could just enjoy life, but instead she felt that HIV had control of her life. One important lesson she learned is that she had to face her own limitations and let go of the desire to do everything.

> Basically my weeks are full. Plus work. You know, I don't have any time for myself. And sometimes it is hard to miss time with family. I do help take care of my grandchildren, and sometimes I want to do other things too, but I can't. I can't do it all. I wish I could. I wish I could go to the health club, but I have these things to do. It's very very hard. Very very hard. Yeah.

Crystal, too, was coping amid difficult medical, emotional, and financial stresses. Crystal was unemployed, but relied on her husband's income and on governmental-assistance programs to get by. She had a strong network of physicians and social workers who helped her navigate the complicated, frustrating, and slow-reacting government programs. Crystal had also learned to be her own self-advocate, but this was exhausting.

> I get mad when they make me wait too long to see the doctor. That's my problem over there, because she's always backed up. That can be frustrating. Sometimes I have to wait a few hours. If my appointment is at nine o'clock, for example, I'll arrive early just to be sure, and sometimes she can't see me until after eleven o'clock. That can happen. That doesn't happen too often. But when it does happen I have to ask God for patience because I'm not too good on the patience. One of my pet peeves is punctuality.

Crystal used to be surprised and even offended by this disregard, but over time she became appreciative that she had health care at all. She told me that God helped her to be patient and not resentful and to have the extra determination and the courage to speak up for herself.

> I do have the personality where when I want something done I try to do it. Like if I've got papers that need filling out, I'll say, "Can't you fill this out for me now?" And they'll say, "We've got to go through the ten-day process." But I know that a nurse can do it for me right now. She already told me that in the room. If all you got to do is Xerox it right now, why I gotta wait ten days? So that can be frustrating because I want it now. But that's all me. That frustrates me, but that's all me. That's not on anybody else. That's something I have to work on. [Laughs]

Crystal's frustrations with a slow and broken system are understandable, and one can imagine that her experiences are not unique to HIV-positive women. While working within any system might require patience, which she admitted she was working on, it would be problematic if over time she became so worn down by the same answers that she ceased to push for help. Her nurse's "ten-day process" was not something that Crystal wanted to accept. But she seemed sensitive to the power dynamics at work here.

Crystal noted that her inability to pay for medications was another challenge in her life. She was required to pay co-payments for doctor visits and for prescription drugs. Even though she had a very helpful social worker who could assist her in developing a payment plan, she still admitted that "sometimes I don't think it's going to catch up to me like it does, but it does." Sometimes Crystal was simply unable to pay the bill. "So that can get to be frustrating, when you can't [pay]. And sometimes I don't want to say 'I don't have it [the money],' but I don't have it. But I need to see you. Because I got something going on with me. But thank God that they do not not see you, you know, when you can't pay it."

It was difficult for Crystal to admit that she could not afford the co-payments. Crystal's husband did have a full-time job, but they lived below the poverty line. His paychecks did not cover all of their expenses so Crystal relied completely on state and federal programs for her health care and medications. This meant that she frequently had to wait for long periods of time to see her doctors, that some care was off-limits, and that she sometimes encountered people who did not appreciate her dire financial situation. When this happened she tried to remain assertive and confident even if providers did not understand her financial situation.

On the day we spoke she was frustrated because she could not pay for one of her prescriptions that morning. "I didn't have the money at the pharmacy. If you go there they want their money right there." Crystal told me how she felt when this happened: "It makes me feel degraded. Less than. You know? See because, you know, I'm going to tell you something. A person will say, 'Oh, you ain't got a dollar?' You know what I'm saying? And that make you feel real little. No, I don't have a dollar. I don't have a dollar this time. Some people just don't have a dollar."

Crystal explained that many of the providers she encounters mistakenly assume that all patients have some financial means to pay for their medical needs. Some look at her with suspicion when she admitted that she was unable to pay.

> Crystal: See, when people say that, you know they look at you, they're like, "Well, you should have this and you should have that," and "Blacks, they don't want to work."
> *ERB: Have people said that to you?*
> Crystal: Not to me, but I hear it. I hear it. That we lazy. Everybody think that we should have something, even when people are struggling on public aid or state money. So what, I don't have a dollar? People make you feel like cause you don't have a dollar or two dollars, you know, you're lower than life, you supposed to be indigent, is that the word, when you don't got a dollar? Some kind of word they use when you don't got a dollar. But like I said, I'm just grateful, in spite of. Whatever space I'm in, in this time in my life, I'm just grateful.

Even though Crystal felt "lower than life," she believed she must bear this indignity and continue to assert her needs and ask for help. For Crystal, survival required advocating for herself so that she could get the care and medicines she needed, even if she had to admit her lack of means or experience blatant racism in the process. Although she remained grateful for the care she was able to receive "in spite of" these struggles, her story carried an undertone of anger and resentment.

All of the women I interviewed have been on antiretroviral (ARV) drug cocktails under the supervision of their infectious-disease (ID) physicians. Some participated in experimental drug trials for new HIV drugs. All challenged themselves to learn more about HIV, especially how it affects their bodies, and became experts decoding the medical terminology, from CD4 counts to viral loads to opportunistic infections to names of medicines.

In addition to this new knowledge, they mastered a myriad of governmental programs in order to figure out the assistance available, from programs that focus on prescriptions (like AIDS Drug Assistance Program, or ADAP), to programs that assist HIV-positive persons with housing (like Housing Opportunities for People with AIDS, or HOPWA), to the Ryan White CARE Act, which has a number of programs contained within it, and more comprehensive medical plans like Medicare and Medicaid and insurance plans. While bogged down by the number of pills and schedules of doses, calendars full with appointments and meetings, and systems of health care based in a capitalist economy, one can become lost in paperwork, frustrated by the complexity of the bureaucracy, and overwhelmed by everything that an HIV diagnosis brings. The women experienced these frustrations on a spectrum. Some relied on insurance plans and paid out-of-pocket premiums and co-pays, all-the-while feeling anxious about increased costs. Some experienced total dependence on governmental-assistance programs, though this brought a different kind of anxiety since these programs usually have to be renewed every year, and the political will is unpredictable at best. Without the support of a partner, a helpful social worker, access to a support group, fluency in English or assistance of a translator, what would happen? For these HIV-positive women in Chicago, it took an enormous amount of personal determination just to get through the day.

"AIDS COMES BETWEEN US": HOW HIV AFFECTS INTIMATE RELATIONSHIPS

In these interviews I asked my collaborators many questions about their intimate relationships, especially their marriages, but also their parenting and grandparenting relationships. Not surprisingly, an HIV diagnosis changes intimate relationships in significant ways and creates new and unique kinds of vulnerability. Sometimes this vulnerability went hand-in-hand with the woman's experience of support from her spouse, while at other times it heightened a sense of loneliness. Each woman experienced feelings of fear, guilt, and confusion in intimate relationships, and this added yet another entire dimension of stress to their lives. Sue, who is in a serodiscordant marriage, explains:

> I've lost the freedom to feel, uh, not fearful, in my personal relationship with my husband. Because I'm the one with the gun right now, so to speak. My biggest fear is infecting him. So this affects the way I look at myself too. And it affects the way we relate, because I want to protect him. Even though now we use protection, it is such a great fear, that really I would say I have lost that great freedom to feel as one. AIDS comes between us. It's always really hard because we always have to use protection. You know, it's just always something that we have to think about, that we never did before. It's really hard because I miss that relationship.

Sue's use of the image of a gun to describe the threat of HIV in her marriage is telling. She was deeply afraid of killing her husband, not with violence, but with a virus that she carries in her blood. This shaped not only their sexual loving, but—in her words—the way she looks at herself too. In this way, HIV is unique among modern diseases. Sue was not the only one to describe her sense of self as a danger to loved ones.

Lettie was also married to a man who is not living with HIV. When she first found out she was positive, she told her family right away:

> And I brought in my kids, and my sister and my niece, and Cesar, and they were all told what I had. And they accepted me. Cesar, he said, "I am with

> you." So, he stood by my side, and he's been good to me. A lot of help, a lot of support. Now, none of my family mentions my illness, but when I get sick, they are with me. When I told them, my family accepted me. And that made me feel good. Mentally and spiritually, they help me, they help me a lot. So I think it was very positive for me to go ahead and let them know right away. Because if I wouldn't, then I don't know what would have happened.

Lettie's family was supportive of her, and her husband Cesar was especially supportive. But sometimes Lettie just wished things could be the same as what they were before, especially their sex life.

> Yeah, it has changed a lot, yeah. Definitely, it has changed. I don't feel safe. At all. That would be the word, safe. So, if I don't feel safe, I don't enjoy my sex life. Because he's not positive, thank God. He didn't catch the virus. So he's negative. Which, I am happy for that, because it would have been sad if, cause, well, that's what I want to protect him from. Because if he wasn't before, he can't be now, so. [Becoming emotional, agitated.] I don't enjoy my sex life anymore. And after I had my cancer operation for my cervical cancer, now I can't take hormones, and so I'm dry. So when I have sex now, it is painful. The doctor told me that is because I'm scarring. The scar is kind of low. So my passage is not that big. Which, before, I never had any problems. I was very happy. And that makes me sad. That makes me really sad. Because I know—even though he doesn't complain—I don't know, cause he doesn't penetrate all the way, sometimes he just does it outside. But it just isn't right. And besides, he's younger than me. So I feel bad about it. And I feel guilty.

Lettie's description of her marital love-making was filled with the need to be safe, by which she meant that she did not want her husband to become infected with HIV. Lettie also had side effects from HIV-related infections that prevented her from feeling pleasure in vaginal intercourse, and this added another level of physical pain as well as emotional frustration to their sexual intimacy. While marital intimacy is not only about sexual intercourse or physical displays of affection, she clearly described this as a loss in their marriage, a loss that saddened her and made her feel "bad" and "guilty" because she could not make love with her husband as before.

> He does tell me, "I wish we could make love the way we used to." And, [starting to cry], I just keep quiet. I don't say anything, but I know why. It's because, I think, being HIV-positive is a trauma for me regarding sex. And then all the side effects that I have had with my medication, that's another thing. I mean, like I said, from 100 percent, it turned around. I mean, there is nothing, nothing, like before. Nothing, nothing at all. And I don't think we can ever go back to the same thing, because even though he says, "I don't care, I don't care, I don't care," I have to say, "Well, I do care. I do care." Yeah. I will never do it without protection. Never. Regardless. If he wants to leave, fine. [Voice cracks] I mean, as much as I care for him, I will never put him in that

> position. No, I would never forgive myself. [Cries.] I think he's a good man. I don't think I deserve him.

Almost in passing, Lettie says that Cesar is a good man and "I don't think I deserve him." She has a sense of being broken, and unworthy of the attention he gives her. Living with HIV has made Lettie feel "dirty." Sometimes it became a barrier to other feelings of intimacy with her husband. She also told me that she regrets her bad temper, and was sorry for the times she took out her frustration on her partner. "But there's no other person for me to get mad at, to take it out on, which is not right, and I realize that. And I feel bad. And I admit I have problems. But he's with me." Lettie's vulnerability was unsettling for her. She felt guilty for losing her temper with Cesar when, deep down, she knows that they love each other deeply. Her fears, guilt, and sense of unworthiness compounded her emotional pain. The stress of other areas of her life, including her difficult work schedule and meetings, only increased her anxiety at home and the strain on their marriage relationship.

Unlike Sue and Lettie and their partners, Diva and her husband, Lamar, were both HIV-positive, so their relationship had an added level of intimacy because they both shared these pains and struggles. They met after each discovered their status, and their relationship was grounded not only in mutual love but also in the desire to take care of each other. Diva's husband, Lamar, was already AIDS-diagnosed, and his health had already begun to deteriorate. She expected that she would have to care for him but did not fear that this would become too burdensome. "Some days he goes through things where, you know, he can't get out of bed. I have to bring him something to eat and stuff. I've got to take care of him. He's my spouse." Diva felt equipped to care for Lamar because she worked as a nurse's aide. "I have worked in nursing homes. I have dealt with elderly people. I have dealt with the dying. I've dealt with hospice. You know? Nothing really turns my stomach or makes me queasy. I guess that's just one way that God prepared me, you know?" While she believed she could handle the demands of caregiving for her husband, Diva hoped that Lamar would remain healthy for a long time.

Diva told me that even though she had been married before, she had never experienced this kind of love and support before.

> Lamar's very nice. He's very compassionate. He does anything he can for me, and I do anything I can for him. He's very loving. He goes everywhere I go. Sometime we go places and he'll be the only man. We are in each other's corner. When I ache, he aches. When I'm down, he's down. He cooks, he cleans, he washes, he can do whatever a woman can do. He is a companion, and I guess I was looking for that in my early years, my other marriages. I needed love. I need to be loved.

For Diva, marriage provided her love and companionship. Lamar even helped her with day-to-day chores to show her his love. They engaged in simple acts of companionship as touchstones of what the marital relationship is all about: accompanying one another to doctor appointments, going to church together, reminding each other to take medicines, caring for the home together. These day-to-day acts of mutual love are reminders that partnership and fidelity are not abstract theological terms. Partnership and fidelity must be lived out daily. For Diva, sharing a similar HIV status as her husband was life-giving, because they could share in one another's hopes as well as fears, companioning each other in good days and bad. It is worth noting that Diva and Lamar met after their HIV diagnosis, so their relationship carries no burden of one having infected the other, which would present different dynamics of intimacy, blame, anger, and possible regret.

Lamar was concerned for Diva's health and encouraged her to take care of herself. "For example, he doesn't want me to do any heavy lifting, because he's concerned for my heart and my lungs. But we have a good understanding. He's a very good companion to me. And sometimes I'm mad at him. Sometimes he doesn't move fast enough for me, but that's my stuff, my problems coming out." Married life is not free of imperfections or sins, and Diva did not only paint a rose-colored picture of her marriage with Lamar. She admitted that she had her own problems with which she continued to wrestle and that sometimes she failed to be patient and generous with her husband. But Lamar accepted her in spite of any imperfections, and they had a "good understanding." Diva described her marriage as built on companionship, and she named concrete ways in which they were companions to each other.

Diva was especially grateful that Lamar loved and cared for her children, and she in turn cherished his grown children too. HIV can affect not only marriage relationships but also parent-child relationships. While Diva accepted her illness, and was open and honest with her husband, she was afraid to tell her children that she is HIV-positive. She became emotional in the interview as she explained this struggle.

> I told my family that I had cancer, you know. And to this day I haven't told my children, you know, that I'm HIV-positive. So, I'm still working on that too, you know what I'm saying. And they're not babies. It's nothing like that. I just haven't figured out how to sit down and tell them. I got this, I don't know what you call it, this, this way I'm carrying myself. That right now I wouldn't want my children to know that I'm HIV-positive. [Voice cracking] You know, they know I did drugs and stuff like that. But I feel ashamed, I would say, to let my children know that I am HIV-positive. They know about all my other medical issues, but they don't know that I'm HIV-positive. So I'm like in denial with them. That's something I'm working on. And it's hard for me.

While Diva was involved in two support groups, and in some safe circles was very open about her status, she could not bring herself to tell her own children. It was something that haunted her. She wanted to seem strong for her children, and she worried that in telling them the truth, they would worry for her health. It was certainly a difficult discernment and Diva had been thinking and praying about this problem for years. She kept asking God for the strength and wisdom to tell them and was hoping for the right time to present itself. Diva remained anxious about her inability to disclose her status to her children and feared that she was not being a good parent by withholding that information.

In addition to the medical and financial struggles these women faced, their lives were complicated in other profound ways by their HIV-positive status. There is a stigma to HIV, because of its nature as a sexually transmitted disease and the cultural and social metaphors attached to it,[5] which complicates the ways that HIV-positive women experience their intimate relationships. Why was Diva willing to tell her children that she had cancer, but not willing to disclose her HIV status? Why were Sue's and Lettie's experiences of sexual intimacy clouded by feelings of fear, loss of libido, and a lost sense of safety and freedom? Out of love they did not want to expose their partners to the virus, but they also internalized a sense of feeling not just "sick" but also "dirty." In some way HIV-positive women can relate to the women of the Bible whose menstrual fluids were declared "unclean," or to the lepers of the New Testament who were marginalized because of their illness.[6] For my collaborators, living with HIV brought new challenges to their understandings of their own identity.

Social stigma and feelings of shame that HIV-positive women internalize can have dramatic effects on their intimate relationships. This dilemma is about much more than condom use. Little attention has been given to the ways that an HIV diagnosis strains one's intimate relationships. Sue and Lettie wanted to protect their husbands from infection. Each woman thought of herself as a threat to her partner's health. This added another level of pain and confusion to their marriages. While Diva's husband was already HIV-positive, still their sexual lovemaking had a degree of risk; they had to be careful because they did not want to transmit drug-resistant viral strains between the two of them.

"WHY ME, GOD?": CHALLENGES TO FAITH

An HIV diagnosis can shatter one's sense of faith in God's providence, and yet these women all found a way to reconcile their faith in God with their real feelings of anger, fear, confusion, and frustration. Six of the women grew up Catholic, and two converted as adults although they had previously identified as Christian; most attended church services regularly, but three did not. All described ways in which their faith—both in God and in the church—had been challenged by their living with HIV.

Sue encountered a great deal of ignorance, stigma, and fear from people in her parish. The people in her church community acted out of ignorance and fear in hurtful ways, but Sue's family helped her to stay strong. She explains:

> I think the first time I felt discrimination was when I was first diagnosed and I was in the hospital with PCP[7] and somebody found out that I was sick, and it was announced in another church on Easter Sunday, my name and what was the matter with me. And I started to get phone calls from people who started to think that I was going to commit suicide. And they wanted to come out and pray for me. I had never felt that kind of rejection and reaction from anybody. That went on for about six months.

An HIV diagnosis can be shocking and stressful enough for the person diagnosed and for her family, but in Sue's case the responses of church members made her situation even worse. Sue was angry that her HIV diagnosis was made public in church, even though it was in the context of liturgical prayers of petition. While some of her acquaintances from the parish may have had good intentions by wanting to pray with her, Sue interpreted these prayer requests as implying that something was wrong with her. Some even assumed that Sue's despair would be so great that she would be a suicide risk. Sue was hurt by this reaction, and angry that her privacy had been violated. But her sense of violation did not end there.

> Then my youngest son, who was about fifteen years old at the time, got a call from another kid at school who said: "We know what's the matter with your mom, and you're not going to have any friends at school this year." And that's when I started to speak at schools. Because it wasn't my sons who were sick and it wasn't my husband. It was me. And I couldn't make anyone else sick. But people just didn't know. So those were really hurtful times.

Sue's description reveals how ignorance of the facts of HIV transmission can breed suspicion, stigma, and violence. She was upset because of the discrimination and rejection that her family faced, even though they were not infected. This ignorance continues even among people of faith. Sue was told by her pastor to sit in the back of the church if she wanted to receive communion under both species during the Eucharist (even though HIV cannot be spread by drinking after an infected person). She was also asked to leave a Catholic bookstore when she tried to post an advertisement for an AIDS family camp on the public bulletin board. Sue says that these are typical things that happen. Sue has had to face the reality that people in her church are afraid of her and think of her as a threat to their own health and a threat to the well-being of their community. While she has tried to raise awareness among children in the schools and among her fellow parishioners in her church, her fight against stigma has been an uphill battle. Because of these struggles, Sue's faith in the church has been shaken.

Despite all of this, Sue explained that her relationship with God remained strong. "It's during those times that I hurt the most that I feel closest to God. If I didn't have my faith, I know I'd be dead by now." Sue relied on personal prayer to get through each day, and she believed God loves her and cares for her. She felt God's presence with her when she spent time with her granddaughter, and when she felt peace and hope. She described God as "powerful, compassionate, loving, nurturing, kind, gentle, always there to pick me up."

But while Sue's personal faith remains strong, she believes the church can do a better job of bringing God to people in HIV-affected families by "accepting us" and "acting more Christ-like." In Sue's interpretation of the gospels, the "good news" of Jesus is God's inclusivity, forgiveness, and mercy.

Despite the many times Sue felt hurt or discrimination in her Church, she told me in 2006 that she continued to attend regularly and that she tried to raise awareness about AIDS issues in her faith community. The priests knew Sue's positive status but she continued to feel isolated and in need of support. That is why Sue traveled to Chicago for meetings, to reach out to the support network in Chicago that was unavailable in her rural town. Her faith in God remained strong, and she prayed often, despite her frustrations with her local church community.

Unlike Sue, Carmen never told her pastor of her HIV-positive status. Like Sue, Carmen felt hurt and rejection in church, but she still prays to God and she believes that when she prays by herself in her own house, God can hear her and God understands her and comforts her. Carmen's descriptions are in the long Judeo-Christian tradition of lamentation.[8]

> I beg my God, where nobody can see me, in a little corner where nobody see me, beg Him, and tell Him everything that bothers me—everything to my God, speak with Him by myself, you know? Praying by myself, rather than telling a priest. That's my opinion. I feel more at ease telling on my own and speak with Him all alone, because I feel that He is listening to me, do you understand? Than telling a padre. I go to the church because it's, like being Catholic, I go to church, you know? But I prefer to pray by myself, or confess by myself, than telling a padre. Not all priests, right, are the same, but I feel that, priests are religious people, but they are not God, did you understand me?

While Carmen did not confide in her priest, she was able to tell God everything that bothered her. In private prayer she felt more at ease and she really believed that God was listening to her. Carmen described a beautiful and intimate relationship with God. While a priest, who is "not God," might not understand her or might judge her, Carmen can pray to God and know that God hears her. Carmen also explained that she has devotions to many saints and to the Virgin Mary. These personal devotions, combined with her personal prayers directly to God, sustain her spiritual life. Even though Carmen felt hurt by the church, she continued to attend regular services. But she was most animated about her private prayers; it is in private prayer that Carmen tells God about everything in her life.

Lettie also attended Mass every week, and she knew her parish priest, but she said that there was no support for her at her church, and so she remained involved in the support groups recommended by her case manager. Lettie admitted that she felt distant from God sometimes and had a difficult time praying.

> You know what, I think I, to be honest with you, I tell myself I don't know how to pray. And I forget to pray. But, sometimes I do pray at night. I just say one prayer, and then that's it, and I go to bed. I guess I'm not really a pray-er. I wish I was because I like to pray. But I don't know how. I don't know how.
> *ERB: Did you ever pray before you found out your HIV-status? Is that something that makes it difficult to pray, or is that unrelated, do you think?*
> Lettie: Yes, my grandmother taught me how to pray, and we used to pray every night. And I used to pray with my kids. But then I lost it. It's not that I don't believe in God, and it's not that I've lost faith in God. But I wish that he would read my mind. Instead of me saying it aloud. Or just always asking for it.

Lettie believes in God, and she attended church regularly, and enjoyed going to church with her grandchildren and her husband, but she struggled to know what to say to God. In some ways she was comforted by attending church and by her faith in God. She confessed that she does not know how to pray, and sometimes forgot to pray, and that she wanted God just to read her mind. It is another way that she was admitting her vulnerability and even her fears and questions. Prayer also takes psychological energy and active hope; perhaps it was difficult for Lettie to muster both when she struggled with the daily grind of living with HIV.

Sue, Carmen, and Lettie asked God many times, "Why me?" And while these questions emerged from their suffering and anger, even in their anger, they had faith that God listened to them.[9] Sue and Carmen found great comfort in personal prayer. All three women attended church services regularly to be nourished by the sacrament and, in Sue's case, to try to make a difference in her parish community's response to HIV/AIDS.

Grace's story presented some contrasts. Grace previously felt support through the church, and especially through the support of a particular priest, but in 2006 she told me that she had become less involved with her church community. When she and her boyfriend Sam first found out that they were HIV-positive, they went to Father Karl, a priest Grace knew.

> So what I did, my very first, right after I found out, the first person I went to was my priest. I went to this Jesuit priest I knew, and I was really worried that I wasn't going to be allowed to get married. Because I didn't want to say that I was open to having children, because at that time, there was no hope for that, you were told you could never have children, so he helped us through that, and he married us. And he buried Sam.

Grace told me that she was fortunate to have known priests in college who were "open to talking about difficult issues face-to-face, up front." Her priest friend helped her to examine her life and to accept the consequences of her actions.

> I mean, I definitely had feelings of guilt around my status. Having had premarital sex when the Church says it's wrong. And I was just really lucky to have Father Karl who listened to me and walked with me during that time. He said, "It's not that you aren't open to having children, if there's a way in the future, you're open, you're not saying that." He said, "The Catholic Church would never condemn you." He was just so wonderful.

Grace explained that during this period in her life, it was very comforting to know a priest who helped her to look honestly at her situation and to discern the right thing to do. Father Karl did not condemn her, but instead described for her a church that modeled inclusivity and love. Father Karl also helped Grace and Sam prepare for the sacrament of marriage. They completed a premarital class, took the required inventory surveys, and confided in Father Karl about their hopes and fears. Grace felt lucky to have met such a compassionate priest who helped her during that difficult time. "I don't think that everyone's experience is like that in the church, at least I hear horror stories, of unfortunate ways that people in the church have treated people with HIV. But I was really lucky."

When Father Karl served as the church's witness as Grace and Sam married each other, he really got to know them and made the ceremony very special.

> You know, Father Karl was so great. We wrote our own vows, and they were very reflective of the possibilities of death in the future. Promising to love and care for one another through diminishment and dying. We both had in our mind that this may not be forever, here, you know, but we would love one another until death. I think that, well, I remember them blessing us [holds out her hands], everyone holding their hands out and blessing us. And I remember

> that power, that sense of peace. It was really moving. [Crying] But a happy day. Very.

As Grace remembered her wedding day, she relived the powerful moment in which the community blessed them, and fondly recalled that faith-filled ceremony.

But Grace admitted that over time her spiritual life was greatly challenged by her relationship with Sam and the struggle of watching him die. She no longer felt comforted by her faith or by participation in liturgies. She became angry with God for a long time. When we spoke in 2006, Grace confided that she did not attend Mass regularly. While Grace continued to pray on her own, she also said that she lived her prayers through her work. As a social worker and program director in public health, Grace has worked in a variety of AIDS-related agencies. As she met and befriended more people affected by AIDS, she told me that she started to hang out with a wider group of people, including more gay and bisexual friends. And they talk about God too. Grace explained that she started to get increasingly frustrated and annoyed by church teachings about sexual orientation and public health policies and she drifted away from the institutional church.

Grace has traveled a long and winding road since she first went to her priest friend with the knowledge or her HIV status. She became a young HIV-positive widow when Sam died, and her spiritual journey was difficult because of her grief and loneliness. When we met in 2006 Grace was in a serious relationship with a man who is Buddhist, and she was learning about his faith as she explored her own again. She was active in advocacy work and educational outreach, and her commitment to justice motivates her in her job. She described her whole life as her prayer to God. But, unlike Sue, Carmen, and Lettie, Grace rarely attended church services and was not a member of a specific parish.

While each woman's spiritual journey was deeply personal, unique, and complex, these women described how their faith in God has given them support and encouragement and how they also questioned God or become angry with God because of the struggles in their lives. I witnessed professions of faith that revealed my collaborators' deep sense of security and trust in God, and in God's providence and love. I also witnessed my collaborators' grief-stricken lamentations and descriptions of their anger toward God and their fears for their futures. For these women, the church was a place of comfort and support as well as a place of stigma and isolation.

"I'M GOING TO HAVE TO TAKE CARE OF MYSELF": THE NEED FOR SELF-CARE

Sue, Carmen, Lettie, Diva, Cheryl, Crystal, Keesha, and Grace were each forthright about the struggles they have endured since the day they first received their HIV-diagnosis. For most, their struggles began long before that day. In describing patterns of ignorance and unnecessary risk-taking in their lives, some of these women blamed themselves for neglecting their own self-care prior to their infection. For most of the women, their struggles with self-love and self-care became easier over time, as they sought support through networks of HIV-affected groups in Chicago. But the stories of their diagnosis usually highlighted difficult past struggles. HIV-diagnosis, for Diva, Cheryl, Crystal, Lettie, and, to a lesser degree, Grace, became a wake-up call that spurred them to reconsider the direction of their lives.[10] Social workers became partners in their attempt to put their broken lives back together. Their ability to access this support highlights the paradoxical nature of the analysis of self-neglect and the need for self-love: for while self-neglecting behaviors led to HIV infection, for these five women, acceptance of their HIV diagnosis led to self-care. Social and medical resources were instrumental in helping them to access supports that enabled their self-care after their diagnosis.

In reflecting on their lives, five of the eight women were candid in describing the personal behaviors that resulted in their HIV-infection, and this was a dominant theme in their self-reflection. But we must consider not only the women's descriptions of their own personal responsibility, but also the social contexts in which the women struggled. As both agents and victims, the women's own stories demonstrate both their legitimate personal responsibility and wider social forces that thwarted their power to act responsibly. Patterns of ignorance and risk-taking emerged in their stories but that risk-taking must be understood in a broader context because of factors that limit their full responsibility.

The first level of self-neglect in these women's lives prior to their infection can be seen in the limited awareness they had of HIV and AIDS before their own diagnosis. All eight women confessed that they did not have full knowledge of HIV and AIDS prior to their diagnosis and did not perceive themselves to be at risk for HIV infection even as they engaged in risky behaviors. This lack of awareness contributed to their difficulty in accepting their diagnosis when their illness was first discovered. For Cheryl, Diva, Crystal, Grace, and Lettie, awareness of HIV could have enabled them to understand their risk of exposure and could have enabled them to protect themselves;[11] their lack of awareness instead contributed to behaviors of self-neglect.

But one is not born with knowledge of HIV and AIDS. Could these women have known better? Is this a failure of personal responsibility or is their ignorance of HIV attributable to limited educational opportunities, ineffective sexual education within their families, schools, and churches, or a failure of the media to give accurate information about HIV and AIDS? Failures on personal and social levels are evident; each woman told me that she *should* have known better, but also described reasons why she did not have full information.

At the time of their infection, Diva, Cheryl, Crystal, and Lettie thought of AIDS as a male homosexual disease.[12] While Grace was more aware of HIV and other sexually transmitted infections, and knew that women could be exposed to HIV through unprotected sex, she did not believe her partner was infected and so did not perceive herself to be at risk.[13] In the cases of Diva, Cheryl, Crystal, Lettie, and Grace, the only way they could have known that their partners were living with HIV was to ask them to be tested before engaging in sexual activity. By not requiring that their sexual partners take the HIV test and by not having an open and honest conversation about prior sexual experiences and drug use (when relevant), these women engaged in behaviors that can be considered risky or dangerous. Though such conversations require vulnerability and honesty from both partners, and can be difficult in dating relationships, avoidance of these discussions is irresponsible, especially when persons are sexually active in these dating relationships.

Lack of awareness about HIV/AIDS is both a personal and social problem. If a woman had access to full and accurate information that she resisted, overlooked, or rejected, then clearly she must bear some responsibility. But formation of one's identity as a sexual person is influenced by broader familial, social, and cultural forces. To care for oneself while dating in our contemporary context, one must resist many cultural pressures. Many young people feel invincible and do not think of their own health and safety as high priorities in their social lives. Additionally some women who struggle with self-esteem may feel incomplete if they are not in a relationship—as if they are not whole human beings on their own. Girls and women who learn about Christian values through church settings also absorb other kinds of messages about embodiment, identity, and morality. If Christian women do not believe in their inherent dignity, and do not have a deep sense of being cherished by God, they may look to dating relationships in order to feel cherished by someone. They may struggle to care for themselves in these relationships because of the patterns of their social formation as girls and women. Barbara Blodgett explains:

> As many women develop capacities for mothering, many girls develop capacities for compliance, idealization of the other, disavowal of self, attentiveness, and connection. These become girls' capacities for erotic relating; or, to put it

> another way, they constitute "erotic" behavior for girls in our culture (the way that caring and nurturing constitute mothering). For many girls, then, that "eroticism" is defined by intense romantic intimacy, pleasing a partner, dreamy visions of blissful union, perhaps even submission . . . These images are not only picked up from popular culture (though they certainly find reinforcement there), but they also represent the way girls are psychologically primed within their family life to think about erotic relationship.[14]

The capacities for erotic relating that Blodgett describes are a part of the cultural landscape for women in the United States. While the desire to please a partner or experience emotional intimacy with a lover is not bad in itself, when women ignore their own self-care in order to please a partner or maintain a dating relationship, something is wrong. The aspects of one's socialization that Blodgett describes might make it difficult for women to perceive self-neglecting actions as risky. If a woman has been formed by cultural messages that include disavowal of the self, and has had limited exposure to accurate information about sexuality and about sexually transmitted diseases, these may prohibit her from taking full responsibility for ignorance about HIV.[15]

In addition, some interpretations of Christian discipleship as self-renunciation also contribute to this self-understanding of the erotic for Christian women. These Christian influences are in addition to many others, to be sure. But if a young woman accepts some cultural and religious messages that promote self-sacrifice or the need to give of oneself to please a partner, she might ignore her own self-care by putting off a conversation about HIV testing or by agreeing to engage in unprotected sex in order to please her mate who does not want to use a condom.

An inability to perceive one's risk for HIV infection does not eliminate one's risk of becoming infected. Ignorance remains a moral problem. But this moral problem has both personal and social dimensions.

Cheryl, Diva, Lettie, Crystal, and Grace also engaged in behavior that put them at risk for HIV-infection, even though they may not have perceived the enormity of the risk at the time. Lettie and Grace engaged in unprotected non-marital sex. They were both in dating relationships, and were at risk for HIV infection because their sexual partners carried the disease, even though they were unaware of this fact. Their sexual partners both died of complications from HIV infection.[16] Cheryl, Diva, and Crystal engaged in unprotected sex and also shared needles during intravenous drug use. Alcohol abuse also contributed to their risk behaviors.[17] Cheryl, Diva, and Crystal sought help; in 2006 Cheryl and Diva were in stable supportive marriages and both had been drug-free for over two years. Crystal, who had a history of drug and alcohol abuse, attended regular AA meetings and was working with a case manager. Crystal was the only collaborator who continued to struggle in an abusive relationship. She explained to me that her abuse was part of God's will and that it taught her how to forgive others as God has forgiven her. This understanding demonstrates that her self-neglect persisted in ways that contrasted starkly with other collaborators' experiences, a point that will be examined in greater detail below.

Through limited awareness of HIV/AIDS, combined with their own actions (including unprotected sex, drug use, and alcohol abuse) these five women neglected their own well-being.[18] Grace and Lettie, who were exposed to HIV through unprotected sex, did not perceive this sex to be risky at the time. Instead, they assumed that since they were in monogamous heterosexual relationships, sex with their partner was safe. While they were not married, Grace and Lettie trusted their partners and believed they were in love.[19] In these dating relationships, Grace and Lettie believed that sex was a way to show their affection for their partners.[20]

Both Grace and Lettie admitted regret over these actions and took responsibility for them. Their descriptions came close to acknowledging these acts as self-neglectful. Grace told me that she "had feelings of guilt around [her HIV-positive] status, having had premarital sex when the Church says it's wrong." She continued, "I never blamed [Sam]. I always felt I made a choice. I knew the risk of sex without a condom, and he didn't know he was positive, you know. It was just like we were both responsible for what happened." While Grace did not know that Sam was HIV-positive, she did know that unprotected sex was risky and could have harmful consequences.

Lettie said she "should have known" that unprotected sex with her boyfriend could have negative consequences, but that "it didn't hit [her] until later." Lettie felt "guilty" about her HIV-positive status because of the possibility of exposing her current husband to the virus. Lettie regretted staying with her first (abusive) husband for so long, she regretted having unprotected sex when dating, she regretted not getting tested earlier, and she regretted that she was so unaware of HIV prior to her diagnosis. Lettie interpreted these actions as personal failures; she believed she could have left her first husband earlier, she could have avoided unprotected sex, she could have gotten tested earlier, and she could have learned more about HIV prior to her own diagnosis.

In naming these acts of unprotected sex as failures of personal responsibility, Grace and Lettie understood that they must accept the consequences of these actions. While each also wrestled with feelings of guilt, they seemed to have reached a healthy sense of perspective on their past actions. Each struggled to forgive herself and accept herself so that she does not only dwell on her regrets from the past but also can care for herself in the present and on into the future. Lettie told me that she felt sadness about her diagnosis and especially about the limitations that this imposes on her husband. Grace and Lettie did not interpret themselves as victims but instead accepted that they made poor choices and have to accept the consequences of those actions. In addition to accepting these consequences, they also had to accept themselves and forgive themselves.

Crystal, Diva, and Cheryl also accepted some degree of responsibility for their past actions, even as they shared the wider pictures of their stories to help put their own actions into perspective. Their descriptions reveal a complicated web of forces that prevented them from making good choices. Each accepted some blame for her drug use and unprotected sex, but they did not only blame themselves.

All three women described a sense of despair in their lives prior to their drug use. Cheryl explained that she had no positive role models in her life and turned to drug use when she lost hope in having a good life. Cheryl knew that drug use was not really going to fix anything in her life, but thought it would be a way to escape and feel good. Things began to spiral out of her control when she became involved with a group of users and lost her housing. As an addict, everything she did was for the sake of one more high. Even when she was first diagnosed with HIV, she could not believe it and continued to use drugs and alcohol. At this time in her life, she was still in denial. It took another hospitalization for Cheryl to accept her status, when a nurse took time to explain what HIV infection means and helped Cheryl find a social worker. Cheryl accepted some blame for her drug use because she knew that drug use would not solve her problems; but the fact that she names some wider problems (unstable family, poverty, despair, no sense of opportunities for fulfilling work) as contributing factors to her drug use meant that she did not accept blame for all of these problems herself.

When Diva started using drugs at the age of thirty-eight, she began with cocaine. At the time, Diva was unemployed and divorced, and fell in love with a man who had a stable income. He introduced her to drug use. She said she "liked the fast lifestyle, glimmer, glitter, stuff like that." She used heroin only once, but drank heavily for many years, and her cocaine addiction worsened over time. During this part of her life, even though she had children at the time, she said, "the drugs came first." Diva explains that when she was hospitalized before her diagnosis, she "didn't know a thing and was just dumb." While admitting that she was "dumb" seems to be a way that Diva accepted some blame, she also tells me that her partner was blameworthy. She says: "We were druggin' together. That's who I contracted it from. Now that I look back on it, he was cheating on me and that's how I got it." Diva tells me that her partner became infected through another relationship and then exposed Diva to his viral load when they engaged in unprotected sex. Later Diva tells me that she was in search of a loving relationship because her family background was less than ideal.

> I was looking for a father figure because my father wasn't with me. I needed love. I need to be loved. And that's why I had so much anger in me. I didn't

> get enough love from my mother and my grandmother. That's why I was going from man to man and different things. I was looking for love, as the song says, in all the wrong places.

In looking for love through a string of short-term relationships and drug use, Diva did not find true happiness.[21] It was not until she "hit rock bottom" that she decided to take care of herself. She went through rehabilitation programs twice and in 2006 was drug-free. She told me that thinking about her past life of drug use and life on the streets, and then her experience of hitting rock bottom, was "enlightening": "I can talk about all of the mistakes that I've made, and hear myself say it out loud. And yet I see that God has always been there, part of my life," Diva said. She thus named drug use and her "fast lifestyle" as "mistakes" and showed regret for this part of her past.

For Crystal, drug use was a way to escape from the pressures and tragedies of her life. She is a rape survivor, left college when she became pregnant with her first son, struggled to take care of him, and moved in with her mother who eventually raised both of her sons as Crystal was "dead into the drugs." She had moments of clarity, even during periods of drug use when she realized she could change her life. "I just wanted it to stop, I just wanted the life I was living to stop, because I wasn't raised that way and I was better than that." Looking back on her life, she claimed responsibility for her drug addiction. "Throughout it all, I mean, I know I did some things. So I would never say, 'Poor me, why me?' To God, I mean. I say instead, 'Well, why not me?' I still am blessed. I'm living. [HIV] hasn't stopped me from doing anything yet." Crystal wanted to take responsibility for her actions, and regretted her failures as a mother, but also admitted that her sexual history is fraught with violence, and she told me she did not always feel empowered to do what she believed was right.

Cheryl, Diva, and Crystal did not only blame themselves for their situations. An understanding of some of the wider social forces that constrained their agency can challenge moral theologians to understand that the burden of responsibility and blame lies not only on the women who have made these choices but also on the wider community. Within the stories told by Cheryl, Diva, and Crystal, we find descriptions of social injustices that contributed to their loss of hope and creeping despair prior to drug use. Diva even admits she was "looking for love," to no avail, when she fell into drug use. Drug use masked the harsh realities of life and offered a method of short-term escape. In such circumstances, one wonders what kind of freedom these women really had. Could they have acted responsibly? What kinds of power and determination would that have required?

Cheryl, Diva, and Crystal were agents who nevertheless experienced compromised moral agency because of these structural injustices in their lives. Human health depends not only on biological factors but also social, economic, and environmental conditions in which people live.[22] Although behavior change is certainly necessary to stem the tide of HIV infections, addressing the social factors that contribute to self-neglecting behaviors, including neighborhood decay, racism, drug use, homelessness, and violence against women is also necessary. Deteriorating inner-city neighborhoods provide the context for a range of traumatic experiences for urban American women, including sexual violence, gang violence, exposure to drug use and drug deals, unstable housing resulting from development and gentrification projects, and unemployment.[23]

Some of my collaborators described experiences of trauma rooted in their unstable social settings. All of my collaborators whose history included drug abuse are African-American and describe growing up amid unstable family networks. Chicago's African-American community struggles with the legacy of slavery and segregation, which persists in both overt and covert racism today, and whose dehumanizing influence is still felt widely.[24] While many neighborhood-revitalization projects are underway in Chicago, attention to persistent racism and corresponding social ills is absolutely necessary in order to contextualize my collaborators' stories.[25] Poverty, unstable families, and violent neighborhoods certainly contributed to their lost sense of power, but even more fundamental was the conviction that no one else cared about them, making it more difficult to care for themselves. As Diva put it simply, "I need to be loved." In such testimonies, it is clear that some of my collaborators did not believe that they could have a life of flourishing; they hoped instead to survive, to get by with what little they had.

One must also look at the experiences of gender-based violence within this context of economic and social distress. Feminist ethicists have called for renewed attention to the problem of violence in our world, and to the realities of women's disproportionate victimization in this ongoing violence.[26] Violence against women remains a widespread problem that too often goes unnoticed, unmentioned, and neglected in Church communities. Violence against women is not a small problem that only occurs in some pockets of society, but rather is a global public health problem of epidemic proportions.[27] Experience of violence and the threat of future violence also form part of the larger picture of my collaborators' HIV risk. [28] Lettie and Cheryl both experienced intimate-partner violence in prior marriages, and were able to leave their abusive partners.[29] Keesha and Crystal are rape survivors and additionally engaged in multiple risk behaviors, including unprotected sex, IV drug use, and alcohol abuse. Unlike Cheryl and Lettie, their relationships remained unstable, and they both struggled with drug and alcohol addictions.[30] Crystal accepted her husband's violence, albeit with reservations, and believed that as a Christian she should forgive her husband. Crystal had been married for two years, and her husband was also a recovering drug addict and alcoholic. They were together for three years before they married. Crystal admitted that it had been a difficult relationship. "He has a bit of an anger problem, to tell you the truth. Sometimes he's been physically abusive. But we're still together, trying to work it out. And he's getting help for that. See, I don't believe in divorce. I made a commitment to God to stay married."

When asked to describe her marriage, Crystal offered insight into her own understanding of expectations between husband and wife. In contrast to Diva's description of her marriage as a companionship in which her husband also helps her cook and clean, Crystal had a different view of her role and of her husband's role in their marriage.

> Crystal: See, I believe like in the Bible, God takes care of man, and man takes care of woman, and woman takes care of children and the house. I know today that women work, so if I work and he works, we're both gonna look after the house. But if I don't want to work, I believe man's supposed to take care of me. And that's what he does. Now, occasionally I have worked, but he has no problem taking care of me. My children are grown, so. So God takes care of man, and he [God] takes care of me too, but you know what I'm saying, and man take care of me. That's the way that it's written in the Bible. I don't believe in this 2006 Split Down the Middle–type thing. Now, I'm supposed to obey my husband, I know that, but, uh, I get caught up with that sometimes. [Pause] But I have no problem allowing him to lead me.
> *ERB: When you say you get caught up with that sometimes—*
> Crystal: I get caught up.
> *ERB: in obeying, is that what you mean?*
> Crystal: Well, you know sometimes. See, I'm close to my mother. My son lives with my mother, and I want to go over there and spend the night sometimes, and I used to do that a lot before I met him. And he'll be like, "eeehhhh, you can't spend the night there, you're married now." And I'm like, "But Ray, I'm not gonna be with anybody, I go over there sometimes, and I stay and I have good times with my mother and my son, I don't see them that often anymore, and I used to see them more before we were married," and I just get tired of having to say stuff like that. And he'll say, "You can't go over to your momma's house."

Crystal described her husband as controlling and abusive. Studies document that domestic violence is motivated by the perpetrator's desire for control over the victim and humiliation of the victim.[31] Crystal's husband accomplished this control over her in daily manipulations, not only on the days he beat her. His forbidding her to see her mother and sons was one example of this control and manipulation. In contrast, Crystal described her relationship with her sons as very close. As if anticipating future violence in her marriage, she mentioned casually that her sons would protect her if necessary. "I have a nice rel—a better than I could ever dream of relationship—with both of my sons. You know, they love me to death, they don't have any problems. If my husband wants to rear up, they'll be there. They'll straighten that out. So I'm blessed." Crystal is grateful that her sons will look out for her well-being.

Pain and resilience can be heard in Crystal's voice. Certainly she is a victim of sin. While it may seem that she was punishing herself for past failures, and was perhaps too accepting of her suffering and even abuse, she also told me that, given her unemployment, her marriage offered her protection that she would not have if she were alone. At the same time, she described her own need for self-love and self-care. Crystal wanted to be dependent on God and on her husband to take care of her, but the reality was that her husband was unpredictable, controlling, and had a history of beating her. She told her support group and health-care providers about her marriage problems, and this was an important first step and an aspect of self-care, but Crystal seemed to be struggling to know how to care for herself better within her difficult circumstances.

Crystal told me that God forgives her when she asks for forgiveness. But she also interprets her ongoing marital abuse as part of God's will for her life and part of her Christ-like call to self-sacrifice. Crystal's understanding of herself is rooted in her Christian faith but failed to emphasize self-love. Her own understanding of being "Christ-like" required following biblical mandates and "doing [God's] will by any means necessary." She sacrificed her own joy in order to submit to abuse and forgive others' wrongdoings. She explained God's will:

> Being kind to my neighbors no matter what it takes, following the Ten Commandments to the best of my ability and then some. And loving my husband, loving other people, basically the love thing. No matter what. That's what God basically wants. My husband has stolen from me. My husband has beaten me, and I still love my husband unconditionally.

Crystal has taken seriously the Christian call to self-sacrifice and forgiveness of others. Her understanding of love—which she named as the central Christian virtue—is complete self-giving. But while her understanding of self-giving love is rooted in biblical understandings of sacrifice and attentiveness to one's neighbor, Crystal does not seem to have an understanding of her own identity as precious to God, worthy of love, and belief in her own dignity. Thus she did not resist abuse, but rather challenged herself to forgive her abuser.

Implicit in Crystal's belief are interpretations of the Bible that sanction her husband's power and violent acts. She believed that she should submit to her husband out of respect for both his authority and divinely sanctioned power and her Christian duty to obey authority and forgive when sinned against. Crystal has adopted a view of herself in relation to her husband that is very close to traditional patriarchal interpretations of the Pauline text of 1

Corinthians 11.[32] She believes that women were created "for man" and that she was supposed to obey her husband, even though she "gets caught up with that sometimes" and looks to her grown sons for protection from her husband's abuse. This seems to imply that, deep down, Crystal recognized that she should not have to endure this abuse.

In Crystal's case we see how some Christian scripts—love one another, forgive seventy times seven times, love your enemies—when combined with brutal social forces that constrain her freedom of choice, including poverty and violence, can be misinterpreted to mean that she should care for others while neglecting care for herself. When reflecting on her experience through the lens of her religious commitments, Crystal has inherited both life-giving and problematic interpretations of biblical scripts. While God was a source of strength in her life, she also saw herself as weak, sinful, and unworthy of mutual committed nonviolent love. In this context some Christian women fail to see themselves as precious to God and worthy of respect.

Crystal is not the only collaborator who described difficulties with self-care—both with regard to acts of self-neglect prior to one's infection and also difficulty of prioritizing one's own needs after discovering one's status. Self-love and self-care did not come easily for these women. Contrary to popular beliefs about the human being's natural survival instincts, self-care requires an enormous amount of determined action and cannot be assumed. Even prior to HIV infection, a majority of my collaborators described struggles with drug and alcohol abuse (Diva, Cheryl, Keesha, Crystal) and experiences of rape and intimate-partner abuse (Keesha, Crystal, Lettie) that contributed to their sense of themselves as "dirty" and "worthless."

Misunderstandings of Christian teachings on sin reinforced these feelings and additionally made women feel ashamed of their bodies and in need of forgiveness. Marie Fortune explains that for marginalized people, who are often the victims of sin, if the sin is immoral sexual activity, the victim/survivor might focus on him/herself as the source of suffering, ignoring the agent of harm who abused, assaulted, or violated him/her.[33] Thus in addition to noting the ways in which Church participation has given much needed community to my collaborators' lives, we also can see the damaging effects of some dominant interpretations of themes of Christianity.

Some of these women admitted in the course of our conversations that they were not always sure of their own self-worth, and had a difficult time affirming their own dignity and attending to their own needs. Lettie, for example, did not share everything going on in her life with her family because she does not want to burden them with her problems. "Sometimes I don't let them know what is going on. Because I don't want to put a burden on their shoulders. So I keep it to myself. There's a lot of things I don't tell them. And I've noticed that, I don't know if it's because of my condition, but my mood, it changes just like that [snaps her fingers], just like that." While

Lettie might withhold this sharing from her family members because she does not want them to see her identity exclusively as "sick" or "HIV-positive," or because she wants to protect her family from her pain, in doing so she alienates herself from the support of people who love her. Lettie had a difficult time letting others see this vulnerability and tries instead just to press on with her life and not burden anyone else.

But some collaborators have already learned that they need to care for themselves. While their lives before their HIV infection were filled with threats to their own dignity, including experiences of sexual violence, unstable family backgrounds, lack of access to comprehensive health care, drug and alcohol abuse, and poverty, some described the moment when they finally accepted their HIV-positive status as a turning point in their life. This experience was particularly true for Cheryl and for Diva.

When Cheryl was in the hospital in 1999 with severe flu symptoms that would not go away, she did not believe the nurse who told her she had tested positive for HIV. It was not until she ended up back in the hospital with pneumonia that she accepted her status.

> Then I really hit rock bottom. I ended up in the hospital again, with PCP, and I really thought I was going to die. I didn't know where I was; I was incoherent and stuff. They even told my mother, "She's not going to make it." All I can say is, by the grace of God. Cause my temperature started going down, and I started coming out of it. And I started getting better and better, and I came out all right. While I was in there, and this was 2000, I came to the conclusion that I was HIV-positive. And that I'm going to have to take care of myself or else the next round I would not come out of there. I still have all sorts of health problems, but I'm taking better care of myself.

Cheryl decided that she would need to take care of herself, and started by entering a drug-treatment facility. She completed a residential drug-rehabilitation program and attended AA meetings regularly. She was proud that she has been drug-free since 2003. After the first period of denial, Cheryl sought help and began to advocate for herself to get the care she needed. While it took a near-death experience for her to realize she wanted to live, she is now in a stable marriage relationship, and despite the many stresses in her life, she had a firm belief in her own dignity and knew what she needed to do to take care of herself.

Diva, too, experienced a period of denial when she was first diagnosed with HIV. She said she did not feel sick, and could not understand how she could have the virus. When she was told she was HIV-positive, she continued to drink as an escape. Diva saw her marriage to Lamar as part of her new path to take better care of herself. She was with a partner who loved and supported her, and in contrast to earlier parts of her life when she was "looking for love in all the wrong places," she was with a partner who respected her and cared for her.

While Diva and Cheryl went through drug-rehabilitation programs and attend AA meetings regularly, they continued to face many difficult challenges. The stresses they had before they became HIV-positive were in many ways still part of their lives, especially poverty. While to some extent they gained a greater sense of their own dignity since they began to seek medical treatment and became involved in the support groups, they still faced threats to their dignity on a daily basis.

Cheryl, Diva, Sue, Grace, Carmen, Lettie, and to a lesser extent Crystal and Keesha, have learned since they became HIV-positive that it is necessary for them to care for themselves. Some aspects of their self-care that have emerged already include self-acceptance, forgiveness of self, self-advocacy with doctors and social workers, honesty with one's partner, treatment for drug and alcohol abuse, taking medications, attending support groups, and accepting the love and sacrifices that others make on their behalf.

CONCLUSION

Four themes emerged from my collaborators' stories: determination to survive, threats to intimacy, challenges to faith, and the need for self-love. In fact, the need for self-love is an undercurrent that runs through all of these themes. The decision to survive and advocate for oneself despite enormous social obstacles is one way my collaborators demonstrated self-love after their HIV infection. Vulnerability in intimate relationships intensified loneliness and shame for some, which compounded the challenge to love oneself. Fear and stigma thwarted their ability to love themselves fully, and faith communities both reinforced shame and offered comfort and support to contrast it. In descriptions of gradual self-acceptance and care for one's body after HIV infection, my collaborators modeled self-love.

However, a majority of my collaborators also described actions that harmed themselves, especially prior to their HIV infection, including drug and alcohol use, denial of HIV risk, acceptance of intimate-partner violence, and unprotected marital and non-marital sex. I have examined these behaviors and beliefs contrary to self-love, focusing especially on risk-taking and acceptance of abuse, and my collaborators' own self-evaluations of these behaviors. Some of these women are the victims of poverty, sexual violence, neighborhood decay, and poor education, which constrained their freedom of choice. Yet each of them also named ways in which they admit and take responsibility for some of their failures to care for themselves.

In listening to their stories I heard struggles for basic survival, not stories of flourishing lives. Their stories indict a broken educational system, broken health-care system, and a broken church. These women are both agents and victims. To the extent that they are victims, we need to draw attention to the agents of harm, including both individuals and social systems. But as human persons they had some degree of agency, and as such may share blame for some self-neglectful behavior. One must tread very carefully in this analysis, however. It would be unjust and counterproductive to blame the women alone or to judge their actions with certainty. Pope Francis has reminded Christians of the important distinction in Catholic ethics between *objective* harm and *subjective* responsibility.[34] This distinction might help us to name some of my collaborator's actions of self-neglect as objectively harmful, even without then simplistically asserting that they bear full responsibility for this harm. Certainly a larger issue that requires further consideration is whether women are encouraged to care for themselves in intimate relationships. What does love for God, self, and neighbor look like in everyday life? One of the ongoing challenges for Christian theology of marriage is how to rightly balance the obligation to love one's neighbors with the obligation to love and care for oneself. This question is explored in the next chapter.

NOTES

1. These struggles can be true for anyone with a serious chronic illness.

2. According to the website maintained by the federal government, some of the ways that the Affordable Care Act helps people living with HIV/AIDS include: ensuring coverage for people with pre-existing conditions; expanding Medicaid coverage; providing more affordable private health coverage; lowering prescription drug costs for Medicare recipients; ensuring coverage of preventive services, including HIV testing; ensuring coverage of essential health benefits; and increasing coordinated care for people with chronic health conditions. For more information, see "The Affordable Care Act and HIV/AIDS," http://aids.gov/federal-resources/policies/health-care-reform/ (Accessed July 9, 2014). The AIDS Foundation of Chicago maintains the website HIVHealthReform.org to educate HIV-affected persons about the Affordable Care Act. See http://www.hivhealthreform.org/top-ways-to-learn-about-the-new-health-care-law/ (Accessed July 9, 2014).

3. National Center for Health Statistics, *Health, United States, 2007* (Hyattsville, Maryland: National Center for Health Statistics, 2007), 4. In 2011, the United States spent $7,326 per capita on health care, according to the National Center for Health Statistics, *Health, United States, 2013* (Hyattsville, Maryland: National Center for Health Statistics, 2014). http://www.cdc.gov/nchs/hus/at_a_glance.htm (Accessed December 26, 2014).

4. Drew Desilver, "Who's Poor in America? Fifty Years into the War on Poverty." Pew Research Center Report (January 13, 2014). Summary available online: http://www.pewresearch.org/fact-tank/2014/01/13/whos-poor-in-america-50-years-into-the-war-on-poverty-a-data-portrait/ (Accessed July 9, 2014).

5. See, for example, Susan Sontag, *AIDS and Its Metaphors* (New York: Farrar, Straus, and Giroux, 1988), and *Illness as Metaphor* (New York: Farrar, Straus, and Giroux, 1977).

6. Lev 11–15, 20; Col 2:16; Acts 10:14; Rom 14:14; Mk 7:3–4; Gal 4:10; 1 Cor 11: 5–16; Mk 5:25–34.

7. *Pneumocystis carinii* pneumonia (PCP) is the most common HIV-associated pneumonia and a leading cause of death among people with AIDS. It is often the first AIDS-defining illness to occur in people infected with HIV, usually developing in adults when CD4 counts drop below 200. See Darrell E. Ward, *AmFAR AIDS Handbook: The Complete Guide to Understanding HIV and AIDS* (New York: W. W. Norton, 1999), 149–150.

8. Denise M. Ackermann, "A Voice Was Heard in Ramah: A Feminist Theology of Praxis for Healing in South Africa," in Denise M. Ackermann and M. Bons-Storm, eds., *Liberating Faith Practices: Feminist Theologies in Context* (Leuven: Peeters, 1998), 96.

9. This was true also for Cheryl, Diva, Crystal, and Keesha, as can be seen in the brief descriptions from the previous chapter. Cheryl, Diva, and Crystal describe daily prayer as a comfort in their lives. Keesha asks God for strength and protection from harm. All believe that God hears them when they pray.

10. Here I exclude Sue, Carmen, and Keesha. Sue and Carmen told me they acquired HIV through tainted blood products during surgery. This source of infection is now rare in the United States, but was a serious problem around 1980, and remains a problem in less developed countries that do not have a stable blood supply. Recall from chapter 2 that Carmen's doctors believe she was infected through heterosexual sex, and that she did not become sick until years after her first exposure. Carmen denies this and claims that these doctors were protecting themselves from lawsuits because they are to blame; she is adamant that they infected her with the virus when she was admitted for a tubal ligation surgery. I exclude Keesha because she did not describe having a similar "wake up call." Keesha was infected through coerced sex and declared that she still cannot accept her HIV-positive diagnosis. She continued to struggle with multiple addictions. Each woman's story was given greater attention in the previous chapter.

11. While Sue, Carmen, and Keesha all described their ignorance of HIV prior to their diagnosis, they also did not accept responsibility for their exposure to the virus, since Sue and Carmen told me they were exposed through surgery, and since Keesha told me she was exposed through coerced sex.

12. In the United States context in the 1980s, HIV *was* most prevalent among men who had sex with men. But the CDC never claimed that heterosexual persons (men and women) were free from risk. The gay community did mobilize in very public demonstrations to demand from the US government more resources for prevention of HIV and care for AIDS patients. Additionally, early media coverage contributed to the interpretation of HIV/AIDS as a "gay" disease. Randy Shilts, *And the Band Played On: Politics, People, and the AIDS Epidemic* (New York: St. Martins Press, 1987).

13. Among sexually transmitted infections, HIV is unique in that HIV-positive persons do not "look sick" and may not know they are infected, because the virus can lie dormant in the body for as long as fifteen years. In the United States, the average time from the initial infection to the development of advanced disease (AIDS) is ten years in an untreated person. Darrell E. Ward, *The AmFAR AIDS Handbook: The Complete Guide to Understanding HIV and AIDS* (New York: W. W. Norton, 1999), 49.

14. Barbara J. Blodgett, *Constructing the Erotic: Sexual Ethics and Adolescent Girls* (Cleveland, OH: Pilgrim, 2002), 152.

15. A growing body of research documents the daily threats to women's well-being and widespread messages that demean and degrade girls and women in the advertising, television, film, and music industries. Scholars and activists like Jean Kilbourne, creator of the documentary series *Killing Us Softly*, have been raising serious concerns about persistent misogyny in mainstream US culture. In her book *Cinderella Ate My Daughter*, Peggy Orenstein explains that our hypersexualized culture is socializing girls into thinking of themselves as sexual objects of boys. Girls are groomed to want to please boys. The hypersexualization of girls' culture begins with three- to seven-year-old girls, the target audience for the Disney Princess line. According to the American Psychological Association, the girlie-girl culture's emphasis on beauty and play-sexiness can increase girls' vulnerability to: depression, eating disorders, distorted body image, and even risky sexual behavior. Orenstein explains that even brief exposure to the typical, idealized images of women that we all see every day has been shown to lower girls' opinion of themselves, both physically and academically. In her book, *Pornland: How Porn Has Hijacked Our Sexuality*, feminist and anti-porn activist Gail Dines argues that even if you have never used or paid for pornography, you have been affected by it. Dines argues that mainstream media images have begun to groom young women in our culture so that they will act like "porn women." Young women today are socialized in this culture and internalize messages about the world and about themselves. Since pornography has become normal and mainstream in our culture, it is changing the way that women think about them-

selves and how women relate to men. Dines explains, "By inundating girls and women with the message that their most worthy attribute is their "sexual hotness" and crowding out other messages, pop culture is chipping away at their self-esteem." See the website of Jean Kilbourne for more information about her books and documentaries: http://www.jeankilbourne.com/ (Accessed June 30, 2014). Other notable organizations including About Face workshops:http://www.about-face.org/educate-yourself/for-adult-advocates/our-workshops/ and Sex Signals by Catharsis Productions: http://www.catharsisproductions.com/sexsignals.php (Accessed June 30, 2014); Peggy Orenstein, *Cinderella Ate My Daughter: Dispatches from the Front Lines of the New Girlie-Girl Culture* (New York: Harper, 2012); Diane Levin and Jean Kilbourne, *So Sexy So Soon: The New Sexualized Childhood and What Parents Can Do To Protect Their Kids* (New York: Ballantine Books, 2009); and Gail Dines, *Pornland: How Porn Has Hijacked Our Sexuality* (Boston: Beacon, 2011), xxiii–xxiv.

16. Here I am describing premarital sex (in Grace's case) as non-marital. Grace and her partner became married before his death. Lettie and her partner dated for three years but never married. When he died in the early 1990s, Lettie knew very little about AIDS and did not know she had been infected by him. In 2006 Lettie was married to another man who was not HIV-positive. Chapter 2 describes their journeys in greater detail.

17. Alcohol use increases risk of unprotected sex because it lowers inhibitions and impairs judgment. This indirectly increases risk of HIV infection.

18. While there is a pattern of self-neglect in their testimonies, one must probe their own interpretations of these behaviors in order to understand more fully how they came to act in these ways. This gives a more complete, though still individual and personal, account of their self-neglect and its impact. A more comprehensive social analysis is required in order to understand fully how these actions are embedded in formative social structures (and to understand the impact of poverty, urban decay, neighborhood violence, broken families, intimate partner abuse, dependence on public welfare, and a weak public-education system). While I attend to these in part, a full analysis of these structural injustices is beyond the scope of this project.

19. Grace and Lettie were in dating relationships. They both considered these relationships monogamous. Even if they had previous sexual partners (as in Lettie's case because she had been married prior), these relationships can be called "serial monogamy," since each successive relationship was monogamous but both partners may have had previous sexual experience.

20. Neither mentioned the Catholic Church's official teaching on birth control as a factor in influencing their decision to engage in sex without using a condom. Strictly speaking, the sexual nature of these dating relationships was in violation of the Catholic Church's official position that only married persons should engage in sexual intercourse, and within marriage sexual intercourse is for the dual purposes of unitive love and procreation. Paul VI. *Humanae Vitae* (*On the Regulation of Birth*), (July 25, 1968), Found online at: http://www.vatican.va/holy_father/paul_vi/encyclicals/documents/hf_p-vi_enc_25071968_humanae-vitae_en.html (accessed June 13, 2007). Six of my collaborators have children (Keesha and Grace do not). Diva, Cheryl, Lettie, Crystal, Carmen, and Sue all had children before they discovered their HIV-positive status. Thus they did engage in procreative sex (for Diva, Cheryl, Lettie, Carmen, and Sue, this was within marriage). All affirmed that they believe condom use should not be prohibited by the church. Only Carmen described the "ideal" relationship as faithful procreative marriage, as when she said, she believed that "the only safe sex" is "that everyone stays with their partners, and stay faithful to them . . . and not to think of anybody else." But even Carmen explained that she believes the Church should allow condoms for other kinds of relationships. All eight collaborators explained to me that, despite official church teaching, they follow their doctors' orders and use condoms with their current partners (both those whose partners were infected—Diva, Cheryl, Crystal, Grace, Carmen—and those whose partners were not infected—Sue, Lettie, Keesha). Thus they have carved out space within which they self-identify as Catholic while at the same time they disagree with and disobey "official teaching."

21. As often happens, Diva's family is an example of multigenerational poverty and instability. While Diva explains that her drug use had roots in her unstable family situation and absentee father, she seems to be unaware, or unreflective upon, the fact that she has repeated this experience for her own children. When Diva was addicted to drugs, her children lived with

her mother and extended family members. Will Diva's children also grow up to complain that their behavior is rooted in their absentee father and mother who could not love them enough? The cycle of violence, poverty, and broken marriages is debilitating for many urban families (and no doubt some rural ones).

22. While for many years the Centers for Disease Control and Prevention, or CDC, in the United States has tracked HIV prevalence in groups based on geography, gender, age, sexual orientation, and ethnicity, a growing number of social scientists are beginning to point out that socioeconomic status has a greater impact on a person's risk for HIV infection. Paul Farmer and his colleagues claim that these women are vulnerable to AIDS through *social* processes: "the economic, political, and cultural forces that can be shown to shape the dynamics of HIV transmission." According to Farmer, "for women most at risk for HIV infection, life choices are limited by racism, sexism, political violence, and grinding poverty." See Paul Farmer, Margaret Connors, Janie Simmons, eds., *Women, Poverty, and AIDS: Sex, Drugs, and Structural Violence* (Monroe, ME: Common Courage Press, 1996), xix, 23, 33, 96. See also United Nations Department of Economic and Social Affairs, *Population, Development, and HIV/AIDS with Particular Emphasis on Poverty: The Concise Report.* (New York: UN Publications, 2005), 49; *UNFPA State of the World Population 2004* (Geneva: Switzerland: United Nations Publications, 2004), 63.

23. In the first year of research for this project, the *Chicago Tribune* reported that thirty-four Chicago Public School students were killed, including, Schanna Gayden, who was buying a snack from a vendor at the Funston Elementary School playground when rival gangs began to fire against each other across Central Park Avenue in Chicago. The thirteen-year-old Schanna was fatally struck. See John Keilman, "Church Packed for Slain Girl's Funeral," *Chicago Tribune Online Edition.* July 1, 2007. http://www.chicagotribune.com/news/local/chi-both_gayden (accessed July 1, 2007). See also Asam Ahmed, Deanese Williams-Harris, and Carlos Sadovi, "3 Kids Die, 5 Hurt in Rash of Shootings," *Chicago Tribune,* Metro, 1 (March 4, 2008). The violence has continued. For a recent report, see "One Dead, At Least Twenty Wounded in Overnight Violence." *Chicago Tribune* July 5, 2014: http://www.chicagotribune.com/news/local/breaking/chi-chicago-shootings-july-4-weekend-20140704,0,6022291.story (accessed July 7, 2014). For more on urban violence, the documentary *The Interrupters* provides insight into Chicagoland violence and offers a compelling portrait of community members who work to resist this violence. (Kartemquin Films, 2011). The film was broadcast February 12, 2014, by PBS Frontline: http://www.pbs.org/wgbh/pages/frontline/interrupters/ (accessed July 7, 2014). See also Rodrick Wallace, "A Synergism of Plagues: 'Planned Shrinkage,' Contagious Housing Destruction, and AIDS in the Bronx," *Environmental Research* 47 (1988): 1–33; Mindy Thompson Fullilove, "Death and Life in the Great American City," *International Journal of Mental Health* 28, no. 4 (1999–2000); Robert E. Fullilove and Mindy Thompson Fullilove, "HIV Prevention and Intervention in the African-American Community: A Public Health Perspective," in *The AIDS Knowledge Base,* ed. P. T. Cohen, M. A. Sande, and P. A. Volberding, 3rd ed. (Philadelphia, PA: Lippincott Williams and Wilkins, 1999); Jon C. Teaford, "Urban Renewal and Its Aftermath," *Housing Policy Debate* 11, no. 2 (2000): 443–465.

24. For example, predominantly African-American neighborhoods have, in comparison to White neighborhoods, less homeownership, increased street violence, more transitional housing units, greater levels of unemployment, fewer businesses, fewer public parks, lower performing public schools, and an infrastructure that is more rapidly decaying. To search the online database of reported crime in the City of Chicago, see Chicago Police Department, CLEAR (Citizen Law Enforcement Analysis and Reporting) Geographic Information System. http://gis.chicagopolice.org/ (accessed July 1, 2007). For analysis on crime and development trends with special focus on race and ethnicity, see William Julius Wilson and Robert J. Sampson, "Toward a Theory of Race, Crime, and Urban Inequality," in *Crime and Inequality,* ed. John Hagan and Ruth D. Peterson (Stanford, CA: Stanford University Press, 1995); Jeffrey Morenoff and Robert J. Sampson, "Violent Crime and the Spatial Dynamics of Neighborhood Transition: Chicago 1970–1990," *Social Forces* 76 (1997): 31–64; Arnold Hirsch, *Making the Second Ghetto: Race and Housing in Chicago, 1940–1960* (Cambridge: Cambridge University Press, 1983); John M. Hagedorn and Paul J. Goldstein, "Murder and Drugs in the Information

Age: An Urban Political Economy Approach to Variation in Homicide Rates," *Great Cities Institute* (Chicago, IL: University of Illinois-Chicago, 1999).

25. The Project on Human Development in Chicago Neighborhoods (PHDCN) reports that a typical African-American resident lives in a neighborhood that is 78 percent Black, while a typical White or Mexican-American resident lives in a neighborhood that is approximately 85 percent non-Black. Blacks in the study were more likely than Whites or Mexican-Americans to live in Chicago neighborhoods with concentrated economic disadvantage and high reported rates of cynicism about law enforcement. According to this study, having married parents or having a large percentage of professionals in a neighborhood will reduce a youth resident's chances of engaging in violence. Thus community initiatives, such as increased economic investment in African-American communities, together with programs that support family stability, could help to decrease violence in these neighborhoods. Robert J. Sampson, Jeffrey D. Morenoff, and Stephen Raudenbush, "Social Anatomy of Racial and Ethnic Disparities in Violence," *American Journal of Public Health* 95 (2005): 224–232.

26. See M. Shawn Copeland, "Wading through Many Sorrows: Toward a Theology of Suffering in Womanist Perspective," in *Readings in Moral Theology No. 9: Feminist Ethics and the Catholic Moral Tradition,* edited by Charles E. Curran, Margaret A. Farley, and Richard A. McCormick, S. J. (New York: Paulist, 1996), 136–163; *Violence against Women and Children: A Christian Theological Sourcebook,* edited by Carol J. Adams and Marie M. Fortune (New York: Continuum, 1995); *Christianity, Patriarchy, and Abuse: A Feminist Critique,* edited by Joanne Carlson Brown and Carole R. Bohn (Cleveland, OH: Pilgrim Press, 1989); Christine E. Gudorf, *Body, Sex, and Pleasure: Reconstructing Christian Sexual Ethics* (Cleveland, OH: Pilgrim, 1994), 170–204.

27. A report from the World Health Organization presents for the first time a systematic review and synthesis of the body of scientific data on the prevalence of intimate partner violence as well as the effects of this violence on women's physical, sexual, reproductive, and mental health. Overall, 35 percent of women worldwide have experienced either physical and/or sexual intimate partner violence or non-partner sexual violence. Worldwide, 30 percent of all women who have been in a relationship have experienced physical and/or sexual violence by their intimate partner. In some regions, 38 percent of women have experienced intimate partner violence. The evidence shows that women experiencing intimate partner violence are significantly more likely to experience serious health problems than women who have not experienced such violence. In this report, physical violence is defined as: being slapped or having something thrown at you that could hurt you, being pushed or shoved, being hit with a fist or something else that could hurt you, being kicked, dragged, or beaten up, being choked or burnt on purpose, and/or being threatened with, or actually, having a gun, knife, or other weapon used on you. Sexual violence is defined as: being physically forced to have sexual intercourse when you did not want to, having sexual intercourse because you were afraid of what your partner might do, and/or being forced to do something sexual that you found humiliating or degrading. While the researchers recognized that intimate partner violence can include emotional abuse, they excluded emotional abuse from this analysis of prevalence and effects because there is no scientific consensus on how to measure emotional abuse. Women who have experienced intimate partner violence are 16 percent more likely to have a low-birth-weight baby. They are twice as likely to experience depression, and they are 1.5 times more likely to acquire HIV as compared to women who have not experienced partner violence. World Health Organization, *Global and Regional Estimates of Violence Against Women: Prevalence and Health Effects of Intimate Partner Violence and Non-Partner Sexual Violence* (2013), 6, 2, 6, 7, 10, 31.

28. Many studies have shown that violence against women increases their vulnerability to HIV-infection. Violent men often use both physical force and psychological and emotional manipulation as methods of control over their partners. Violence or the threat of violence increases the inability of women to negotiate safe-sex practices like condom use. It also increases the possibility for open sores, thereby increasing the likelihood of HIV transmission during unprotected sex. Survivors often have little power to resist this violence in the future. See UNAIDS, *Women and HIV/AIDS: Confronting the Crisis, A Joint Report by UNAIDS/UNFPA/UNIFEM* (New York: United Nations Publications, 2004).

29. Cheryl admits that before marrying her second husband, she should have paid more attention to his abusive behavior. Lettie also stayed with an abusive partner for many years before leaving him and ending her first marriage. While these relationships were surely complex, the ability of these women to look back on them and name the violence against them as unjust shows that in their gradual recovery from this trauma they have begun to take steps toward caring for themselves more deeply.

30. Keesha and her husband of nine years were separated, and Crystal described ongoing abuse in her marriage for which her husband had sought help through anger-management therapy.

31. Crystal's history of violence makes her a more likely candidate for future violence. Research shows that women who have been battered for many years grow to expect further abuse and no longer think of themselves as having dignity and power to resist abuse. In the cycle of battering, there is usually a period of time after an episode of abuse when the perpetrator "is nice" and even admits guilt. This is sometimes called the "honeymoon" phase of the battering cycle. Victims of battery look forward to this reconciliation period, and might remain in the abusive relationship because they do not feel the power to resist it. See Rape, Abuse, and Incest National Network (RAINN), "Battered Woman Syndrome," Online article found at http://www.rainn.org/effects-of-rape/battered-woman-syndrome.html (accessed June 13, 2007).

32. "I want you to know that Christ is the head of every man, and a husband the head of his wife, and God the head of Christ . . . .[man] is the image and glory of God, but woman is the glory of man. For man did not come from woman, but woman from man." 1 Cor 11:1,7–9. Recall Crystal's description: "See, I believe like in the Bible, God takes care of man, and man takes care of woman, and woman takes care of children and the house."

33. Marie M. Fortune, "The Conundrum of Sin, Sex, Violence, and Theodicy," in Andrew Sung Park and Susan L. Nelson, eds., *The Other Side of Sin: Woundedness from the Perspective of the Sinned-Against* (Albany, New York: State University of New York Press, 2001), 109–142, at 124.

34. Pope Francis, *Evangelii gaudium*, nos. 172–173. Available online: http://w2.vatican.va/content/francesco/en/apost_exhortations/documents/papa-francesco_esortazione-ap_20131124_evangelii-gaudium.html (Accessed July 9, 2014).

Chapter Four

Self-Care and Christian Discipleship

> And a voice came from heaven, "You are my Son, the Beloved; with you I am well pleased."
> Mk 1:11

Many Christians, including some of the women interviewed for this study, believe that selflessness is holy and pleasing to God and that Christian discipleship is characterized by sacrificial love and uncritical acceptance of suffering. These messages are reinforced by theological claims such as the need to take up one's cross or abandon self-concern in order to follow Jesus. Christ-like self-sacrifice is too often promoted in such a way that self-love is abandoned.

When women internalize these problematic scripts from parts of the Christian tradition, their flourishing is thwarted. Messages which fail to emphasize self-love can be especially problematic for women, who are also subjected to sexist messages that do not affirm their dignity.[1] Such an interpretation is problematic and contrary to the heart of the gospel, where discipleship is summed up in the love commandment: love God, love yourself, and love your neighbor. Love for God *requires* love for self and love for neighbor.

But how are these loves—for God, self, and neighbor—related in the moral life? My collaborators' stories illumine how these loves do compete at times. Thus my task in this chapter is not only to elaborate on the need for self-love in the moral life but also to show how one can feasibly balance self-love, love for God, and love for neighbor in real life. This account must be both faithful to the gospel and faithful to the experiences of my collaborators.

LOVE FOR GOD

We are to love God with all our heart, all our soul, all our mind, and all our strength.[2] In the early Christian community, this was a way of saying we should love God with our whole being. Every aspect of our personhood can love God. Benedict T. Viviano comments that because Jesus is citing Deut 6:5, we are to interpret love of God not primarily as a feeling but as "covenant fidelity, a matter of willing and doing."[3] For Jesuit theologian Edward C. Vacek, the language of *acceptance* and *affirmation* is more apt.[4] Our faithfulness to God can be affirmed both directly (as when we affirm belief in God, when we pray to God, when we accept God's love, when we participate in ritual worship and thanksgiving) and indirectly (as when we love self and others in God and cooperate in God's love in the world). To love God with our whole personhood means we seek communion with God and all that God loves in our concrete lives and strive to be aware of God's presence in our lives. While love of God may lead to love of neighbor, the two loves are distinct and should not be collapsed.[5]

LOVE FOR SELF

For Christians, self-love is a response to God's prior loving of us. The Psalmist offers praise to God that suggests a deep appreciation of God's gift of life: "You formed my inmost being; you knit me in my mother's womb. I praise you, so wonderfully you made me; wonderful are your works! My very self you knew."[6] As beloved children of God, we know we are cherished by our loving Creator. When Christians fail to believe that God loves them, they may also lose their own sense of purpose and reason to care for themselves. Conversations with the study participants reveal the need for greater attention to be paid within Christian communities to the fundamental theological anthropology of the person as loved by God. For a Christian woman to accept God's love for her will mean that she can begin to challenge some cultural messages that tell her she only has value or only deserves respect when she has status, beauty, and economic power. For women struggling in situations of dehumanizing poverty or in violent relationships, for women who feel dirty and who fear infecting their spouses, or for women who rely on government assistance programs, to hear and accept this message of God's unfailing love will likely not, in itself, shield them from stress or pain; nevertheless, the acceptance of God's love can give one a sense of dignity and, perhaps, with time, the power to resist violence, the power to reject feelings of shame, and the courage to try again to make a way for oneself. God's initiation calls for a response from us. Our response can begin with love for God and lead to radical self-acceptance and love for others.

In Christian faith, self-love begins with an affirmation that I am a creature in relationship to the Creator, created in love and sustained in love. By recognizing my identity in relationship to God, I affirm the goodness of my being, my dignity as a child of God, and myself as an irreducible end. A number of theologians have explored this important aspect of Christian discipleship.[7] We cannot earn God's love by anything we do, but God loves us simply because we are. To see God in this way is to see God as a Lover and to see oneself as special and precious to God, no matter what. Henri Nouwen emphasized this radical self-acceptance as necessary component of Christian discipleship when he reflects on the baptism of Jesus: "In those days Jesus came from Nazareth of Galilee and was baptized by John in the Jordan. And just as he was coming up out of the water, he saw the heavens torn apart and the Spirit descending like a dove on him. And a voice came from heaven, 'You are my Son, the Beloved; with you I am well pleased'" (Mk 1:8–11). Just as God was pleased with Jesus, Nouwen claims that God is pleased with Christians today, and that we too should hear this message:

> Yes, there is that voice, the voice that speaks from above and from within and that whispers softly or declares loudly: "You are my Beloved, on you my favor rests." It certainly is not easy to hear that voice in a world filled with voices that shout: "You are no good, you are ugly; you are worthless; you are despicable, you are nobody—unless you can demonstrate the opposite."[8]

When we explore self-love through the lens of the love commandment, we find that self-love should be affirmed together with love for God and love for one's neighbor. The first and greatest commandment given in the Gospels of Matthew and Mark is love for God.[9] The second in these accounts is "You shall love your neighbor as yourself."[10] Luke's account places these two commandments together without explicitly naming love of God as greater, though it is given first.[11] In these accounts of The Great Commandment we are called to love our neighbors *as we love ourselves,* implying a distinct love for self. That this self love is inferred does not mean it is less important than love for neighbor. Does this mean that love for self is secondary to love for God? Even if this is the case, this still does not imply a devaluing of self-love. Love for God is a response to God's prior initiative. In that initiative of God's love, creation is affirmed and given value in God. Our self-love says *yes* to God's prior valuing and loving of us.

Self-love is multidimensional, experiential, holistic, and aimed toward well-being. This means it seeks the well-being of the totality of our selves as multidimensional persons—bodily, intellectually, spiritually, emotionally. Self-love requires being honest with oneself, accepting oneself, valuing oneself, and forgiving oneself. Because self-love is open to deeper self-awareness and strives for authenticity, it is a process of continuing openness and becoming. In this awareness we accept our finitude and vulnerability and admit the ways we have failed to love ourselves and God. Self-love requires caring for oneself by eating, sleeping, working, learning new skills, protecting oneself from harm, setting personal goals, and fostering supportive relationships.[12] Self-love also requires that we allow others to care for us, attend to friendships that nurture us, ask for support from friends and loved ones, and even that we accept praise.

Jesus is a model of self-love for Christians. He allows others to care for him,[13] attends to friendships, asks for help and support,[14] and accepts praise from others.[15] He honors his embodiment by taking time to eat and rest, honors his friendships by dining and conversing with his followers, and he honors God through his prayer and his ministry in the name of God.[16]

Jesus prioritizes his relationship with God, whom he addresses as Abba, Father, and seeks to follow God's will in his life. Jesus' relationship with God does not necessarily imply a rejection of self-love, since self-love is properly a response to God's love. At a time when these loves seemed to clash, as in Gethsemane, Jesus submitted his will to God's: "Abba, Father, all things are possible to you. Take this cup away from me, but not what I will but what you will."[17] If we interpret Jesus's agony as a model of the love commandment, we see that he prioritizes love for God by trusting in God and choosing to remain committed to God. He petitions to God to take away the cup of suffering. We do not see Jesus lose faith in God or reject God.[18] Jesus does not ask God to send suffering into his life. He is willing to accept the consequences of his decision to remain committed to God, including suffering and death. Jesus remains honest and self-aware. He continues even amid this conflict to seek integrity and authenticity. Jesus is not a mere victim in this scene. He is not being pushed or controlled by outside forces. Instead, he deliberates and decides that his full personhood can best be affirmed through remaining committed to God.

Because self-love is most properly thought of as a response to God's prior loving and affirmation of the self, self-love from a Christian perspective can never be construed as selfishness or arrogance. Selfishness is grounded in an inability to see one's integral good as related to the good of others. At its core, selfishness is contrary to self-love because the selfish person sees other persons and the world as existing for her benefit alone. Everything and everyone else exists for her use and pleasure. This attitude is sinful, not because the self is unworthy of love and attention, but because the self exists in a web of relationships to God and others, and these relationships demand mutual affirmation. Christian love for self does not necessarily lead to self-centeredness. One can affirm and care for oneself even in relationship to others. As one is an inherently social person, one's true integral flourishing occurs precisely in our mutual relationships. But if I am an end in myself, called to love and cherish myself, and at the same time a relational being situated within a web of relationships, how am I to negotiate these multiple loves?

LOVE FOR NEIGHBOR

Our love relationship with God spills over into the other relationships in our lives when we begin to respond to God's command to care for others. Love for the neighbor is a central theme of Jesus' preaching and, like self-care, is a concrete way that Christians cooperate with God in the world. In his preaching, Jesus called his followers to love not only their family and friends, but also the outcast, the sick, and the weak. Mercy and compassion for others are not optional for the Christian, who is called to feed the hungry, give drink to the thirsty, welcome the stranger, clothe the naked, care for the ill, and visit the imprisoned.[19] In Luke's account we hear Jesus tell his followers that there is personal cost to discipleship.

> Do to others as you would have them do to you. For if you love those who love you, what credit is that to you? Even sinners love those who love them. And if you do good to those who do good to you, what credit is that to you? Even sinners do the same. If you lend money to those from whom you expect repayment, what credit is that to you? Even sinners lend to sinners, and get back the same amount. But rather, love your enemies and do good to them, and lend expecting nothing back; then your reward will be great and you will be children of the Most High, for he himself is kind to the ungrateful and the wicked. Be merciful, just as your Father is merciful.[20]

For the early church these commands to show mercy to other persons summed up the identity of the Christian community.

Mercy and compassion remain essential components of the Christian life of discipleship. When we accept our own finitude and vulnerability, and also see ourselves as loved and cherished by our Creator, we can understand that God calls us to empathize with our neighbors' vulnerabilities and affirm them as beloved of God. The early Christian community thought of this command as central to discipleship, uniting love of God with love of neighbor. In the gospels, love for one's neighbor means love for family, dependents, strangers, and even enemies. But in his preaching Jesus does not tell us how to negotiate any conflicts that arise from these loves. It is important to explore how these loves are related to one another.

Some theologians characterize sacrificial agape as *the* radical Christian love to which Jesus called his disciples. These authors tend to give the impression that we can and should choose between love of self and love of neighbor, and some go so far as to name self-love as sinful.[21] Other theologians have been concerned about the problems of subordinating self-love to love for others and have rightly identified problems with excessive self-surrender.[22] Surely the Christian life requires love of neighbor, but the question is how one should rightly balance the obligation to love one's neighbors with the obligation to love and care for oneself.

CHRISTIAN LOVE IN REAL LIFE

The love commandment, which is the central call of the Christian life, contains overlapping moral obligations to love God, oneself, and one's neighbors. But how is one balance Christian love for God, self, family, community members, strangers, and even enemies? What happens when a parent struggles to love her children while also caring for herself? How can marital love for a spouse be compatible with care for oneself? When one barely has enough quality time with one's own family, how is one to welcome the stranger? Which stranger? These hard cases demonstrate the need for continued reflection on the compatibility of these loves in the moral life.

These questions surfaced in the stories of the women interviewed for this study; in some cases, these women modeled the balance of love for God, self, and others, despite enormous tensions in their lives. Their experiences reveal a deep paradox within the problem of self-love; that is, self-giving love can be life-giving for the one who loves even as it requires some donation of self felt as loss. But this paradox does not mean that self-giving love should automatically be validated or recommended over self-love. Let us further examine this problem in the lives of Carmen, Grace, Sue, Lettie, Cheryl, and Diva.[23] Their insights into the compatibility of love for self and love for others can inform a grounded theology of mutuality that leads to flourishing-in-relationship.

Carmen: A Mother's Sacrifice

In Carmen's life, we see that parental love can be life-giving even when it requires service and attention to the needs of others. Carmen has struggled for many years with self-esteem and self-care. When Carmen struggled to accept her HIV-diagnosis, she lost hope in the value of her own life. She battled depression and had suicidal thoughts, but fulfilling her role as mother by caring for her daughters helped her to stay alive. She told me, "If I didn't have my daughters, I wouldn't be here speaking with you today. If I hadn't had my daughters, I would have taken my own life a long time ago." While she is progressing toward the radical self-acceptance representative of self-love, she begins to see her value and dignity precisely in relationship, because others depend on her. Her daughters' dependence upon her makes Carmen feel that her life is worth preserving. This affirmation is a first step toward self-love.

Carmen tells of how it has been difficult for her to accept the way her body has changed because of the strong medications she has been taking for so long. She used to be proud of her beautiful figure and now struggles to see herself as beautiful. Coming to terms with the changes in her body has been difficult but over time, through prayer and caring for her children, she gradually came to accept herself, to cherish her body, and to begin to take care of herself by taking her antiretroviral medications.

In part, by taking care of her family, Carmen regained belief in her own dignity. Her daughters helped her to see that she has a lot of special gifts. She gained confidence in her ability to provide for herself and her children, to advocate for their best interests in their schools, and to provide a loving and nurturing environment for them at home. She is especially proud that her daughters are bilingual. She tells me that in focusing on their care, she forgets things that used to bother her about herself. She is able to put all of her problems in perspective. Her life remains busy and even overwhelming at times, but her care for her daughters is life-giving for her. Carmen tells me that she wants to take care of herself so that she can be healthy for her children and continue to be a positive example in her daughters' lives. She sees her own flourishing in relation to her daughters' flourishing. They are interdependent and mutually affirming. While it would have been preferable if Carmen had understood her own dignity and value prior to her daughters' needs to depend on her, Carmen did not recognize the need to love and care for herself until she felt she mattered to others. Now she balances these loves in her life and does not neglect her own self-care.

Grace: A Wife's Sacrifice

Grace also found that in caring for a dependent family member—her spouse, Sam—she experienced not only fatigue and emotional heartache but also peace and an even deeper love and appreciation of him. Grace told me that she felt many burdens when she was caring for Sam before his death. In this time she put so much energy into his care that she thought of his needs before her own. Only six months after they got married, Grace took a leave of absence from her job so she could be the primary caregiver for Sam as his health deteriorated. She learned how to give him home infusion treatments, and her life was focused on Sam's care. Even when she had to go back to work, she spent a great deal of time before and after work taking care of him.

In caring for Sam, Grace sacrificed out of love for him and in honor of their relationship. Grace arranged for hospice nurses to help Sam in their home as he was dying. She also invited her family to help take care of Sam, especially in his final days, so that she would not have to help him alone. But she says that if she had to do it all over again, she would do it the same way. By caring for her dying spouse, she was able to spend precious time with him, even when they were just watching a movie together. She was able to process her own grief while she was caring for him. Sam often shared his gratitude with her, and this affirmed her and made her feel she was doing the right thing. In making him feel as comfortable as possible, she was able to begin to let go of him, even in small ways.

In caring for Sam during his illness and dying, Grace's priorities did not emphasize her own flourishing. She sacrificed advancement in her career, part of her income, and the bulk of her free time. But these decisions were not coerced. Grace freely chose to show her love for her spouse by giving up these aspects of her own fulfilling lifestyle. In doing so, she felt she was honoring her husband and their marriage. In turn, she felt affirmed by her husband and remembers his dying months not only as sad and emotional times but also as precious time in their relationship where she was able to accompany him in his difficult journey. In those moments that were the most overwhelming, when she knew she could no longer care for Sam by herself, she reached out to family and organized hospice care so she would not have to accept the burdens of Sam's care giving by herself. In doing so Grace cared for herself by honoring her own limitations. She sacrificed a great deal, but managed to let others help her and care for her during this difficult time.

In this case, as in Carmen's, Grace's good was intimately linked with the well-being of her loved one. It would be wrong to say Carmen should neglect her daughters to focus on herself, or that Grace should ignore her dying husband to focus on her own self-care. But there would be harm if—within their roles of caring and providing—Carmen and Grace did not also protect, at least in some way, their own well-being. These are examples of positive self-giving; had Carmen not sought help in therapy for her depression, and had Grace not sought help from her family in Sam's care, they might not have been able to achieve this delicate balance between care for the self and care for dependent loved ones. But because of their interdependence, Grace could not focus on herself without thinking of her husband; Carmen's own flourishing depends on the flourishing of her children. In caring for others Carmen and Grace found increased meaning in their own lives, deeper personal satisfaction, and a more intimate communion with their family members.

Sue, Cheryl, and Diva: Admitting Vulnerability and Accepting Love

In Sue's case we see that one aspect of self-care is that one must accept the love and sacrifices that a spouse makes on your behalf. Sue tells me that she feels both guilty and grateful when she recalls the sacrifices that her husband has made on her behalf. Sue explains that financial burdens make it very difficult for her to care for herself. "There have been a lot of times where we had to choose between medicines or food. Or medicines or paying our electric bill." She has had to rely on her husband's financial and emotional support and frequently feels that she cannot return his love to the same degree. She is dependent on him, and it is a challenge for her to accept the sacrifices that he makes for her—from long hours of work to driving her to doctor visits, to the constant emotional support. Sue's experiences reveal the foolishness of interpreting equal giving in marital love as identical giving and show us that sometimes self-love requires welcoming and accepting the sacrifices that others make for us.

In her marriage, Sue has had to admit the many ways that her illness makes her vulnerable. She feels especially vulnerable in her sexual intimacy with her loving husband. Additionally, Sue often feels tired, she gets sick easily, she is less able to help with chores at home, has frequent doctor appointments, and is unable to work full-time. All of these commitments put added pressure on her husband. Sue struggles to accept her limitations and feels frustrated, but also feels safe, grateful, and cherished because of her husband's love.

Cheryl and Diva both describe how their marriages model the possibility of the unity of self-love and self-gift. Cheryl remembered a time when her husband showed special concern for her after she underwent surgery. "He was so worried; he called and checked up on me." That meant a lot to Cheryl, who explained that the companionship she feels in her marriage helps her to bear her illness with dignity and hope. "We aren't perfect, nobody is perfect. You have your good days and your bad days, but we are in this thing together, me and him. And we support each other. This is a big process, a big struggle, HIV. So I think being married helps you deal with it." For Cheryl, part of her own self-care has required that she accept her husband's help and companionship.

Diva, too, explains that her marriage to Lamar has given her strength that helps her handle her life with HIV.

> [Lamar] does anything he can for me, and I do anything I can for him. He's very loving. He goes everywhere I go. Sometime we go places, and he'll be the only man. We are in each other's corner. When I ache, he ache. When I'm down, he down. He cooks, he cleans, he washes, he can do whatever a woman can do. He is a companion, and I guess I was looking for that in my early years, my other marriages . . . . He's very concerned for me.

For Diva, as for Carmen, Lettie, Sue, and Cheryl, intimate relationships provide the locus for love that requires both self-donation and acceptance of another's sacrifice on their behalf. In their lives we see that they are given strength to love themselves because of intimate support from their loved ones. In their stories, the sacrifices that were life-giving for giver and recipient were so because they were freely chosen (not coerced) and because they either reduced suffering or the one who sacrificed accepted the suffering as a consequence of their desire to love and not for its own sake.[24] These real life cases of mutual love convey both the difficulty and the necessity of self-love within mutual relationships aimed toward flourishing.

Overlapping Moral Obligations

Self-love in my collaborators' experiences required attention to both their own flourishing and the flourishing of their loved ones.[25] While some named ways in which they had neglected to love themselves in their past (as in the experiences of drug use and unprotected sex analyzed earlier), they try now to forgive themselves, accept themselves, value themselves, and take good care of themselves. Some have demonstrated this self-regard through adherence to a drug regimen (despite uncomfortable side effects); some have left abusive partners in order to care for themselves. Some are involved in HIV-advocacy campaigns so they can have their voices heard by lobbying for policies that would offer them direct benefits. In all cases, their descriptions of self-love had were not simply private or personal but reflected the ways that they are embedded in multiple relationships. The challenges they faced involved caring for themselves without losing sight of their responsibilities to others, and their interdependence with others.

Love for self and love for others frequently overlap. Because human beings are social and relational beings, our experience of self-love is fostered and made possible in human community. Catholic social teaching has emphasized this inherently social view of the human person.[26] As an inherently social person, one cannot seek one's own good without attention to relationships that contribute to the self's flourishing and, necessarily, to the good of others.[27] Nevertheless, Christian life is messy and sometimes Christians do experience conflict among these loves and demands. How might the love commandment inform a Christian woman's discernment about such a dilemma?

Sometimes neighbor love requires a gift of self that is experienced initially as a loss to self, as when parents chose frugal living in order to save for their children's higher education, or when a woman cares for her dying spouse. Not all neighbor love is reciprocal, and it may not be immediately mutual even if it has the goal of eventual mutual relationship, as a pregnant woman's love of her child *in utero* can have the goal of mutuality even while her sacrifices are unrewarded. But sacrificial love for the other, if freely chosen and affirming of one's total self can be good and moral. We can interpret sacrifice—for family members, for example—not as the goal *per se* of Christian life, but as a means to fulfill loving care and devotion to children and spouse, as Jesus' acceptance of suffering was not intended for its own sake but was accepted as a consequence of fidelity to God.

Christians should not seek out opportunities for suffering. But some suffering can be accepted within a larger love relationship. Still, the Christian life does not require total renunciation of the self. Meaningful relationships are built upon mutuality and reciprocity, but we will never discover a mathematical solution to achieve perfect balancing of receiving and giving. Rather, in patterns of giving, caring, sharing, and relating to others, persons establish trust and enable deeper life-giving connections with others. A relationship of mutuality requires "sharing of power—with, by, and among all parties in the relationship in a way that recognizes the wholeness and particular experience of each participant toward the end of optimum flourishing of all."[28] This understanding of interconnected obligations relies on a relational anthropology and an interpretation of the life of Jesus as a call to transform relationships of oppression into relationships of mutual obligation, justice, and flourishing.

Mutuality affirms the person as beloved of God but does not wholly reject the place of self-sacrifice in loving relationships. Instead, as theologian Dawn Nothwehr claims, "only when one chooses self-denial toward a goal of greater mutuality (or of mutual love) is sacrifice healthy."[29] Margaret Farley explains how self-sacrifice can be a part of love, but that not all self-sacrifice is loving:

> [We have] a moral obligation not to relate to another person in a way that is truly destructive of ourselves as persons. It does not mean that we ought never to sacrifice our own welfare—sacrifice even our home, our health, our security, our reputation, our professional future, our very life.
> What it does mean (to say that we must not relate to others in ways destructive of ourselves as persons) is that while we may sacrifice everything we have, we may not sacrifice everything we are. We may not sacrifice in a final sense our autonomy. We may not sacrifice our capability for union and communion with God and human persons.[30]

Christians should not sacrifice to the point of despair, desperation, or loss of identity as a person loved by God with inherent dignity. Social constraints that demand this kind of dehumanizing sacrifice are not of God.

Don Browning instructs that sacrificial love has an "unavoidable role in the Christian life and Christian families."[31] But with Andolsen and Farley, Browning asserts that self-sacrifice has limits, and should work in the service of mutual love. "Love as equal regard is not something that one individual expresses unilaterally toward another. It is something that people create together . . . through successive attempts to communicate needs and desires, to listen and to understand, to empathize with, hold, and accept, and then to live their mutual agreements."[32]

Browning describes self-sacrifice in the context of mutual relationships, the ongoing process of establishing trust, of communicating one's needs, and of knowing that one's love for the other will be accepted, cherished, and reciprocated.

Christian life does require sacrifice and self-gift but these are not incompatible with self-love. Christian ethicists should continue to probe the gospels for resources of this healthy self-gift modeled in the life of Jesus. When the Christian story of salvation focuses narrowly on Jesus' death while excluding the loving care of God the Creator, and rejecting the import of Jesus' own proclamation of the love commandment, the ensuing message of sacrifice and self-renunciation fails to be life-giving. Indeed, if it is to be salvific at all, the Christian story of salvation must be life-giving for Christians. For too long Christian women have heard and internalized messages that fail to affirm their dignity as beloved daughters of God. The Christian gospel of God's affirming love does offer profound resources for women's acceptance of God's love. It is increasingly important for pastoral ministers to make distinctions between healthy and unhealthy sacrifice so that marginalized persons are not subject to messages that over-simplify this important aspect of Christian discipleship.

CONCLUSION

The love commandment reveals the heart of the radical call to discipleship—to follow the one who revealed to humanity the fullness of God's love, we are to respond by loving God, by loving ourselves, and by loving our neighbors. For Christians, the starting point is acceptance of God's love. Each person is loved by God and precious to God. Each person is unique and has inherent dignity as a child of God. From this experience of God's love, the person is called to see herself as beloved. She is called to affirm herself, forgive herself, love and care for herself. This self-love, in turn, prepares her for mutual relationships with others. Self-love requires that she seek relationships of mutuality. In relating to others she will need to continue to guard her own self-care, maintain her identity, protect herself from victimization. But over time, as trust builds in mutual relationships, she can become more vulnerable with loved ones and in deeper intimate relationships.

The love commandment itself establishes the criteria according to which we judge the adequacy of any calls to self-sacrifice that appear to contradict self-love. Self-sacrificial love for one's neighbor, to be moral, must coincide with love for God and must irrupt from radical self-acceptance. Thus sacrifice can be promoted only if it is willingly chosen, preserves love for God, and is self-affirming. Neighbor love can be mutual, not in the sense of equal amounts of self-gift (as if this could even be measured), but united toward a goal of mutual affirmation in relation to God.

Messages that affirm self-sacrifice without the saving message of God's affirming love are not only inadequate but also harmful. Christians should not be taught to die to self, to take up one's cross, or to submit and obey like Jesus. These scripts misrepresent the love commandment when they imply that a Christian should not care for herself, or should not see herself as precious to God. In my collaborators' lives, such messages were sometimes interpreted as validation of the need to accept manipulation by others, to accept emotional, physical, or sexual violence, to accept degrading work, or to neglect self-care such as fighting one's substance abuse. A message of self-love, in contrast, responds by affirming the person, even in all her brokenness and vulnerability, as a beloved daughter of God who is called to a life of flourishing. Mutual sharing in relationships, when they require self-gift or sacrifice, should always affirm the person as loved by God, cherished by God, and called to full and integral flourishing.

NOTES

1. The literature on sexism in Christianity is extensive. Two representative works on the topic include Rosemary Radford Ruether, *Sexism and God-Talk: Toward a Feminist Theology* (Boston, MA: Beacon, 1983) and Elizabeth A. Johnson, *She Who Is: The Mystery of God in Feminist Theological Discourse* (New York: Crossroad, 2000).

2. Mk 12:30; Mt 22:37; Lk 10:26; Jn 13:34–35 implies this love in the "New Commandment" to love one another.

3. Benedict T. Viviano, O.P., "The Great Commandment (Mt 22:34–40)," in *The New Jerome Biblical Commentary,* ed. Raymond E. Brown, S. S., Joseph A. Fitzmeyer, S. J., Roland E. Murphy, O.Carm (Upper Saddle River, NJ: Prentice Hall, 1990), 666.

4. Edward Collins Vacek, *Love, Human and Divine: The Heart of Christian Ethics* (Washington, DC: Georgetown University Press, 1994), 126–149.

5. Ibid., 141–146.

6. Ps 139:13–14.

7. Theologians have begun to emphasize the importance of self-love in recent years. According to Darlene Fozard Weaver, self-love is an independent moral obligation based on regarding all human beings as equals created by God in God's image. See Weaver, *Self-Love and Christian Ethics* (Cambridge: Cambridge University Press, 2002), 47–77, 131-166. James Keenan writes about self-esteem or self-care as a "cardinal virtue," or a "bottomline moral task" sought for its own sake. Keenan proposes four cardinal virtues: justice, fidelity, self-care, and prudence. See Keenan, *Virtues for Ordinary Christians* (Franklin, WI: Sheed & Ward, 1999), 70–75, at 72; "Proposing Cardinal Virtues," *Theological Studies* 56:4 (1995): 709–729. See pages 726–728 where Keenan draws heavily on the theology of Thomas Aquinas. Though Aquinas does not name self-care a cardinal virtue, Aquinas' *Summa* is rich in discussion of self-care, especially because of his anthropology of the human person as created for union with God. Aquinas thus claims in the *Prima Secundae* that all nature seeks its own perfection (1.5.1, 48.1), that it is natural to prefer oneself to others (27.3), that it is impossible to hate oneself (29.4); and argues in the *Secunda Secundae* that self-love belongs in the order of charity and is prior to neighbor love (25.12, 26.4). Thomas Aquinas, *Summa Theologica,* Trans. Fathers of the English Dominican Province (Allen, TX: Christian Classics, 1948). Stephen Pope calls for renewed attention to a relational anthropology in order to counter the cultural views of self-love as expressive individualism. See Pope, "Expressive Individualism and True Self-Love: A Thomistic Perspective," *Journal of Religion* 71:3 (1991):384–99. Maria Cimperman offers three helpful markers of self-care in terms of HIV-AIDS: commitment to growth, relationality, and

self-acceptance. Cimperman affirms the need for responsibility for oneself, and, like James Keenan, names self-care as a virtue that should be held in balance with both fidelity and justice. See Cimperman, *When God's People Have HIV/AIDS: An Approach to Ethics* (Maryknoll, NY: Orbis, 1995), 50–52. Cheryl Townsend Gilkes remarks that self-love is "probably the most critical task we complete" in our commitment to human wholeness. Cheryl Townsend Gilkes, "The 'Loves' and 'Troubles' of African-American Women's Bodies: The Womanist Challenge to Cultural Humiliation and Community Ambivalence," in Emilie M. Townes, ed., *A Troubling in My Soul* (Maryknoll, NY: Orbis, 1993), 232–249, at 247.

8. Henri M. Nouwen, *Life of the Beloved: Spiritual Living in a Secular World* (New York: Crossroad, 1992), 26.

9. Mt 22:36–38; Mk 12:28–30.

10. Mt 22:39 and Mk 12:31.

11. Lk 10:25-28.

12. For a more sustained treatment of basic goods for human flourishing, see Cristina L. H. Traina, *Feminist Ethics and Natural Law: The End of the Anathemas* (Washington, DC: Georgetown University Press, 1999), 44–48.

13. Mk 14:3–9; Mt 26:6-13; Lk 7:36–38.

14. Mt 26:36–46; Mk 14:33–34; Jn 12: 1–11, 11:2–3, 17–44.

15. Jn 12:13–15, 18:36–37; Lk 19:35–40; Mt 21:9–11.

16. Mk 1:12, 1:35, 14:32–42.

17. Mk 14:36.

18. In two of the four gospel accounts, as Jesus is dying on the cross, in excruciating pain, having been humiliated, tortured, and taunted, Jesus cries out in a loud voice, "My God, my God, why have you forsaken me?" (Mt 27:46, Mk 15:34). These are difficult words to interpret. On the one hand, the expression could mirror the questions of the disciples who wondered how God could let this happen to Jesus. Some also interpret Jesus's final words on the cross as his expression of doubt or abandonment. I interpret them instead as lament, an outpouring of anguish and desolation, a human cry of sense-making, but not despair. These words echo the psalmist's cry in Psalm 22:1, concerning the suffering of a righteous person. Assuming the gospel authors were aware of the psalm, which ends in an act of faith declaring "dominion belongs to the Lord," (Ps 22:28), one can interpret the reference to Psalm 22 as the evangelists' way of showing Jesus to be a righteous servant of God.

19. Mt 25:31–46.

20. Lk 6:31-36. See also 1 Jn 3:17–18.

21. Søren Kierkegaard, *Works of Love,* trans. Howard and Edna Hong (New York: Harper Torchbooks, 1962), 62–63; Anders Nygren, *Agape and Eros* (Chicago, IL: University of Chicago Press, 1982); C. S. Lewis, *The Four Loves* (San Diego, CA: Harvest/HBJ, 1960); Gene Outka, *Agape: An Ethical Analysis* (New Haven, CT: Yale University Press, 1972); Bernard V. Brady, "Christian Love is Sacrificial Love," in *Christian Love: How Christians through the Ages Have Understood Love* (Washington, DC: Georgetown University Press, 2003), 194–209; Reinhold Niebuhr, *Love and Justice,* ed. D. B. Robertson (Cleveland, OH: World Publishing Co., 1967), 38 and *Moral Man and Immoral Society: A Study in Ethics and Politics* (New York: Charles Scribner's Sons, 1960), 74–75. Reinhold Niebuhr is known for "Christian realism," which was closely associated with "political realism" in the context of the Cold War. Scholars of Niebuhr caution against overemphasizing his analysis of pride and the need for self-sacrifice. Rebekah Miles explains that some feminists have mischaracterized and oversimplified Niebuhr's understanding of sin, pride, and self-sacrifice. See Miles, *The Bonds of Freedom: Feminist Theology and Christian Realism* (Oxford University Press, 2001), 28–89, 147–153; Robin W. Lovin, *Reinhold Niebuhr and Christian Realism* (Cambridge: Cambridge University Press, 1995), 142–147.

22. Martin D'Arcy, *The Mind and Heart of Love* (New York: Meridian Books, 1956); Barbara Hilkert Andolsen, "Agape in Feminist Ethics," in *On Love and Friendship: Philosophical Readings,* ed. Clifford Williams (Boston, MA: Jones and Bartlett, 1995), and "Elements of a Feminist Approach to Bioethics," in *Feminist Ethics and the Catholic Moral Tradition,* ed. Charles E. Curran, Margaret A. Farley, and Richard A. McCormick, S.J. (New York: Paulist, 1996), 341–381; Valerie Saiving (Goldstein), "The Human Situation: A Feminine View,"

Journal of Religion 4/1960, reprinted in *Womanspirit Rising: A Feminist Reader in Religion*, ed. Carol P. Christ and Judith Plaskow (New York: Harper & Row, 1979), 25–42.

23. Crystal and Keesha are excluded because there was insufficient evidence in their interview transcripts that they do model this balancing of self-love and love for others. In their descriptions of intimate relationships, self-giving loves were not consistently life-giving. Their stories are given greater attention in previous chapters.

24. While I did not interview my collaborators' spouses, one can imagine them affirming that their sacrifices were ways that they showed deep love and commitment to their spouses, and that when they were able to offer physical assistance, emotional support, or simple companionship, they also, even in their self-donation, felt rewarded because the mutual relationship benefited.

25. See Rebekah Miles on the tension between "freedom" and "boundedness" in *Bonds of Freedom*, 3–27; 147–156.

26. See *Catholic Social Thought: The Documentary Heritage*, ed. David J. O'Brien and Thomas A. Shannon (Maryknoll, NY: Orbis, 2001), Charles E. Curran, *Catholic Social Teaching 1891–Present: A Historical, Theological, and Ethical Analysis* (Washington, DC: Georgetown University Press, 2002), and John Paul II, *Familiaris Consortio* (On the Family) (Washington, DC: United States Catholic Conference, 1981), 21.

27. See David Hollenbach, S.J., *The Common Good and Christian Ethics* (Cambridge: Cambridge University Press, 2002).

28. Dawn M. Nothwehr, *Mutuality: A Formal Norm for Christian Social Ethics* (Eugene, OR: Wipf & Stock, 1998), 233.

29. Ibid., 221.

30. Margaret Farley, *Personal Commitments: Beginning, Keeping, Changing* (San Francisco, CA: Harper & Row, 1986), 106.

31. Don Browning, Bonnie Miller-McLemore, Pamela Couture, K. Brynolf Lyon, and Robert Franklin, *From Culture Wars to Common Ground: Religion and the American Family Debate* (Louisville, KY: Westminster John Knox Press, 1997), 127.

32. Ibid., 276.

Chapter Five

A Pro-Life Approach to HIV Prevention and Care

> They do not practice what they teach. They tie up heavy burdens, hard to bear, and lay them on the shoulders of others; but they themselves are unwilling to lift a finger to move them.
> Mt 23: 3b–4

While there is much we do not know about how the historical Jesus self-identified, many scholars believe there is clear evidence that Jesus thought of himself as a good Jew whose mission was to begin a reform of his own religious tradition.[1] In Matthew's version of the gospel story, Jesus is a law-giver in the tradition of Moses and the other great figures of Jewish theological history. Jesus repeatedly challenges dominant interpretations of the law by retrieving a forgotten or misunderstood law from the Jewish canon. The three-fold love commandment is one example, and one can find many such examples, not only in the synoptic gospels but also in John. The story of the woman threatened with stoning in John 7:53–8:11 provides a case from John's Gospel. There, the "law of Moses" is invoked to condemn the woman to stoning. But Jesus invokes a different law, the law of mercy: "Let anyone among you who is without sin be the first to throw a stone against her."

This pattern of teaching in the ministry of Jesus may provide welcome relief to women and men hungry to experience the church today as a community of inclusion, mercy, and solidarity. Theologians who construct a Christian ethical response to HIV and AIDS are in some ways faced with the same methodological question that the historical Jesus faced: what laws from our tradition should we recover and privilege in this new situation? What teachings have priority when applied to this new moral problem? How is God inviting us to respond in this new moment? Conceiving of the theological task in this way helps us to recognize that theology is more art than science; while there is a place for deductive argumentation, before we know how to apply a principle or law we must decide which principle or law best fits the case at hand. Thus, inductive analysis often precedes deductive analysis—and often this inductive analysis involves thinking with the heart as well as with the head.[2] It requires immersion into the moral problem to discern what is going on, and then reflection on the variety of approaches from the tradition through a kind of attunement and discernment of the values at stake until one arrives at the best approach for the given problem. Even then, the application of a principle is not self-evident but must be explained and defended. Often, every step in this process is contested. Now certainly magisterial texts have applied a variety of legal and methodological frameworks in their pronouncements on official church teachings on HIV and AIDS. We will see those in the analysis to follow. But one of the problems is that in the interests of reasserting official church teachings on sexual morality, other important laws from our tradition have been neglected or undervalued. Theological ethicists have an obligation to mine the tradition for resources that may prove to be life-giving for persons affected by HIV and AIDS. This chapter contributes to that goal, both at the level of raising up principles from the tradition and offering normative applications.

As I interpret Jesus's approach to the law, I see his concern for those most vulnerable and his attention to their flourishing. Jesus did not use the law to demean the person but instead to inspire, heal, and to bring about right relationship. "Salvation" means to be freed from oppression, to be made whole. In both Greek and Latin, the root word means to make safe, to deliver or protect, to heal or make well.[3] A Christian response to HIV and AIDS, then, must think critically about whether our words bring healing, freedom, and wholeness. Do we tie up heavy burdens on the shoulders of others and then look on to see how they manage? Or does the church's message inspire, heal, and foster right relationship?

In the United States, AIDS was first recognized as a public health threat that affected gay men, hemophiliacs, and intravenous drug users.[4] Now, almost thirty-five years after the first cases were reported, women represent a growing percentage of new cases of HIV infection, and a majority of these cases are from sexual transmission. While the public's response needs to remain multifaceted, this chapter's analysis will propose a Christian HIV prevention strategy that builds on the stories of the women in this study. What community interventions would have been welcomed during their most difficult struggles? How can the church learn from their stories, adapt its responses, and better address the needs of other families in similar situations? I propose that the church counteract stigma with hospitality, counteract ignorance with increased sexual education initiatives, counteract rising infection rates with specific HIV prevention recommendations, and counteract social apathy with renewed attention to the demands of social justice.

STIGMA AS SIN

The Catholic Church remains a locus of stigma for many AIDS-affected persons throughout the world. This pervasive and overwhelming problem contributes to the marginalization and invisibility of many AIDS-affected Catholics. Their complex needs for spiritual nourishment, communal support, and social services go unmet. Some of the women who participated in my study experienced stigma within their faith communities that prevented them from seeing themselves as beloved of God. While Lettie bemoaned the silence about HIV and AIDS in her parish, Carmen complained of inaccurate information in homilies, and Sue was explicitly told to sit in the back of the church if she wished to receive communion. Their experiences help to illumine the challenges facing parish communities today.

On the one hand, silence is not the solution. The church must be a place where christians can talk openly about the facts of HIV and AIDS, including the behaviors that put persons at risk, the fact that no cure exists, and available methods of prevention. But on the other hand, these discussions pose the risk of contributing to fear of HIV-affected persons and of increasing blame and shame. If the only message from the pulpit is that "AIDS kills," this hardly offers hope for persons already living with HIV. But by drawing on the rich theological resources of our faith, the Catholic Church can resist this disintegration into blame and shame by naming stigma as a sin and by counteracting that sin with the gospel value of hospitality.

Ironically, since the beginning of the HIV epidemic, Catholic caregivers have been first responders to the suffering of those living with HIV and most especially to those dying of AIDS. Even now, the Catholic Church's direct outreach to HIV-affected persons is unmatched by any other religious group.[5] Yet when communities retain sin-talk and judgment of affected persons instead of welcoming them in solidarity, then the church thwarts their flourishing.

We see the dehumanizing effects of stigma in the US context in that 19 percent of American adults who responded to a 2000 national survey agreed with the claim that "people who got AIDS through sex or drug use have gotten what they deserve."[6] Such overt claims of personal responsibility tend to construe HIV-infection as a personal moral failure. This construal results in experiences of stigma and shame among those infected and affected.

Erving Goffman defines stigma as a mark of social disgrace which arises within social relations and disqualifies the stigmatized person from full social acceptance.[7] The stigmatized person retains a "spoiled identity" and is devalued in social relations.[8] Harriet Deacon describes stigma as a social process of "othering, blaming, and shaming" that contributes to but should not be conflated with discrimination, the effects of stigma that result in behavior against a specific stigmatized group.[9] Stigma is a social process that results from ignorance, fear, and unequal social power relations. Deacon explains: "Stigmatizing discourse allows people to distance themselves and their self-defined in-groups from the risk of infection by blaming the contraction of the illness on characteristics normally associated with out-groups, who are classified as deviant and 'other.'"[10]

The presence of the stigmatized person can evoke disgust, fear, or discomfort among those in the non-stigmatized group.[11] Health-related stigma follows a specific pattern:

1. Illness is constructed as preventable or controllable;
2. "Immoral" behaviors causing the illness are identified;
3. These behaviors are associated with "carriers" of the illness in other groups, drawing on existing social constructions of the "other;"
4. Certain people are thus blamed for their own infection; and
5. Status loss is projected onto the "other," which may (or may not) result in disadvantage to them.[12]

This pattern is especially discernible for HIV-positive persons who are stigmatized because of the presumed behaviors that exposed them to the virus. All of the women whom I interviewed explained that upon disclosing their HIV status, they are frequently asked "how they got it." Sue became so frustrated by this question that she tries not to answer it any more. "Because that's how it starts," she said. "First they want to know how you got it and then they know whether to respond with compassion or not. But why don't they respond to everyone with compassion? Even though I was infected through a blood transfusion, that doesn't mean I deserve more compassion than someone infected through drug use."

Within church communities, stigma often results from the association of sexual activity and drug use with sin and with HIV-infected persons as sinners.[13] Othering, blaming, and shaming of HIV-infected persons within church communities constitute stigma. Resulting acts of discrimination can include silence, social exclusion, insults, or verbal abuse, all of which can make the stigmatized person feel ashamed, worthless, excluded, and physically vulnerable.[14] Because of stigma, people are then more likely to delay HIV testing, to withhold disclosure of positive status from family members and to delay access to treatment.[15] Thus stigma has concrete and potentially death-dealing effects.

The concrete effects of stigma surfaced in the stories of the women in this study, as when Lettie explained why she did not disclose her HIV status at work, even among close friends, and when Diva explained that she had not disclosed her status to her adult children. Stigma can also be discerned as a factor in the stories of the women who went through a long period of denial after they were first diagnosed, including Diva, Cheryl, and Carmen. These three women continued to engage in risky behaviors during their period of denial, at a time when they could have accessed treatment and support; in that sense, stigma works against self-care because it adds to the sick person's fear and robs one of motivation to take care of oneself. Today, one of the most common reasons given by people at risk for HIV infection for not getting tested is that they would rather not know their status. In the face of very real stigma perceived not only by those infected but also by those at risk of being infected, ignorance can mask itself as a beneficial coping strategy. But ignorance of one's status causes more harm than good, both personally and socially.

With regard to HIV and church communities, the language of sin has been misused. In describing persons living with HIV as sinful, or in describing illness as a punishment for sin, some church communities have contributed to the suffering and stigmatization of people living with HIV. It is *this harm*, the stigma itself, and corresponding acts of discrimination, that should be clearly named as sinful.

Stigma is sinful at both personal and social levels. At the personal level, it results when one ignores one's own sin and judges another, oftentimes without knowing the unique context of the other person's struggles. At the social level, stigma functions as an instrument of social control. Social groups define their values, in part, by imparting messages about who fits and who does not, what actions are permitted and what actions are not. Those who are stigmatized by a social group are seen to be outside the boundaries of that group's norms. A person's social group, whether cultural or religious, socializes him or her to accept these messages about people and behaviors deemed "misfits." Social systems that institutionalize oppression, domination, and privilege are sinful. The US Catholic bishops have explicitly and directly named such patterns of exclusion and marginalization as violations of human dignity and as social sin.[16]

Catholic theologian Bryan Massingale challenges the church to reevaluate any teachings that seem to justify stigma in the name of God. In his interpretation of the Second Commandment, it is a violation of God's law to make God an accomplice in human evil. This is to blaspheme. Instead, "whenever a religious belief or practice supports or leads to the marginalization or exclusion of any human community, it is not and cannot be of God."[17] The Global Consultation of the World Council of Churches is also explicit:

> As churches, we must now take up the responsibility to overcome stigma and discrimination within our own structures, while being a voice of moral

> strength demanding that our communities, nations, and wider society respect the rights and dignity of people living with HIV/AIDS and condemn acts that stigmatize. The truth is that we are all made in the image of God. This means that discrimination is a sin, and stigmatizing any person is contrary to the will of God.[18]

How can church communities combat such stigma and discrimination? Since the narrative of stigma follows the pattern of othering, blaming, and shaming, a Christian response must correspond to each of these levels. Instead of othering, Christians need to recognize persons living with HIV as part of the body of Christ. As members of the body of Christ, what ails a group of Christians ails us all. To disrupt the pattern of othering, Musa W. Dube, Professor of Theology at the University of Botswana, challenges church communities to see that as members of the Body of Christ we are already affected by AIDS.

> The church has AIDS, for many of our members are infected, sick, dead, or dying of HIV/AIDS and because if one of us has it we all have it, it means that Jesus Christ himself has AIDS, for the church is the body of Christ (1 Cor 12:27). It is my contention therefore, that we do not have to wait until the judgment day to hear Jesus saying, "You saw me sick with AIDS." Today Jesus Christ stands amongst us saying, "Look at me, I have AIDS."[19]

Some theologians have repeated these powerful words in different contexts in order to elicit compassion and solidarity among members of the Body of Christ.[20] This claim—that the Body of Christ has AIDS—can arouse our emotions and call us to solidarity. Indeed, it has been fruitful in calling churches to hold communities accountable to the faces of Jesus in our midst. For HIV-positive persons, too, this claim can function as an affirmation of *imago Dei*, the recognition that one is created in God's image and that God desires one's full flourishing.

To combat the narrative of blaming, faith communities must recognize the wider social problems that constrain individual agency and encourage the spread of HIV infection. By drawing attention to the social processes—the economic, political, and cultural forces—that shape the dynamics of HIV transmission, social analysis can help us to see that for many HIV-positive persons, their infection is not simply their own fault.[21] Since human personhood is marked by sociality and relationality, we are formed as moral agents within the wider social contexts of family, community, social institutions, church, and nation. Poverty, gender inequality, neighborhood decay, sexual violence, racism, and myriad other social factors can contribute to an individual person's risk for engaging in drug use, unprotected sex, or other risky behaviors. For example, Keesha's experience of broken family relationships, rape survival, and witnessing of neighborhood violence contributed to her sense of despair, resulting drug use, alcohol abuse, and now, her own marital separation. The question of fault in a complex life story like Keesha's is not at all simple. While she is not without some personal responsibility, it is a disservice to blame her current situation exclusively on her own moral failings. In telling her story, she displayed resilience and determination. When Keesha asks God for strength to "beat the demons away," she is not only fighting against her personal weaknesses or sins, but also against the social demons of poverty, racism, and gender violence. When as a church we begin to understand this more complex picture of moral responsibility, "the blame game" will look simplistic and unjust.

Finally, church communities need to combat the third aspect of the narrative of stigma—shaming. Shaming tells the HIV-positive person, "you aren't good enough," "you don't deserve God's love," or "you are dirty and do not belong to this community." Nothing could be further from the truth. God's love for every person tells us that no matter what we have done, we are invited into the forgiving love of God. If our God is indeed like the father in the story of the Prodigal Son, or the shepherd who celebrates when finding the lost sheep, or the woman who rejoices when she finds her lost coin—if these parables describe our God—then Christians must face the reality of God's compassion and forgiveness and begin to model that inclusivity within everyday praxis.[22] As a community that proclaims this faith, the church should affirm all persons as created in the image of God and beloved of God. Parishes should explicitly welcome those affected by AIDS in the church community. To do so is to live according to the principle of hospitality, an ethic proclaimed in the ministry of Jesus both in his preaching and in his ministry to the marginalized within his world: women, the sick, and those accused of sinful behaviors. If the church is to be the body of Christ on earth, the church simply must be welcoming. To be otherwise risks an incoherent ecclesiological message. Pope Francis repeats this message in *Evangelii Gaudium*: "The Church is called to be the house of the Father, with doors always wide open."[23]

Catholic ethicist Christopher Vogt reminds Christians that "at the heart of the practice of hospitality is the conscious development of attentiveness to the presence of the 'least of these' in our midst and the establishment of a relationship of solidarity with them."[24] Feminist theologian Beverley Haddad remarks, "Perhaps the biggest challenge that HIV/AIDS poses to the Christian church is the call to become a true community where acceptance, love, and belonging flourish."[25] In Haddad's experience, Bible study groups in Church contexts can become a place of solidarity for women and can provide an example to the wider Church.[26] Such a community of acceptance, love, and belonging can be a "foretaste of salvation" for persons living with HIV and AIDS,[27] a place of support and care, "an oasis of the hospitality of God."[28]

How might parish communities become this "oasis" of God's love? Catholic theologian Kevin Kelly proposes that an important first step is to take away some of the association of AIDS with sin. "It is not strictly accurate to say that the AIDS virus is being spread because of immoral behavior. It is being spread mainly because people who have the virus are having sex with people who are not infected. That is a medically accurate reading of the situation."[29] This "medically accurate" definition tries to eliminate the initial judgment and blaming that can occur when discussing various risk behaviors. Similarly, Catholic physician and ethicist Daniel Sulmasy notes that drug addiction is "almost universally considered by modern medicine to be a disease, and one that dramatically impairs the will of the addict, whether actively intoxicated or not."[30] Sulmasy questions whether, in light of this understanding of disease, it would be better to consider addicts sick persons instead of sinners, and he finds precedent in the moral manuals' treatment of alcoholism.[31] Further, activists within the AIDS-affected community discourage the use of descriptors that convey fear or contagion because language matters. Church communities should not only discourage sin-talk but also should discuss "persons," not "victims" or "infected patients."

The challenge to faith communities is significant. Parishes will need to walk a fine line: clearly attacking ignorance by discussing the facts of HIV transmission and the serious nature of the disease while simultaneously considering the ways that such facts are heard and internalized by persons already living with HIV. They should also offer a welcoming community, commitment to solidarity, and a message of hope grounded in God's love to those living with HIV and AIDS. Catholics should not be afraid to discuss sex, disease, or death; neither should such discussions contribute to othering, blaming, or shaming of persons already affected by HIV and AIDS. Individual communities can attend to these needs by encouraging voluntary HIV testing, by advocating for local, state, and national legislative concerns, by celebrating AIDS Compassion Sunday to raise awareness of HIV and AIDS, and by encouraging age-appropriate comprehensive sexuality education for all persons. Parishes could normalize HIV testing by inviting the local health department's mobile testing bus to the church parking lot after Sunday Mass or by organizing a group of parishioners to walk in the annual AIDS Walk. Had Lettie experienced this kind of support in her church, perhaps she would not have needed to attend two weekly support groups miles away from her home. Perhaps Keesha and Grace would have attended church more regularly. When stigma in church communities makes people feel unwelcome, they are then more likely to cut themselves off from the grace of the sacraments. While certainly regular church attendance should also expose a believer to challenging messages, church attendance should not be demeaning or demoralizing on a regular basis; when it is, the value of participation is thus in tension with the value of self-care.

SEX EDUCATION PROGRAMS

Each woman interviewed for this study was shocked to learn of her HIV status upon diagnosis. Even women who had engaged in risky behaviors thought, "It couldn't happen to me." After learning their HIV status, those women who continued to attend Mass became very sensitive to messages about HIV and AIDS. Diva said that the lack of information was startling. "There are a lot of people in the dark about this disease," she told me. When I asked Sue how the church community could better respond to her needs, she answered, "Accepting us. Acting more Christ-like. Because Christ is in all of us. Education too. AIDS is an isolating, lonely, ugly disease. And we need our church to be there too." Eventually Sue decided that she could be part of the change she wanted to see, and Sue began to work in AIDS educational outreach to public and private schools, including Catholic schools.

HIV is a preventable infection. In combating HIV and AIDS the church needs to examine with renewed attention curricula of sex education within and outside of church-sponsored settings. What messages do young people, and especially young women, hear in sexual education? Are they encouraged to recognize their own dignity and equality, empowered to care for themselves? Is the curriculum based in fear, in idealized notions of self-fulfillment or happiness, in purity, or in responsibility?

Education involves a process of formation and empowerment, through which one learns how to recognize values, negotiate competing values, assert one's own goals, make choices that conform to those goals, and make more over-arching lifestyle decisions. Sex education should assist women in recognizing appropriate and inappropriate levels of vulnerability, in resisting peer pressure and violence and, when not constrained by social factors that impede them, in taking responsibility for their actions.

Curricula in schools and church communities vary widely. Some primarily attend to biology and health, while others promote fear by explaining the negative consequences of sexual activity. Still others offer idealistic or romanticized messages about self-fulfillment through sexual activity. Theologian Christine E. Gudorf names three problematic aspects of contemporary sexual education in the US context:

> One is the assumption that the goal of sex education is sexual abstinence among adolescents. Another is the assumption that sex education is primarily cognitive, designed to promote rational, informed decision-making. These two are, of course, related, in that the assumption of most educators is that rational, informed decision-making will lead to sexual abstinence among the young. The third assumption is that sexuality is essentially private.[32]

Gudorf refutes each of these assumptions. First, she argues that the goal of sex education—both by parents within the family and by educators within the school system—should not focus exclusively on abstinence but on giving the student the resources and skills for constructing a "responsible, satisfying sexual life for her/himself both in the present and into the future."[33] According to Gudorf, an exclusive focus on abstinence during the teen years, even if that is successful, still does not prepare adults for sexually intimate relationships. And with a growing body of evidence that suggests abstinence-only sex education is not effective, this type of curriculum unduly limits the effectiveness of sex education and may cause more harm than good.[34]

Gudorf also critiques the assumption that sex education should focus exclusively on biology and cognition, that is, the facts of human reproduction, contraceptive methods, and sexually transmitted diseases. It would be more effective, she argues, for sex education to focus on the meaning of sexual relationships and the values that inform healthy relationships. Such a framework would articulate for people (young and old alike) the power of sexual activity, which can promote and sustain just and loving intimacy in relationship. It would also highlight the ways that sexual activity can increase vulnerability, with special attention to how sex can be used as a tool of exploitation or harm.[35] It is important for educators to pay attention to student critiques of curricula that are perceived as "boring" or "irrelevant." Gudorf explains that a fact-based curriculum can be boring for students "because there are no clues as to what the information really means—that is, how it relates to the goals and ambitions, the activities, emotions, and relationships of the individual."[36] Students want to make sense of the confusing messages they hear.

Third, Gudorf refutes the claim that sex is essentially a private matter. Frequently in community discussions of sex education curricula, this objection from parents serves to limit the exposure their children have to a wide range of educational materials. The thought is that since sex is a private decision between two persons, it does little good to discuss private matters in public. Accusations of scandal are sometimes lobbied as well. But Gudorf argues that "when we insist that sexuality refers to the private bodies of individual persons, we close off critical attention to existing sexual power structures and relationships."[37] Sex education is a public matter because the formation of sexual identity happens in the context of multiple familial and peer relationships, and because sexual behavior has social implications. For example, two possible consequences of sexual behavior—pregnancy and the transmission of a sexually transmitted infection—create obligations not only for the sexually active couple but also for their medical providers, friends, and family members.

Sex education that promotes empowerment, self-care, and responsibility for women as well as men will require that adults reject some culturally prevalent scripts. It will mean rejecting the socialization that splits teenage girls' identities into either "virgin" or "whore."[38] It will mean that we encourage, not discourage, questions about sexual orientation, sexual pleasure, romantic attachment, intimacy, body image, self-esteem, vulnerability, consent, fear, cultural pressure, guilt, and violence. Such a broad range of issues—coupled with adult reluctance to engage in sexual discourse—means the task of revamping sexual education is a difficult one.[39] But church communities have an important part to play in this necessary educational formation. First, they should be willing to engage in open dialogue about sexuality. Second, church communities should reject oversimplified curricula that fail to engage the whole range of issues (curricula that refuse to discuss condom use, for example). Third, churches should continue to affirm that sexual education should remain not only concerned with genital sex but also with the psychological and spiritual areas of human fulfillment that gives meaning and significance to intimate relationships. Catholic educator Jennifer Mertens reflects on the urgency of this task and the importance of a method that seeks to be both realistic and encouraging:

> We need to enter the storm. We need to listen more than speak. Ask more than preach. Standing for and with our teens, we must empower them as faithful stewards of their own bodies and sexuality. Rule books aren't enough. Young people need more. They need parents, teachers, clergy, coaches, and mentors who are willing to be real. They deserve candid, honest information. Safe spaces for all the tough questions. We must learn to see their world: not black and white, but gray. Trekking it together, we must offer discernment tools for the journey, resources that equip teens to consciously and prayerfully set boundaries for themselves. Teach them how to say "no" but also how to declare "yes!" to celebrating their sexuality in healthy, appropriate ways.[40]

The church should not feel threatened by comprehensive sexual education curricula. On the contrary, if we believe in the goodness of sexuality and the power of reason within the human person, then students can learn about all methods of preventing sexually transmitted infections without being thereby encouraged to engage in non-marital sexual intercourse. In age-appropriate curricula, church communities can emphasize a wide range of factors, including these named by one group of US bishops in 1987: "the qualities of mature, loving, and stable relationships; the characteristics of a solid and loving marriage; the development of such qualities as warmth, communication, responsiveness, fidelity, caring, and unselfishness; the fact that people are not to be treated as throw-away items."[41] If the Catholic Church could be known for championing justice for women and fostering a culture of empowerment, care, and responsibility, church communities could better accompany young people in their difficult discernment and would have greater opportunities to hear the liberating messages: "You are God's beloved." "You have inherent dignity." "You deserve respect." These messages could challenge the other messages from pop culture that breed loss of self-esteem. When church communities instead choose fear-based curricula or lessons based on misinformation, these do more harm than good for young people and hardly prepare married couples well for healthy marital sexuality. Sue explains that as an AIDS educator, her goal is to help young people have the courage to make good decisions.

> One thirty-minute class in high school health class is not enough! When I go to schools, I don't push condoms. I tell the students, "You've been given this amazing gift from God: your body. You can say 'no.' You can treat your body with respect. You can protect yourself from disease. You are the gatekeeper. You are special. Think of your body like a giant computer, but smarter. You have the right to say 'no, that is not good for my body.' God wants you to be safe and healthy." So I offer age appropriate but empowering sexual education. I want others to feel empowered. I want them to believe that they are worthy of love.

Sue tells me that she thinks young people crave straight talk about sexuality, and that she sees so much insecurity in their questions and interactions that her heart aches for them. "We have a lot of work to do," Sue says. "But I want to do my part." Sue would be delighted if church communities would begin to implement comprehensive sex education framed in a values-based curriculum.

CONDOM USE

Since sexual transmission of HIV is preventable through sexual abstinence, as well as correct and consistent condom use, some moral theologians have begun to advocate for increased education about latex condoms, increased access to condoms, and encouragement of condom use by sexually active persons who are at risk for HIV infection. While condoms are not a "quick fix" solution,[42] they can be part of a more comprehensive response that includes increased awareness, personal discipline, and harm reduction.

Sexual abstinence is the most effective means of preventing the spread of sexually transmitted infections like HIV. As such, abstinence should be recommended as the ideal behavior for teens and unmarried persons. But for married persons, for whom abstinence is not desirable, condom use can enable sexual lovemaking while also reducing the risk of transmission of HIV. Public health officials worldwide have achieved broad consensus on the effectiveness of latex condoms in preventing the transmission of HIV. The Centers for Disease Control (CDC) in the United States maintains that latex condoms, when used consistently and correctly, are highly effective in preventing the transmission of HIV. Citing scientific evidence of both laboratory studies of latex barriers as well as studies of sexually active couples, the

CDC claims that latex condoms provide an essentially impermeable barrier to particles the size of STD pathogens and that consistent and correct use of condoms within sero-discordant HIV couples provide protection for the partners who are not HIV positive.[43]

Despite this evidence, there is no consensus among Roman Catholic ethicists about whether the church should endorse condom use for the purpose of preventing HIV transmission. While no pope has made an authoritative statement concerning condoms, representatives from various Vatican congregations, bishops, bishops' conferences, and moral theologians have passionately debated condom use. These arguments demonstrate an engagement with the Church's moral tradition in a variety of ways.

Some bishops and moral theologians draw on the 1968 encyclical *Humanae vitae* to argue against the use of condoms in any situation, interpreting that encyclical as forbidding any act of sexual intercourse that is not open to procreation.[44] Germain Grisez, a longtime defender of *Humanae vitae*, argues that only *marital* intercourse facilitates human flourishing, and that *marital* intercourse must remain open to procreation.[45] Others question the effectiveness of condoms. For example, Cardinal Alfonso Lopez Trujillo, President of the Pontifical Council for the Family, has stated that the HIV virus is small enough to "easily pass through" latex condoms.[46] In their 1989 pastoral the U.S. bishops called condoms "technically unreliable," further contributing to misinformation and confusion among Catholics. Other Church officials have argued that Church promotion of condom use would encourage promiscuity, or cause scandal, that is, confusion leading to sin, among the faithful.[47]

In contrast to these rigorist positions,[48] a number of Catholic moralists have applied a variety of principles of Catholic moral theology to offer a more favorable interpretation of condom use. Jesuit moralist James Keenan describes these arguments as "very traditional."[49] According to these moralists, the tradition has always recognized that moral action in constrained circumstances might require the toleration of or cooperation with evil. Principles from the Roman Catholic moral tradition can help Catholics avoid, limit, or distance themselves from such evil by giving specific criteria for morally acceptable accommodation within certain cases.

The first of these arguments to emerge was the use of the principle of toleration in the 1987 letter from the United States Catholic Conference Administrative Board, entitled T*he Many Faces of AIDS: A Gospel Response*.[50] There, the bishops describe the case of a health worker who tells an HIV-positive person to remain sexually abstinent. However, if it is obvious that the person will not do so, then the health worker could advise a form of conduct to "avoid inflicting greater harm."[51] According to the principle of toleration, the evil actions of others can be tolerated if either a greater good or set of goods would be lost if the evil action were not tolerated, or if greater evils would occur were the original evil not tolerated. Keenan describes this moral argumentation thus:

> The USCC appropriated the earlier logic and made an important distinction: they were opposed to the promotion or advocacy of condoms, but when faced with a person who could further spread the disease and whose conduct would not be altered, they tolerated the advice that the patient should use a condom to prevent the spread of the disease. This position allowed the bishops both to resolve the new case and to protect the material principle that sex is illicit outside of marriage.[52]

The document's casuistic logic enabled the bishops to respond to the new case by relying on wisdom from the tradition.

In a separate essay, Keenan reached the same conclusion but invoked the principle of cooperation instead of the principle of toleration.[53] According to the principle of cooperation, the one who cooperates can participate in circumstances that are not essential to the commission of an action (such as recommendation of prophylactics), assuming the action (illicit sexual activity) could occur even without this cooperation, if there is proportionately serious reason (grave harm to sexual partner) and if the danger of scandal is avoided (the proportionate judgment). Use of this principle invites the reflection of proportionate judgment instead of an analysis of any potential "intrinsic evil" resulting from the action in question.

In the case of sero-discordant married persons, as another moralist explained, since the purpose of using a condom would be to prevent infection from one spouse to another, and not to prevent conception (as *Humanae vitae* forbids), then condom use would be licit.[54] This reasoning depends upon an analysis of the intent of the action. Similarly, Bela Somfai reached the same conclusion by arguing from the principle of double effect.[55] According to the principle of double effect, if an action that is good in itself has two effects, one good and intended, and an unintended yet predicted evil effect, the action can be licit if the action is not intrinsically evil, if the direct intention of the agent is to achieve the intended good effect and to avoid harmful effects, if the good effects are not achieved by means of harmful effects, and if the good effects follow from the action at least as immediately as the harmful effects. In this thinking, the use of a condom is not intrinsically evil; rather, the contraceptive intent is. If one uses a condom to prevent infection (direct intention) but one accepts the unintended consequence of the contraceptive effect, then the action is licit.

In 2010, Pope Benedict XVI signaled the possibility of a wider investigation into these moral questions when he made a brief public statement about condoms. He did not promulgate this as official church teaching nor did he elaborate on this teaching in a subsequent encyclical, but in an interview with journalist Peter Seewald, Pope Benedict explained:

> There may be a basis in the case of some individuals, as perhaps when a male prostitute uses a condom, where this can be a first step in the direction of moralization, a first assumption of responsibility, on the way toward recovering an awareness that not everything is allowed and that one cannot do whatever one wants. But it is not really the way to deal with the evil of infection. That can really lie only in a humanization of sexuality.[56]

Seewald then asked a follow-up question of Pope Benedict, inquiring as to whether "the Catholic Church is actually not opposed in principle to the use of condoms?" Pope Benedict responded: "She of course does not regard it as a real or moral solution, but, in this or that case, there can be nonetheless, in the intention of reducing the risk of infection, a first step in a movement toward a different way, a more human way, of living sexuality."[57] In this statement Pope Benedict XVI was drawing on another principle from the moral tradition: the law of gradualism. Moral theologian Richard M. Gula explains that the principle of gradualism comes from the distinction between the objective and subjective poles of morality.[58] "The Catholic moral and pastoral traditions honor the distinction between *ought* and *can*," writes Gula, who then makes a distinction between moral theology (the realm of the *ought*) and pastoral guidance (the realm of the *can*). He explains:

> Pastoral moral guidance, by contrast to moral theology, is the art of the possible. It focuses primarily on the subjective pole of morality, or the individual's conscience, rather than on abstract principles. The subjective pole of morality has to do with the behavior that flows from one's capacity of knowledge, freedom, and emotion to appreciate moral values, to commit oneself to them, and to choose them freely. Pastoral guidance is concerned with the ability of a person to fulfill the objective moral order. In other words, it seeks the best possible expression of basic human goods that this person can make at this time to satisfy what love demands.[59]

Gula grounds this analysis in a Christian anthropology that is sensitive to sin, an anthropology that presumably would have been operating for Pope Benedict as well. Gula writes:

> There is a limit to what can be done by each person at each time in order to live truthfully, compassionately, and respectfully of self and others. To refuse to accept this is to demand perfect love from imperfect creatures. To face the reality of human sinfulness and to accept our limited ability to love is not to dissolve the gospel demand but to recognize that we are still in need of conversion. We are still on the way to the full flowering of love.
>
> Pastoral guidance follows the *principle of gradualism*. This means that a person progresses one step at a time toward a deeper integration of the demands of objective morality. For example, we may not be able to fulfill the demands of justice, honesty, truthfulness, chastity, and courage immediately. The pastoral moral guide must pay attention to what limits a person's ability to fulfill

> moral standards because of where that person may be in his or her moral freedom. Each person moves toward the fullness of being loving only at the pace and to the extent that he or she can.[60]

When Pope Benedict employed the law of gradualism, he said condom use would not be a "real or moral solution," thereby referring to what Gula called the "objective pole," or the "ought." Yet condom use could be a "first step," said Benedict, indicating that condom use could be recommended within what Gula called the "subjective pole," or the "can." In this way of thinking, condom use could indicate a step in the right direction, a step towards a deeper integration of the demands of love and justice. While this action would not conform to the ideals of Christian sexual ethics, nevertheless this approach is consistent with a harm reduction strategy like those found in the application of the principles of double effect and toleration.

Unfortunately, Pope Benedict's selection of a case might not prove to be as helpful for married women as the foregoing implies. Baptist ethicist Melissa Browning evaluates the statement in this way:

> The weakness of [Pope Benedict's] statement lies in the fact that a male prostitute is used as an example. In this way, Benedict XVI continues the current line of thought that sees condoms as needed in casual relationships but not needed within marriage. Marriage is still naively portrayed as a safe space where the "humanization of sexuality" is taken for granted. To his credit, in this statement, Benedict XVI does accept condom use as a temporary measure that can lead us toward more responsibility for life. Extending this argument, we could ask if condoms could be used within marriage as a temporary measure that would give women more space to negotiate the terms of sex with an HIV-positive husband (or a husband who is thought to be HIV-positive).[61]

Ultimately, it would be most fruitful if official Catholic teachings would affirm condom use for the prevention of HIV and other sexually transmitted infections as part of the church's moral theology in addition to its pastoral guidance. If that happens, many may indeed point to Pope Benedict XVI as the pope who initiated this fruitful conversation in Catholic ethics.

The moral principles to which we have already given sustained attention—toleration, cooperation, double effect, and gradualism—still do not exhaust the principles within the Catholic moral tradition that can be applied to the moral problem of HIV prevention. Still other theologians rely on principles from the tradition of Catholic social teaching.[62] Lisa Sowle Cahill provides an analysis of the resources of Catholic social teaching in her essay, "AIDS, Justice, and the Common Good."[63] By situating AIDS in a context of structural sin—including poverty, gender inequality, racism, and an exploitive system of global markets—Cahill argues that human dignity, the common good, and preferential option for the poor are principles that can help

Catholics promote human flourishing in specific contexts. By relying on the principle of human dignity Catholics claim that every person should be respected as a valuable member of society; actions contrary to the dignity of the person are prohibited.[64] Thus, if sex without a condom (thereby risking HIV infection) is "contrary to the dignity of the person," such an act is prohibited. While this does not necessarily imply that condom use is good in itself, it does clearly reject the absolute prohibition of condom use for persons who are HIV-positive or at risk of becoming infected with the virus.

The principle of the common good, which is grounded in an anthropological account of the person as social and interdependent, regards human flourishing as interconnected. Cahill explains that the "purpose of the common good is to enhance the well-being of every single member of society, as well as of society as a whole."[65] Applied to condom use and sexual education the principle of the common good would advocate for programs that increase public health, including advocacy for both abstinence and avoidance of risk behaviors, in addition to methods for decreasing harm by preventing new infections.

Finally, to have an "option for the poor" means that Catholics call special attention to those members of society who are most marginalized, poor, and vulnerable. Bishop Kevin Dowling explains that in his own context, the Diocese of Rustenburg, South Africa, attention to the marginalized, poor, and vulnerable demands that Catholics prioritize human dignity in moral discernment. For Dowling, the promotion of condom use is a pro-life issue and an issue of social justice.[66] Dowling argues that since life is sacred, and condom use can protect and save lives, he believes that the most compassionate response is to promote condom use for those at risk of acquiring HIV through sexual activity.[67] In his context, the poor and marginalized, including sex workers, married women, and single women, need to be able to protect their own health. "We do not live in an ideal world," writes Dowling. "What do we have to say to this *real* world?"[68] According to Dowling the church cannot only preach the ideal of abstinence and fidelity when this ideal is not possible for all church members (for example, when a married woman cannot expect sexual fidelity from her husband).

In addition to these principles from the Catholic moral tradition and from Catholic social teaching, Christian discipleship requires self-care. To care for oneself requires that one accept oneself, resist unnecessary risks, and protect one's health. For many women, self-care will require sexual abstinence. But this is not always the case. For women who fear intimate partner violence, for example, abstinence is not always possible.[69] For married women, permanent abstinence is hardly desirable.[70] Instead, sexual loving in marriage, if precautions are taken, can foster deeper intimacy and mutuality. While both partners retain their vulnerability, still the emotional bond that is renewed in marital sexual love-making can strengthen the couple's mutual pleasure, can re-connect them to some appreciation of their bodies and can lessen anxiety experienced in other areas of life.[71]

None of the women whom I interviewed—women who self-described as Catholic, married, and HIV-positive—had chosen permanent abstinence. Even when women described loneliness, increased vulnerability, physical pain, or fear of infecting their spouses, none concluded that they should abstain from sex completely.[72] All indicated that they agreed with the recommendations of their physicians to use condoms. Carmen reported feeling conflicted, at least to some degree, because while she knew that she and her husband needed to use condoms, she thought the church forbade it.

HIV is a deadly virus, and yet its spread is preventable. When abstinence is neither possible nor preferable, condom use can offer reliable means to prevent HIV infection. In light of these women's experiences and the ongoing research by Catholic moralists, church communities should explicitly advocate for increased education about the usefulness of latex condoms in preventing the spread of HIV. Condom effectiveness depends upon using the condom correctly and consistently. Persons are not born with the knowledge of how to use condoms; indeed, this must be taught. Contrary to some assertions by Catholic bishops, familiarity with condom effectiveness does not necessarily increase promiscuous behavior. Instead, knowledge of condoms can help a person to understand the comprehensive responses possible. For a curious teenager to learn about condom use and effectiveness does not constitute sinful, imprudent, or unnatural behavior. This information can help the teenager to understand the complexity of the decision to engage in sexual activity, including the real risks and dangers of sex. Furthermore, for sexually active persons who are at risk for HIV infection, condom use is a clear directive of the imperative to care for oneself.

SOCIAL PROGRAMS

The twin answers of abstinence and fidelity have been emphasized with great force by Catholic thinkers in response to the AIDS pandemic. The third answer emphasized by public health officials and by some Catholic moral theologians is condom use to prevent new infections. These three answers are often called the ABCs: Abstinence, Be faithful, Condoms. But this tripartite answer is still too simplistic for two reasons. First, the ABC prevention framework focuses only on sexual transmission of the disease, which is just one method of HIV transmission. Secondly, the ABC answer stays too strictly within a personal and interpersonal framework, without attention to the wider social realities that have an impact on an HIV-positive person's life.[73] While behavior change is certainly necessary to stem the tide of HIV infections, urban communities need to address the social factors that contribute to rising HIV infection rates, including poverty, despair, drug use, homelessness, and violence against women. As previously described, some of my collaborators experienced trauma rooted in their unstable social settings, including gender-based violence. Clearly, eliminating violence and empowering women lies at the very heart of addressing HIV risk factors for women. Other concrete items that should be on the church's agenda include advocacy for access to comprehensive affordable health care, needle exchange (clean syringe) programs, and treatment for substance addictions.

The women whom I interviewed depended on a variety of social programs available within the United States, including Ryan White CARE,[74] HOPWA,[75] ADAP,[76] Medicare, and Medicaid, as well as support groups facilitated by social service organizations in Chicago. Yet research has shown that women, more than men, experience social barriers to accessing treatment and services.[77] Four out of ten women living with HIV in the United States have the virus under control; retention in medical care has become a significant concern for HIV-positive women in the United States.[78] Even after the implementation of the Patient Protection and Affordable Care Act, health care reform remains a major social and political concern in the United States, and for reform to be successful, it must attend to the growing disparities in health care access among Americans so that women, and especially poor and marginalized women, can access the care they need.[79]

Four of the eight women in my study—Cheryl, Keesha, Diva, and Crystal—were in recovery for addictions to drugs and alcohol and noted that their risk factors for acquiring HIV infection included both injection drug use and unprotected sexual intercourse.[80] Their experiences surface another key element that is needed in a comprehensive response to the problem of HIV/AIDS: the church must tackle head-on the ongoing drug epidemic in the United States through prevention, education, treatment, and outreach interventions. One part of that comprehensive strategy should be the promotion of needle exchange programs, which are also sometimes called clean syringe programs; these are harm reduction strategies supported by many United Nations bodies including the General Assembly, Joint Programme on HIV/AIDS (UNAIDS), the UN Office on Drugs and Crime, and the World Health Organization.[81] Needle exchanges are community-based programs where drug users can safely dispose of old syringes and exchange them for new, sterile ones. There are at least 221 sterile syringe exchange programs currently operating in the United States in thirty-three states.[82] A report published by the Centers for Disease Control and Prevention explains that persons who inject drugs (IDUs, or injecting drug users) should use a new, sterile needle and syringe for each injection. Syringe exchange programs effectively reduce transmission of bloodborne pathogens, including not only HIV but also hepatitis B virus and hepatitis C virus. Needle exchange programs in community-based clinics frequently also provide HIV testing, referrals for medical care and case management, and referrals for substance abuse treatment programs;[83] thus, the CDC argues that needle exchange programs serve as an effective public health approach for a vulnerable population.[84] Empirical evidence clearly demonstrates that needle exchange programs do not result in increased drug use among participants or the recruitment of first-time drug users.[85] These programs are part of a harm reduction approach to public health, and in that sense they invoke similar principles as seen with advocacy for condom use. While harm reduction policies do not condone illegal intravenous drug use, they seek to limit the harmful effects of this behavior for those who continue to engage in it.

The US bishops rejected needle exchange programs in their 1989 document *Called to Compassion and Responsibility*, instead proposing that "a better approach to the drug epidemic would be increased government support for outreach and drug treatment programs."[86] In the absence of such increased government support, however, the drug epidemic has continued in the United States.

Catholic theologians continue to mine the resources of the moral tradition for principles that could guide our thinking on this complex issue today. Catholic moral theologian Mary Jo Iozzio has drawn upon the principles of human dignity, preferential option for the poor, and social justice in her advocacy for needle exchange programs.[87] Catholic physician and ethicist Daniel Sulmasy invokes the principle of cooperation when he argues that needle exchange programs sponsored by a Catholic organization would constitute remote, contingent, mediate material cooperation, and would be licit.[88] Sulmasy begins by noting that the free distribution of clean needles is not intrinsically evil; the same needles are used by diabetics to administer insulin and opioid medications are effective drugs for treating pain.[89] Sulmasy continues by explaining that harm reduction efforts are not formal cooperation because the cooperator does not share in the actor's intent.[90] He further claims that Catholic participation in needle exchange programs constitutes material cooperation because some addicts will use the supplied needles to inject drugs for the purpose of obscuring consciousness, but that the cooperation is mediate rather than immediate because the needles are often supplied by organizations other than the sponsoring Catholic organization.[91] In his treatment of the risk of scandal, Sulmasy explains that needle exchange programs are not at risk of causing scandal (in the technical theological understanding of scandal). In reflecting on his experiences practicing medicine in Chicago, Sulmasy draws upon the principle of human dignity and the data of social analysis in addition to the principle of cooperation. His analysis coheres with the life stories of the four women in my study who are recovering drug addicts, all of whom are African American/Black women who grew up in Chicago. It is worth quoting his analysis at length here:

> For the church to give scandal by participating in a needle-exchange program, however, it would be necessary to believe that people will thereby be led to think that what the church really believes is that drug abuse is not a serious moral wrong, and that this would lead them to start using injectable drugs to escape life's pressures or to create a false sense of happiness. On the face of it, this seems an extremely far-fetched promise.
>
> In my medical practice, I have treated hundreds of persons dependent on injectable heroin or cocaine, and I do not recall one for whom the opinions or actions of the Roman Catholic Church about anything had the slightest impact on their drug use. The prevalence of injection-drug use is highest among poor persons of color growing up in conditions in which drug abuse dominates their local cultures. Many of these abusers are the children of addicts. Most are high school dropouts. Many begin using drugs at young ages through the influence of older siblings and friends. Their lives are often caught up in and dominated by the world of drugs and the crime associated with drugs before they have had genuine opportunities to escape. And persons addicted to these substances generally die very young. The aim of a needle-exchange program is to help addicts live longer and reduce the harm they do to themselves and their communities, and to give them the time to recover from their addictions and not harm anyone else. Thus, such programs are truly respectful of their human dignity, and aim to treat them as whole, integrated persons.[92]

To treat Cheryl, Keesha, Diva, and Crystal—and women with similar experiences—as whole, integrated persons, sensitive to the trauma of their past and yet concerned for their physical and spiritual well-being in the present, is no easy task for members of the church or for medical professionals. But it seems irresponsible for church leaders to deny drug users who are at risk for HIV infection with the means to prevent HIV infection, especially in the face of mounting evidence of the effectiveness and long term cost savings of needle exchange programs.[93] To simply reassert the ideal of abstinence from drug use without also offering concrete assistance to people impacted by substance abuse risks oversimplification to the point of hypocrisy.[94] Despite the substantial health risks and economic costs associated with substance abuse, only a small percentage of persons needing substance abuse treatment actually receive it.[95] In the midst of ongoing funding cuts to mental health and substance abuse treatment programs in the United States, Catholic leaders must be both compassionate and prophetic, urging politicians and voters to fund effective programs to assist persons facing drug addictions to overcome their dependency on these harmful substances while simultaneously working to address the situations of social decay and fractured lives caused by addictive lifestyles.

It is unfortunate that public debate around AIDS-related issues so often focuses on controversial topics like condom use or needle exchange programs, when there are many more social justice-related concerns on which the Catholic tradition already speaks with profound clarity. Catholic social teaching offers a framework for thinking about the moral dimensions of public policies. If more committed Catholics would advocate for public spending for HIV-specific programs like HOPWA, Ryan White, ADAP, as well as related programs like poverty reduction, housing assistance, and comprehensive medical care for all US citizens, we could give public voice to Catholic social teaching on these important issues.

In addition to public advocacy, Catholic parishes can offer concrete support to HIV-affected persons through formation of church-based support groups and educational outreach initiatives. Support groups are frequently run from social service agencies, hospitals, or clinics, but if church groups began to host these groups then participants could find a place to discuss the inevitable theological and spiritual questions that arise from the reality of suffering from chronic and terminal illness. For my collaborators, their support groups offered them safe places to express fear, anger, pain, and joy with people whom they trusted. In addition to support groups, parishes could offer assistance with meals and rides for HIV-affected persons through voluntary networks, and HIV educational outreach (including information for adult education, teen education, and age-appropriate material for catechetical classes). While educating parishioners about the fundamental aspects of HIV and AIDS would include descriptions of the modes of transmission and symptoms of infection, a more comprehensive picture of the epidemic would also include how social forces like poverty, racism, and sexism impact rates of HIV infection and the principles of Catholic social teaching that demand a comprehensive response to the epidemic.

By re-framing AIDS-related questions in the church as problems of social justice, we can begin to understand better the complexity of the epidemic. But to say that it is complex does not imply that the problem is mysterious or that our situation is hopeless. Indeed, HIV/AIDS is a predictable outcome of interrelated personal decisions and social injustices, including poverty, racism, urban violence, uneven economic development, decaying neighborhoods, and the lack of affordable comprehensive medical care for all. What is needed is determined action on behalf of justice.

When asked to describe what constitutes abundant life for them, my collaborators included descriptions of feeling well, emotional support from family, friends, and loved ones, the ability to care for their children and to provide for their families, respect from medical workers, freedom from violence, the ability to access affordable, comprehensive health care, employment, safe and affordable housing, educational opportunities, and freedom from discrimination. Their descriptions help to elaborate on the work of theologians who have described human flourishing as integral and interdependent.[96] In listening to their stories, I began to understand how their faith remains very important to them, and gives them strength, comfort, and meaning, but yet does not shield them from suffering, fatigue, and financial stress.

In order to best serve these women, church communities can listen to their experiences, welcome their participation, and stand in solidarity with them against the social injustices they face.

CONCLUSION

While these recommendations—for reducing stigma, expanding sex education, advocating for harm reduction strategies like condom use and needle exchange programs, and increasing the church's social action programs—emerge from the stories of eight particular women, their stories and experiences may resonate with a much broader population. While the next chapter will attend in greater detail to the women's experiences as *married* women, here I have demonstrated that their experiences living with HIV can encourage Christians to reconsider our strategies for combatting AIDS while simultaneously addressing the needs of people living with HIV. Recall that the meaning of salvation, drawing from the original Latin and Greek, means to rescue, to heal, to make whole. If Christianity is to be a force for good in the world, a means through which people experience the love of God, a community through which one is saved, then Christian churches must carefully discern those laws from our moral tradition that will helps us to speak a word of loving care to persons affected by HIV and AIDS. The interventions for which I advocate would be pro-life: affirming the inherent human dignity of persons living with HIV and bringing the most accurate scientific data at our disposal to bear on this significant public health crisis.

NOTES

1. In other words, these scholars tell us that the historical Jesus did not necessarily think of himself as starting a new religion. His rebuke of the leaders of his own time—both political leaders and religious leaders—could thus be interpreted as his desire to critique unjust practices towards the aim of reforming first century Judaism. E. P. Sanders, *Jesus and Judaism* (Minneapolis: Fortress, 1985); John Dominic Crossan, *The Historical Jesus: The Life of a Mediterranean Jewish Peasant* (New York: Harper, 1993).

2. Richard Gula explains: "The strict logic of a scientific nature is necessary in morality in order to defend publicly what we have decided. But we do not actually make our decisions in the same logical way that we try to justify them. Ordinarily in the moral life, we lead with the heart. Judgments of rationality follow in a complementary way. They set the outer limits of moral action and they provide reasons for action which are publicly intelligible. As a matter of the reasoning heart, discernment requires the fuller use of the virtue of prudence and the theology of the moral conscience." *Reason Informed by Faith: Foundations of Catholic Morality* (New York: Paulist, 1989), 316.

3. Gerald O'Collins, S. J. and Edward G. Farrugia, S. J., *A Concise Dictionary of Theology*, Rev. Ed. (New York: Paulist, 2000).

4. Darrell E. Ward, "The Emergence and Early Years of the HIV/AIDS Epidemic," in *The AmFAR AIDS Handbook: The Complete Guide to Understanding HIV and AIDS* (New York: W.W. Norton & Company, 1999), 366–385.

5. The works of Catholic Relief Services, Caritas International, Catholic Fund for Overseas Development, and the Catholic Medical Mission Board exemplify these commitments. A report on faith-based organizations explains the impact these and other organizations have had worldwide. Global Health Council, *Faith in Action: Examining the Role of Faith-Based Organizations in Addressing HIV/AIDS*, available at http://www.globalhealth.org/view_top.php3?id=448 (accessed August 29, 2005).

6. Centers for Disease Control and Prevention, "HIV Related Knowledge and Stigma—United States, 2000," in *Morbidity and Mortality Weekly Report* 49:47 (2000):1062–1064.

7. Erving Goffman, *Stigma: Notes on the Management of Spoiled Identity* (Englewood Cliffs, NJ: Prentice Hall, 1963).

8. Ibid.

9. Harriet Deacon, "Towards a Sustainable Theory of Health-Related Stigma: Lessons from the HIV/AIDS Literature," *Journal of Community and Applied Social Psychology* 16 (2006): 418–425. See also G. M. Herek, "Thinking about AIDS and Stigma: A Psychologist's Perspective," *Journal of Law, Medicine, and Ethics* 30(2002): 594–607; H. Joffe, *Risk and 'The Other'* (Cambridge, United Kingdom: Cambridge University Press, 1999).

10. Deacon, 420.

11. Reverend Bryan N. Massingale, "Stigma: The Other Virus," Presentation, National Catholic AIDS Network Annual Clergy and Religious HIV/AIDS Roundtable. June 2, 2006. Loyola University Chicago, Chicago, IL.

12. Deacon, 421.

13. Kari Hartwig, Seelah Kissioki, and Charlotte Hartwig, "Church Leaders Confront HIV/AIDS and Stigma: A Case Study from Tanzania," *Journal of Community and Applied Social Psychology* 16 (2006): 492–497, at 494–495; Laura Van Vuuren, "AIDS Apathy Campaign Debuts: Yet Christian Leaders Say Stigma, Not Neglect, is the Bigger Problem," *Christianity Today* 46:10 (2002):28. For a fictionalized account, see Pearl Cleage, *What Looks Like Crazy on an Ordinary Day* (New York: Perennial, 1997).

14. William L. Holzemer et al., "Validation of the HIV/AIDS Stigma Instrument—PLWA (HASI-P)," *AIDS Care* 19:8 (9/2007): 1002–1012, at 1008.

15. W. R. Wolfe et al., "Effects of HIV-related stigma among an early sample of patients receiving antiretroviral therapy in Botswana," *AIDS Care* 18:8 (2006): 931–933, at 932.

16. Massingale, "Stigma." See also, United States Conference of Catholic Bishops, *Economic Justice for All*, available at http://www.usccb.org/sdwp/international/EconomicJusticeforAll.pdf (accessed 10/31/2007). In the Bishops' 1989 document *Called to Compassion*, they explain "we have all been touched by original sin, and all of us commit personal sins of our own. The story of the prodigal son (Lk 15:11–32) calls each of us to personal conversion and reform." United States Bishops' Meeting, *Called to Compassion and Responsibility: A Response to the HIV/AIDS Crisis* in *Origins* 19:26 (11/30/1989), 421–436, at 431.

17. Ibid.

18. World Council of Churches Global Consultation on Ecumenical Responses to the Challenges of HIV/AIDS in Africa, "Plan of Action," Adopted in Nairobi, Kenya, November 28, 2001. Available athttp://www.oikoumene.org/en/resources/documents/wcc-programmes/justice-diakonia-and-responsibility-for-creation/ehaia/declarations-and-policy-statements-on-hivaids-by-churches-and-faith-based-organisations-2001-2005/2001-ehaia-consultation.html (accessed 10/31/2007).

19. Musa W. Dube, "Theological Challenges: Proclaiming the Fullness of Life in the HIV/AIDS and Global Economic Era," *International Review of Mission* XCI: 363 (2002a): 535–549. Dr. Dube's comments were met with shock, outrage, and accusations of scandal; then the World Council of Churches transformed her critique into a slogan, "The Body of Christ has AIDS." Musa W. Dube, "HIV and AIDS-related Stigma: Responding to the Challenge," in *A Report of a Theological Workshop Focusing on HIV- and AIDS- Related Stigma, Windhoek, Namibia, 12/3/2003* (Geneva: UNAIDS, 2005), 51–62, at 58.

20. Donald Messer, "We Are All HIV-Positive," in *Breaking the Conspiracy of Silence: Christian Churches and the Global AIDS Crisis* (Minneapolis, MN: Fortress, 2004), 19, 27–38; Maria Cimperman, *When God's People Have HIV/AIDS: An Approach to Ethics* (Maryknoll, NY: Orbis, 2005), xi.

21. Paul Farmer with Margaret Connors and Jamie Simmons, Eds., *Women, Poverty, and AIDS: Sex, Drugs, and Structural Violence* (Monroe, ME: Common Courage Press, 1996), 23.

22. These parables are found in Luke 15.

23. Pope Francis, *Evangelii Gaudium* (2013), no. 47. Available online: http://w2.vatican.va/content/francesco/en/apost_exhortations/documents/papa-francesco_esortazione-ap_20131124_evangelii-gaudium.html (Accessed July 11, 2104).

24. Christopher P. Vogt, "Fostering a Catholic Commitment to the Common Good: An Approach Rooted in Virtue Ethics," *Theological Studies* 68 (2007): 394–417, at 412. See also Maureen H. O'Connell, *Compassion: Loving Our Neighbor in an Age of Globalization* (Maryknoll, New York: Orbis, 2009), and Christine D. Pohl, *Making Room: Recovering Hospitality as a Christian Tradition* (Grand Rapids, MI: Eerdmans, 1999).

25. Beverley Haddad, "Reflections on the Church and HIV/AIDS," *Theology Today* 62 (2005): 29–37, at 33.

26. Beverley Haddad, "Living it Out: Faith Resources and Sites as Critical to Participatory Learning with Rural South African Women," *Journal of Feminist Studies in Religion* 22:1 (2006) 135–154.

27. Haddad, "Reflections," 33. Haddad cites Steve de Gruchy, "How Then Shall We Be Saved? AIDS, Community, and Redemption," *Bulletin for Contextual Theology in Africa* 7 (2000): 18–20.

28. Haddad, "Reflections," 34.

29. Kevin T. Kelly, *New Directions in Sexual Ethics: Moral Theology and the Challenge of AIDS* (London: Geoffrey Chapman, 1998), 203.

30. Daniel P. Sulmasy, O. F. M., "Catholic Participation in Needle- and Syringe-Exchange Programs for Injection-Drug Users: An Ethical Analysis" *Theological Studies* 73 (2012): 422–441, at 433. Sulmasy cites *Diagnostic and Statistical Manual of Mental Disorders DSM-IV-TR* (Washington: American Psychiatric Association, 2000). See also Daniel Sulmasy, "Diseases and Natural Kinds," *Theoretical Medicine and Bioethics* 26 (2005): 487–513.

31. Sulmasy cites Bill W., *Alcoholics Anonymous: The Story of How Many Thousands of Men and Women Have Recovered from Alcoholism*, 4ed. (New York: AA World Services, 2002), 344; John C. Ford, S. J. and Gerald Kelly, S. J., *Contemporary Moral Theology, vol. 1, Questions in Fundamental Moral Theology* (Westminster, MD: Newman, 1960), 290; Pontifical Council for Pastoral Assistance to Health Care Workers, *Charter for Health Care Workers* (Vatican City: Vatican, 1995), no. 94.

32. Gudorf, *Body, Sex, and Pleasure*, 155.

33. Ibid., 156.

34. Bruckner, Hannan, and Bearman, "After the Promise: The STD Consequences of Adolescent Virginity Pledges," *Journal of Adolescent Health* (May 2005): 36–38. Norman A. Constantine, "Converging Evidence Leaves Policy Behind: Sex Education in the United States," *Journal of Adolescent Health* 42:4 (April 2008): 324–326; L. Lindberg, "Changes in Formal Sex Education: 1995–2002," *Contraception* 74:2 (August 2006): 186–188; Bobbie Crew Nelms, "Adolescent Sex Education: Making It a Priority," *Journal of Pediatric Health Care* 17:5 (Sept/Oct 2003): 221–222; Lynda Richardson, "Condoms in School Said Not To Affect Teenage Sex Rate," New York *Times* (30 Sept 1997): A1, 33. See also, *Illinois Campaign for Responsible Sex Education*, http://www.responsiblesexed.org/ (accessed October 31, 2007).

35. Gudorf, 53–54.

36. Ibid., 52.

37. Ibid., 158.

38. Barbara J. Blodgett, *Constructing the Erotic: Sexual Ethics and Adolescent Girls* (Cleveland, OH: Pilgrim Press, 2002), Leora Tanenbaum, *Slut! Growing Up Female with a Bad Reputation* (New York: Seven Stories Press, 1999), Peggy Orenstein, *School Girls: Young Women, Self-Esteem, and the Confidence Gap* (New York: Bantam Doubleday Dell Publishing Group, 1994), Lynn Phillips, ed., *The Girls Report: What We Know and Need to Know About Growing Up Female* (New York: National Council for Research on Women, 1998), Carole Vance, ed., *Pleasure and Danger: Exploring Female Sexuality* (London: Routledge and Kegan

Paul, 1984), Sharon Thompson, *Going All the Way: Teenage Girls' Tales of Sex, Romance, and Pregnancy* (New York: Hill and Wang, 1995).

39. Not only are parents reluctant to discuss sex with their children, but parents do not always have medically accurate information about methods of birth control. See Marla E. Eisenberg, Linda H. Bearinger, Renee E. Sieving, Carolyne Swain, and Michael D. Resnick, "Parents' Beliefs About Condoms and Oral Contraceptives: Are They Medically Accurate?" *Perspectives on Sexual and Reproductive Health* 36:2 (2004): 50–57.

40. Jennifer Mertens, "Catholic Sex Ed 101: How Can the Church Empower Teen Girls?" *National Catholic Reporter* (June 20–July 3, 2014), 20.

41. Massachusetts Bishops, "Sex Education: Information or Formation?" *Origins* 17 (12/31/1987): 510–511, at 511.

42. *Called to Compassion and Responsibility* characterizes prophylactics as "quick fixes" that are "technically unreliable," 429.

43. Centers for Disease Control and Prevention, "Are condoms effective in preventing HIV transmission?" http://www.cdc.gov/nchstp/od/latex.htm (accessed May 6, 2006). With "typical" use, condoms are 80 percent effective, while with "correct and consistent use for every sex act" condoms are 99 percent effective. See also Jon Fuller, "AIDS Prevention: A Challenge to the Catholic Moral Tradition," *America* 175 (December 28, 1996): 13–20); DeVincenzi, *New England Journal of Medicine* 331 (1994): 341–346; Y. Laurian, "HIV Infection of Sexual Partners of HIV-Seropositive Patients with Hemophilia," *New England Journal of Medicine* 320:3 (1989): 183; S. K. Hira et al., "Condom and nonoxynol-9 use and the incidence of HIV infection in sero-discordant couples in Zambia," *International Journal of STD and AIDS*, 8:4 (1997): 243–250.

44. Luke Gormally, *National Catholic Bioethics Quarterly*, January 2005, as reported by John Allen, "The Word from Rome: Vatican in Condom Debate," *National Catholic Reporter* 5/5/2006. The Bishops of Metropolitan Washington, USA, stated in 1987: "It is never morally permissible to employ an intrinsically evil means to achieve a good purpose." See "Reaction to AIDS Statement," *Origins* 17:28 (1987): 489-–93, at 490. John Paul II, in his closing remarks to the attendees of the first Vatican-sponsored conference on AIDS in 1989, stated: "It is extremely harmful to the dignity of the person, and therefore it is morally illicit, to support as AIDS prevention any method which violates the authentically human sense of sexuality and is a palliative for those deep needs which involve the responsibility of the individuals and of society: and right reason cannot admit that the fragility of the human condition—instead of being the motive for greater care—be used as a pretext for yielding to a way of moral degradation." (Translated by the Vatican from the Italian). See "Pope Addresses Vatican AIDS Conference," *Origins* 19:26 (1989): 434–436, at 435.

45. Aline Kalbian summarizes Grisez's argument: "Marital intercourse, in Grisez's view, must meet four conditions: (1) It must involve a married couple; (2) it cannot be coerced; (3) it must result in ejaculation by the husband; (4) it must be sexual intercourse, which he defines as follows: 'The male's penis enters the female's vagina and is stimulated by movement and contact until the male's ejaculation occurs.' Thus the husband must ejaculate semen into his wife's vagina. If that fails to happen, as would be the case for a couple using a condom, then the very nature of the act is changed." Kalbian, *Sex, Violence, and Justice*, 85, citing Germain Grisez, "Moral Questions on Condoms and Disease Prevention." *National Catholic Bioethics Quarterly* 8:3 (Autumn 2008): 471–476.

46. BBC interview, 2004, as reported by John Allen, "The Word from Rome: Vatican in Condom Debate," *National Catholic Reporter* 5/5/2006. Archbishop May of St. Louis claimed in 1987 that "safe sex practices are at best only partially effective." See "Reaction to AIDS Statement," *Origins* 17:28 (1987): 489–493, at 490. The US Bishops in their 1989 document "Called to Compassion and Responsibility" claimed that "the use of prophylactics to prevent the spread of HIV is technically unreliable." See United States Bishops' Meeting, "Called to Compassion and Responsibility: A Response to the HIV/AIDS Crisis," *Origins* 19:26 (1989): 421–434, at 429. See also Julie Hoffman, "Bennett and Carey Rap Condom Plan," *National Catholic Register* 68 (31 May 1992):1; Russell Shaw, "Condom Cure Questioned by Top AIDS Researcher," *Our Sunday Visitor* 82 (23 January 1994):3; Jean-Marie Guenois, "Sex, Lies, and Latex: Study Busts Condom Myth," *Our Sunday Visitor* 86 (2 November 1997): 21.

47. *Called to Compassion*, 429.

48. Joseph Howard, "The Use of the Condom for Disease Prevention," *Linacre Quarterly* 63 (1996): 26–30. See also, "Reaction to AIDS Statement," *Origins* 17:28 (1987) 489–93; "Continued Reaction to AIDS Statement," *Origins* 17:30 (1988): 516–522; "Cardinal Ratzinger's Letter on AIDS Document," *Origins* 18:8 (1988): 117–121. See also *Catechism*, no. 2370.

49. James F. Keenan, S. J., in the introduction to James F. Keenan, Ed., with Jon D. Fuller, Lisa Sowle Cahill, and Kevin Kelly, *Catholic Ethicists on HIV/AIDS Prevention* (New York: Continuum, 2000), 14.

50. United States Catholic Conference Administrative Board, *The Many Faces of AIDS: A Gospel Response*, *Origins* 17:28 (1987): 482–89.

51. Ibid, 489.

52. Keenan, *Catholic Ethicists*, 22. See also Keenan, "Applying the Seventeenth-Century Casuistry of Accommodation to HIV Prevention," *Theological Studies* 60 (1999): 492–512; Charles Bouchard and James Pollock, "Condoms and the Common Good," *Second Opinion* 12 (1989): 98–106; David Hollenbach, "AIDS Education: The Moral Substance," *America* 157 (1987): 493–94; Michael Place, "The Many Faces of AIDS," *America* 158 (1988): 141.

53. James Keenan, "Prophylactics, Toleration, and Cooperation: Contemporary Problems and Traditional Principles," *International Philosophical Quarterly* 28 (1988): 201–220. For an overview of these moral principles and their application to health care ethics, see: United States Conference of Catholic Bishops, *Ethical and Religious Directives for Catholic Health Care Services*, 4th ed. (Washington, DC: USCCB Publishing, 2001); Beauchamp and Childress, *Principles of Biomedical Ethics*, 5th ed. (New York: Oxford University Press, 2001); Ashley & O'Rourke, *Healthcare Ethics: A Theological Analysis*, 4th ed. (Washington, DC: Georgetown University Press, 1997). Aline H. Kalbian dedicates a chapter of her book to HIV/AIDS and the condom debate within Catholicism, and analyzes Keenan's contributions to this debate: Aline H. Kalbian, *Sex, Violence, and Justice: Contraception and the Catholic Church* (Washington, DC: Georgetown University Press, 2014), 60–94.

54. David Kelly, *Critical Care Ethics* (Kansas City, MO: Sheed & Ward, 1991), 204–209. See also James Drane, "Condoms, AIDS, and Catholic Ethics," *Commonweal* 189 (1991): 188–192.

55. Bela Somfai, "AIDS, Condoms, and the Church," *Compass* (November 1987): 44. See also Dennis Regan, "Perspectives from Moral Theology," *Dossiers and Documents: The Pandemic of AIDS—A Response by the Confederation of Caritas International* (February 1988), 58–67; James Keenan, "Living with HIV/AIDS," *The Tablet* (3 June 1995): 701; John Tuohey, "Methodology or Ideology: The Condom and a Consistent Sexual Ethic," *Louvain Studies* 15 (1990): 53–69. Some moralists have also relied on the principle of double effect to promote needle exchange programs. See Jon Fuller, S. J., "Needle Exchange: Saving Lives," *America* 179 (18–25 July 1998): 8–11; Jorge J. Ferrer, S. J., "Needle Exchange in San Juan, Puerto Rico: A Traditional Roman Catholic Casuistic Approach," in Keenan, ed., *Catholic Ethicists*, 177–191.

56. Peter Seewald, *Light of the World* (San Francisco: Ignatius Press, 2010), 117–119.

57. Ibid., 119.

58. Richard M. Gula, S.S., *Moral Discernment* (New York: Paulist, 1997), 106–111.

59. Ibid., 108.

60. Ibid., 108–9.

61. Melissa Browning, *Risky Marriage: HIV and Intimate Relationships in Tanzania* (Lanham, Maryland: Lexington Books, 2014), 168.

62. For an overview of these teachings, see Donal Dorr, *Option for the Poor: A Hundred Years of Catholic Social Teaching* (Maryknoll, NY: Orbis, 2001); David J. O'Brien and Thomas A. Shannon, eds., *Catholic Social Thought: The Documentary Heritage* (Maryknoll, NY: Orbis, 1992); Charles E. Curran, *Catholic Social Teaching 1891-Present: A Historical, Theological, and Ethical Analysis* (Washington, DC: Georgetown University Press, 2002); Charles E. Curran and Richard A. McCormick, S. J., eds., *Readings in Moral Theology, No. 5: Official Catholic Social Teaching* (New York: Paulist, 1986).

63. *Catholic Ethicists*, 282–293.

64. USCCB, *Ethical and Religious Directives*, 4–5; Cahill, "AIDS, Justice," 286–288.

65. Lisa Sowle Cahill, "AIDS, Justice, and the Common Good" in *Catholic Ethicists on HIV/AIDS Prevention*, ed. James F. Keenan (London: Continuum, 2000), 282, 288; See also Lisa Sowle Cahill, *Theological Bioethics: Participation, Justice, and Change* (Washington DC: Georgetown University Press, 2005), 158–159.

66. Kevin Dowling, "Let's Not Condemn Condoms in the Fight Against AIDS," *U.S. Catholic* (November 2003): 20–22. Laurie Goering, "A two-front fight: AIDS, The Church—South African Bishop Bucks the Vatican, Argues Condoms are Pro-Life in HIV Battle," *Chicago Tribune* (November 4, 2005).

67. Dowling also relies upon the principle of double effect. See Ibid., 21.

68. Ibid., 21.

69. Microbicides, which are currently in development, would be a woman-controlled preventive measure. The hope is that even if a woman is coerced into sex or engages in survival sex, she would be able to protect herself from HIV infection by using a microbicide jelly or lotion.

70. Christine E. Gudorf, "Why Sex is Good For Your Marriage," *U.S. Catholic* (Nov 1992), 6.

71. See Gudorf, "Sexual Pleasure as Grace and Gift," *Body, Sex*, 81–138.

72. Lettie and Carmen did admit that sex was not a priority in their marriages, but neither affirmed permanent abstinence either.

73. Eileen Stillwaggon, *Ecology of Poverty*; Paul Farmer, Margaret Connors, Janie Simmons, Eds, *Women, Poverty, and AIDS: Sex, Drugs, and Structural Violence* (Monroe, ME: Common Courage Press, 1996), xix, 23, 33. See also United Nations Department of Economic and Social Affairs, *Population, Development, and HIV/AIDS with Particular Emphasis on Poverty: The Concise Report* (New York: UN Publications, 2005), 49; *UNFPA State of the World Population 2004*, 63; A joint report by UNAIDS, UNFPA, UNIFEM. *Women and AIDS: Confronting the Crisis* (Geneva, Switzerland, UNAIDS, 2004).

74. Ryan White CARE (Comprehensive AIDS Resource Emergency). See Patricia D. Siplon, "A New Means for Providing for the Sick: The Ryan White CARE Act," in *AIDS and the Policy Struggle in the United States* (Washington, DC: Georgetown University Press, 2002), 93–110.

75. Housing Opportunities for Persons Living With AIDS.

76. AIDS Drug Assistance Programs.

77. Carole A. Campbell, *Women, Families, and HIV/AIDS: A Sociological Perspective on the Epidemic in America* (New York: Cambridge University Press, 1999). See also Lynellyn D. Long and Maxine Ankrah, eds., *Women's Experiences with HIV/AIDS:, An International Perspective* (New York: Columbia University Press, 1996); Aana Marie Vigen, *Women, Ethics, and Inequality in U.S. Healthcare: "To Count Among the Living"* (New York: Palgrave Macmillan, 2006).

78. Centers for Disease Control and Prevention, "HIV Among Women," Available online: http://www.cdc.gov/hiv/risk/gender/women/facts/index.html (Accessed July 11, 2014). See also Victoria Cargill, "Reaching, Engaging, and Retaining Women in HIV Care." Available online: http://aia.berkeley.edu/media/2013_webinars/Cargill%20Presentation%20Slides.pdf (Accessed July 11, 2014).

79. For an analysis of health care reform within a human rights approach, see Audrey R. Chapman, ed., *Health Care Reform: A Human Rights Approach* (Washington, DC: Georgetown University Press, 1994). Other authors whose work addresses the experiences of marginalized women in the United States include Lisa Sowle Cahill, *Theological Bioethics: Participation, Justice, Change* (Washington, DC: Georgetown University Press, 2005); Emilie M. Townes, *Womanist Ethics and the Cultural Production of Evil* (New York: Palgrave Macmillan, 2006).

80. My study is consistent with national data; substance use and abuse are common among HIV positive individuals, with nearly 50 percent of persons living with HIV/AIDS reporting current or past histories of drug or alcohol disorders. See Bing, Burnham, and Longshore, "Psychiatric Disorders and Drug Use Among HIV-Infected Adults in the U.S." *Archives of General Psychiatry* 58:8 (2001): 721; Rabkin et al., "Mood and Substance Use Disorders in Older Adults with HIV/AIDS: Methodological Issues and Preliminary Evidence." *AIDS* 18

(2004): 43–48; Durvasala and Miller, "Substance Abuse Treatment in Persons with HIV/AIDS: Challenges in Managing Triple Diagnosis," *Behavioral Medicine* 40:2 (2014): 43–52.

81. World Health Organization, *Effectiveness of Sterile Needle and Syringe Programming in Reducing HIV/AIDS Among IDUs: Evidence for Action Technical Paper and Policy Brief* (Geneva: World Health Organization, 2004); UNAIDS, "Call for Urgent Action to Improve Coverage of HIV Services for Injecting Drug Users." March 2010: http://www.unaids.org/en/Resources/PressCentre/Featurestories/2010/March/20100310IDU/ (accessed July 30, 2014). See also Centers for Disease Control and Prevention, "Syringe Exchange Programs: December 2005." Available online: http://www.cdc.gov/idu/facts/aed_idu_syr.pdf (Accessed July 30, 2014).

82. Sarah Barr, "Needle Exchange Programs Face New Federal Funding Ban." Kaiser Health News Online (12/21/2011): http://www.kaiserhealthnews.org/stories/2011/december/21/needle-exchange-federal-funding.aspx (Accessed July 30, 2014). For an updated list, see the website of the North American Syringe Exchange Network: http://nasen.org/programs/ (Accessed July 30, 2014).

83. Durvasula and Miller argue that too often mental health and substance use issues have been set apart from medicalized health care—and this false dichotomy can result in undertreatment and/or disintegrated care. Durvasula and Miller,"Substance Abuse Treatment," 50.

84. Centers for Disease Control and Prevention, "Syringe Exchange Programs, United States, 2008." *Morbidity and Mortality Weekly Report (MMWR)* 59(45) (November 19, 2010): 1488–1491.

85. D. Vlahov and B. Junge, "The Role of Needle Exchange Programs in HIV Prevention." *Public Health Reports* (June 1998) 113 (Suppl1): 75–80.

86. United States Bishops, *Called to Compassion and Responsibility,* 429. Bishop Jose Redrado Marchite, Secretary of the Pontifical Council for Health Care Ministry, publicly rejected needle exchange programs in 2009 when he led the Vatican delegation to the UN Commission on Narcotic Drugs in Vienna, Austria. In an attempt to influence drug policy at the United Nations, Bishop Redrado issued a statement claiming that using drugs is "anti-life" and that "so-called harm reduction leads to liberalization of the use of drugs, to an increase in the number of addicted people and to blurring of consciences, leading also to the loss of one's free will." He instead encouraged delegates to promote strategies that focus exclusively on the "health, dignity, and life of drug addicts." Duncan Campbell, "Vatican Stance on UN Drug Policy Risks Lives," *The Guardian* (February 27, 2009).

87. Mary Jo Iozzio, "Moving beyond the Impasse: Catholics Should Support Use of Federal Funding for Needle Exchange Programs," *Health Progress* 90:2 (2009): 55–57. The Society of Christian Ethics adopted a resolution in support of needle exchange programs during its Business Meeting of January 8, 2000. See also Jorge J. Ferrer, S. J., "Needle Exchange in San Juan, Puerto Rico: A Traditional Roman Catholic Casuistic Approach" in *Catholic Ethicists on HIV/AIDS Prevention*, eds., James F. Keenan, S. J., with Jon Fuller, Lisa Sowle Cahill, and Kevin T. Kelly (New York: Continuum, 2000): 176–91.

88. Sulmasy, "Catholic Participation." See also Jon Fuller, "Needle Exchange: Saving Lives," *America* 179:2 (July 18, 1998): 8–11; and James F. Keenan, S.J., "Applying the Seventeenth-Century Casuistry of Accommodation to HIV Prevention," *Theological Studies* 60 (1999): 492–512.

89. Sulmasy, "Catholic Participation," 425.

90. Ibid., 426.

91. Ibid., 428.

92. Ibid., 432. Sulmasy cites the following sources: Hannah L. F. Cooper et al., "Estimating the Prevalence of Injection Drug Use among Black and White Adults in Large U.S. Metropolitan Areas over Time (1992–2002): Estimation Methods and Prevalence Trends," *Journal of Urban Health* 85 (2008): 826–56; Carl A. Latkin et al., "Neighborhood Social Disorder as a Determinant of Drug Injection Behaviors: A Structural Equation Modeling Approach," *Health Psychology* 24 (2005): 96–100; Joseph Biederman et al., "Patterns of Alcohol and Drug Use in Adolescents Can Be Predicted by Parental Substance Use Disorders," *Pediatrics* 106 (2000): 792–97.

93. Franklin N. Laufer, "Cost Effectiveness of Syringe-Exchange as an HIV Prevention Strategy," *Journal of the Acquired Immune Deficiency Syndrome* 28 (2001): 273–78; Alex Wodak and Annie Cooney, "Do Needle Syringe Programs Reduce HIV Infection among Injecting Drug Users? A Comprehensive Review of the International Evidence," *Substance Use and Misuse* 41 (2006): 777–813; G. Alan Marlatt and Katie Witkiewitz, "Update on Harm-Reduction Policy and Intervention Research," *Annual Review of Clinical Psychology* 6 (2010): 591–606;

94. On the epidemiological nexus of poverty, race, injection-drug use, and HIV, see Victoria A. Cargill and Valerie E. Stone, "HIV/AIDS: A Minority Health Issue," *Medical Clinics of North America* 89 (2005): 895–912; Vivian T. Shayne and Barbara J. Kaplan, "Double Victims: Poor Women and AIDS," *Women and Health* 17 (1991): 21–37.

95. Substance Abuse and Mental Health Services Administration, *Results from the 2009 National Survey on Drug Use and Health, vol. 1: Summary of National Findings* (NSDUH Series H-38A, HHS Publication No. SMA 10-4856). (Rockville, MD: Office of Applied Studies, 2010).

96. Cristina L. H. Traina, *Feminist Ethics and Natural Law: The End of the Anathemas* (Washington, DC: Georgetown University Press, 1999), 43–48; Lisa Sowle Cahill, *Sex, Gender, and Christian Ethics* (Cambridge: Cambridge University Press, 1996); Martha Nussbaum, *Women and Human Development: The Capabilities Approach* (Cambridge: Cambridge University Press, 2000).

Chapter Six

Marriage for Life: A Christian Theology of Marriage in a World with AIDS

> "I came that they might have life, and have it abundantly."
> Jn. 10:10

How should the church define marriage? What is marriage *for*? These questions are as important today as ever, and yet confusion remains about how to best answer these questions in a way that will be life-affirming even for people who experience serious difficulties in intimate relationships. Simply put, couples affected by HIV are raising questions for the church that have not yet been adequately addressed.

In traditional constructions of Catholic theology of marriage, marriage is *for life* in at least two ways: first, marriage is *for life* because the couple is expected to be open to procreation in their marital lovemaking; and second, marriage is *for life* because the couple commits to live together for the rest of their lives. These two dimensions of Catholic theology of marriage—fruitfulness and indissolubility—are core components of Catholic marriage traditions and have justifications in Scripture. For the US bishops, two important symbols of married life arise out of reflection on fruitfulness and indissolubility: the symbol of the marital act (sexual intercourse) and the symbol of the cross.

Unfortunately, the church's defense of these values of marriage, especially the language used and the tone of the church's teachings, seem to lift up children and indissolubility as the litmus tests of what makes a good marriage, without enough attention to the quality of the couple's relationship. Too often this perpetuates a legalistic approach to marriage instead of a personalist approach, a contrast I described earlier as "persons over paperwork." In order to construct a theology of marriage that is life-affirming for women living with HIV, the church must continue to develop a vocabulary for talking about the building blocks of a healthy marriage. Drawing from revisionist proposals in sexual ethics, I will argue that a marriage *for life* should promote the full flourishing of both spouses and that loving care and justice go hand-in-hand in this reconstruction of theology of marriage.

This chapter begins with an overview of official teachings on the purposes of Christian marriage. But the life experiences of the women in this study surface questions and challenges to the adequacy of the church's theology. In light of some of the problems identified, I offer a new interpretation of *marriage for life* that attends to the values of fruitfulness and indissolubility held sacred within the tradition by naming them as ideals that remain unrealizable for some couples. Drawing on resources from the church's own documents, I reinterpret the pro-life dimensions of marital love in such a way as to include the experiences of married couples for whom procreation is not possible, and I argue that, in some limited cases, the dissolution of a valid sacramental marriage promotes human flourishing and is thus reflective of *marriage for life* in a revised understanding of Christian marriage.

WHAT IS MARRIAGE *FOR*? THE PURPOSES OF CHRISTIAN MARRIAGE, RECONSIDERED

Catholic accounts of the purposes of marriage are not static and unchangeable but have in fact developed significantly, even in the last century. While the trajectory of this development moves towards an appreciation of the equality of spouses and the value of mutual love, official teachings retain unhelpful physicalist[1] and legalist strands that should be revised so that Catholic teachings better emphasize the quality of the marriage relationship instead of the legalistic and institutional thrusts of canon law that seem to value paperwork over persons; descriptions of Christian marriage must not alienate Christian couples who are doing the best they can in difficult circumstances. One place to start would be reconsideration of the language used to describe the purposes of Christian marriage.

Catholic accounts of the purposes of Christian marriage prior to Vatican II said little about the affirmation of married women or men as persons beloved of God who are called to care for themselves. Instead, the purposes of marriage focused on marriage as an institution that primarily promoted social stability and procreation, though secondarily it fostered love of others.[2] The 1917 *Code of Canon Law* stated that the "primary" end of marriage is the procreation and education of children, while the "secondary" end is "mutual help and the allaying of concupiscence."[3] Papal teachings prior to

Vatican II assumed and explicitly taught in varying degrees women's inequality and subordination to men.[4] When Piux XI promulgated *Casti Connubii* in 1930, he emphasized hierarchy, order, and stability, in addition to love, as when he stated:

> Domestic society being confirmed, therefore, by this bond of love, there should flourish in it that "order of love," as St. Augustine calls it. This order includes both the primacy of the husband with regard to the wife and children, the ready subjection of the wife and her willing obedience, which the Apostle commends in these words: "Let women be subject to their husbands as to the Lord, because the husband is the head of the wife, and Christ is the head of the Church."[5]

Contemporary readers may find it noteworthy that Pius XI valued "the bond of love," but the fact that Pius XI defended mutual love as coherent with natural gender hierarchy may invite us to reflect on whether the pope was talking about "the bond of love" in the same way that we speak of mutual love as an indispensable component of marriage today.

Casti connubii further stressed stable and complementary gender roles; a married woman's pursuit of a career was considered "debasing of womanly character and the dignity of motherhood."[6] Prior to Vatican II, the "ends" of marriage required self-gift and self-sacrifice for men and women, but especially for women: in procreation of children, education of children, and mutual help between spouses. Roles for fathers were not as developed as role descriptions for mothers. While the husband was called the "head," the wife was the "heart." The woman was respected as valuable, and yet at the same time was limited in her role designations. Particularly jarring for contemporary readers are the encyclical's claims that a marriage of equal partners would be "unnatural" and "to the detriment of the woman herself."[7] The document reasserted magisterial teaching on the indissolubility of the marriage bond, declaring that even in cases of abuse or adultery, the marriage bond remains indissoluble.[8]

The Second Vatican Council's treatment of marriage initiated an important shift in the way that the purposes of marriage were named.[9] The 1965 Pastoral Constitution *Gaudium et spes* describes marriage as "an intimate partnership of life and love" and does not use the terms "primary" and "secondary," even as the Council does retain an emphasis on procreation.[10] The 1994 *Catechism* offers a succinct definition of marriage, drawn from Canon 1055 of the 1983 *Code of Canon Law,* itself reflecting new emphases after the Second Vatican Council:

> The matrimonial covenant, by which a man and a woman establish between themselves a partnership of the whole of life, is by its nature ordered toward the good of the spouses and the procreation and education of offspring; this

> covenant between baptized persons has been raised by Christ the Lord to the dignity of a sacrament.[11]

This synthesis represents a significant shift in teaching from the 1917 *Code*, most notably by including mutual love of spouses as an end in marriage together with procreation and education of children.[12] Todd Salzman and Michael Lawler explain:

> Notice three things: first, it is the *matrimonial covenant* and not *each and every act of intercourse* that is ordered toward procreation; second, there is not specification of either of these ends being primary or secondary; third, as in *Gaudium et spes*, the good of the spouses or *conjugal* love is discussed before procreation and education of children or the fruitfulness of marriage. The Catholic Church changed its canon law to be more in line with its renewed theology of marriage, moving beyond the narrow legal essence to embrace in the very essence of marriage the mutual love and communion of the spouses.[13]

Recent papal teachings no longer affirm male headship or the wife's duty to obey her husband, as described in papal encyclicals prior to Vatican II. Catholic teaching has in fact developed over time. But further development is necessary, especially because some post-Vatican II pronouncements seem to recover a pre-Vatican II anthropology and theology of marriage. Additionally, the continued emphasis on procreation as a purpose of marriage yields confusing expectations for HIV-affected couples.

The US bishops, in their 2009 pastoral letter *Marriage: Love and Life in the Divine Plan* restate Vatican II's description of the two purposes of marriage (above), and yet as they elaborate on this conciliar teaching they describe the two purposes of marriage in such a way as to blur the lines between the two distinct purposes. They do this by emphasizing the inseparability of the two: "the Church teaches that marriage is both unitive and procreative, and that it is inseparably both."[14] In a section titled "How Are the Two Ends of Marriage Related?" the bishops repeat the "inseparable connection" between the two ends of marriage and cite the *Catechism of the Catholic Church*: "These two meanings or values of marriage cannot be separated without altering the couple's spiritual life and compromising the goods of marriage and the future of the family."[15] The bishops claim that the inseparability principle derives from "the very nature of conjugal love, a love that stands under the twofold obligation of fidelity and fecundity."[16] The bishops then further collapse these two distinct purposes of marriage when they assert: "The unitive meaning is distorted if the procreative meaning is deliberately disavowed. Conjugal love is then diminished."[17] Even though the pastoral letter admits that some heterosexual married couples will be unable to bear children because of infertility or old age,[18] the bishops assert that "without its ordering toward the procreative, the unitive meaning of marriage is undermined."[19] They simply do not allow for the possibility of unitive love without openness to procreation. "These are two connected meanings of the same reality" and "two aspects of the same self-giving," according to the bishops.[20]

According to the bishops, sexual intercourse is "the act most symbolic and expressive of the marriage as a whole," and "the whole meaning of marriage is present and signified in each marital act."[21] In the sexual act each partner "gives oneself completely."[22] Drawing on the "theology of the body," authored by Pope John Paul II, the bishops argue that if a couple deliberately uses contraceptive practices to close off an act of intercourse to the possibility of procreation, "the language of the body that is meant to express self-gift becomes mixed with another message, a contrary message—namely, the refusal to give oneself entirely. Thus the unitive meaning of that language is falsified."[23] This analysis—promoted by the US bishops as official church teaching—privileges the procreative over the unitive by asserting that the unitive is "falsified" if the procreative potential is closed off. No exceptions are given within this analysis, and no qualifications are specified. They go on: "The deliberate separation of the procreative and unitive meanings of marriage has the potential to damage or destroy the marriage."[24]

The US bishops thus interpret the conciliar teaching to mean that every married couple must be open to procreation, and that couples who deliberately choose to close the possibility of procreation risk destruction of their marriage relationship. Has procreation become a litmus test for the validity of Catholic marriage? If so, this presents serious problems for women living with HIV infection.

With regard to indissolubility, the bishops explain that marriage is a symbol of Christ's love for the church. Drawing on a legalistic strain of the tradition, the bishops explain that "divorce claims to break the *contract*, to which the spouses freely consented, to live with each other till death."[25] The document cites evidence from the gospel of Matthew, interpreting Mt 19:3–9 to mean "Jesus himself teaches that divorce does not accord with the binding nature of marriage as intended by the Creator."[26] Thus the indissolubility principle is rooted in God's plan[27] for marriage, as expressed by Jesus, and when lived out becomes a symbol for Christian believers of the relationship between Christ and the church, a relationship for which Christ died on the cross. "Christ's love for the Church is a love of complete self-giving," explain the bishops. "This love is most completely expressed by his death on the Cross."[28] When the bishops introduce the symbolism of the cross in marriage, the theme of suffering emerges, but with confusing results. That the cross is seen as a symbol of marriage creates ambiguity because it risks valuing the marriage over the well-being of the people united in marriage.[29] The bishops ground this analysis in a theological anthropology that focuses on self-giving love as the universal human vocation, as when they write: "To say that man [sic] is created in the image and likeness of God means that man [sic] is called to exist for others, to become a gift."[30] From this anthropology of "the gift," the bishops go on to apply an understanding of Christian discipleship and sacramentality to self-giving love in marriage.

> Christian spouses are called to this imitation of Christ, an imitation that is possible only because, in the Sacrament of Matrimony, the couple receives participation in his love. As a sacrament, marriage signifies and makes present in the couple Christ's total self-gift of love. Their mutual gift of self, conferred in their promises of fidelity and love *to the end*, becomes a participation in the *love to the end* by which Christ gave himself to the Church as to a Spouse (Jn. 13:1).[31]

But what happens when a spouse experiences dehumanizing abuse in marriage? Should she *love to the end* and *lay down her life* because of the value of indissolubility? The totalizing language employed here can have the unfortunate effect of valuing the permanence of the marriage bond over the good of vulnerable persons married. To put it simply: What is more valuable—the symbol of marriage or the vulnerable person in an abusive marriage? The pre-Vatican II model of marriage placed greater emphasis on the institution of marriage, but the personalist approach of Vatican II may open the door towards the possibility of a more life-affirming answer to women who have suffered in abusive marriages.

How might the women in this study react to the privileging of procreation and indissolubility in definitions of Christian marriage? From the perspective of women living with HIV, the marital act described by the bishops was an impossible ideal. If Sue had decided to give of herself *completely* and *totally* to her husband during sexual intercourse—without using a condom—her spouse's health would have been endangered. Such an act could hardly be described as loving. Sue remained troubled by the fact that she and her spouse "lost that great freedom to feel as one." The women were candid in their reflections about how sexual loving brought new fears and difficulties, even as condomistic intercourse provided opportunities for shared intimacy and communion. But they also did not focus exclusively on sexual lovemaking as the ultimate symbol of their married love; instead, they described acts of reciprocal love that were not at all sexual: eating fried chicken in the middle of the bed while watching a movie (Cheryl), sleeping under the stars on a family camping trip (Sue), going to church together (Lettie), savoring a gourmet meal together (Grace), or going shopping together (Diva). These were moments of grace in their marriages, times in which each woman felt loved, cherished, and honored by her spouse. Perhaps their stories can serve as a corrective to the bishops' construal of marriage, in that the women's stories alert us to the potential dangers of romanticizing the marital act or discussing sexuality in the abstract, apart from the ordinary messiness of sexual loving in real life. For these women, condomistic sex was loving; while some recognized that it was not ideal (in that they wished they did not have to use condoms), still it was the best they could do in their constrained circumstances in order to experience the good of marital intimacy while also protecting the health of their spouses. Drawing on the law of gradualism, one might say that the women in this study recognized the objective good of procreation in Christian marriage, even while in their own subjective contexts they understood this as an unrealizable ideal.[32]

It is important to note that even though the women I interviewed did not wish to achieve pregnancy, it is possible for a woman living with HIV to become pregnant. This raises different ethical concerns than those previously addressed. Dr. Joel Gallant explains: "Pregnancy is a realistic option for HIV-positive women now that we can treat HIV effectively and prevent women from passing it to the baby. However, pregnancy should be carefully planned and closely monitored in HIV-positive women."[33] Gallant explains that if the HIV-positive woman has an undetectable viral load then transmission to the baby is extremely unlikely. So this requires access to anti-retroviral therapy and the close supervision of a physician. But just because some women *can* achieve pregnancy does not mean that they *should* try to become pregnant (even though some may interpret the bishops' focus on procreation to imply as much). I would affirm the principle forwarded by Margaret Farley, who writes of the need for human responsibility: "No children should be conceived who will be born in a context unconducive to their growth and development in relationships, or unconducive to their ultimately becoming autonomous, morally responsible for themselves."[34] Farley's principle highlights what we find in church teaching on marriage: that it is not simply procreation that is seen as a good but also the education and care of offspring.[35] The decision to be open to procreation in sexual relationships is a complicated one that requires discernment of many practical factors including the physical health of both partners, the emotional and mental stability of both partners, the degree of family and social supports should one partner's health deteriorate, and the couple's ability to lovingly care for the child until the child is self-sufficient. While the bishops find it problematic when a married couple treats as two separate decisions the decision to get married and the decision to have children,[36] the experiences of HIV-positive women demonstrate that these are in fact distinct and valuable discernments that should not be collapsed together. The decision to marry is not the same as the decision to try to achieve pregnancy. A married woman does not relinquish her right to say "no" to sexual activity by saying "yes" to her partner on her wedding day; she must retain control over her decision to consent to sexual acts. Further, in *each and every act* of intercourse, the HIV-positive spouse must reaffirm again her commitment to protect her partner and to care for herself; sometimes this requires that she and her partner deliberately act to prevent the spread of HIV infection while simultaneously preventing the possibility of procreation.

In chapter 5 I addressed the ethical question of condom use in the context of HIV prevention and public health; but here I consider another dimension of this dilemma, this time from the context of reflection on the *purposes* of Christian marriage. The emphasis on procreation as a purpose of marriage continues to place undue burden on women living with HIV and can jeopardize proper self-love for women. Because the virus is spread through bodily fluids, sexual intercourse can be dangerous for women living with HIV and for their sexual partners. Physicians routinely instruct HIV-positive persons to use condoms to prevent the spread of HIV to their sexual partners, but condom use also prevents procreation from occurring in the sexual act.

HIV-positive Catholic persons who wish to marry thus experience a unique challenge. On the one hand, HIV-positive persons are not prohibited from becoming married.[37] But on the other hand, married persons are expected to consummate their love in sexual union.[38] As we've seen, use of artificial birth control within marriage is described as a "lie" by John Paul II and direct contraception is explicitly prohibited in *Humanae vitae*. But marriage is also, by its very nature, "ordered to the well-being of the spouses,"[39] which, together with the law of charity and Church teaching against killing would seem to imply that a married person living with HIV should take all necessary precautions so as not to expose her/his spouse to the virus. Thus, one canonist argues: "It would be immoral for a person who has AIDS or another sexually transmitted disease to enter marriage with a non-infected partner with the intention of carrying on a normal sexual relationship since the inevitable outcome of such a relationship would be the death of the uninfected spouse."[40] A second canonist presents a more restrictive obligation by demanding permanent abstinence: "It appears to be irrefutable according to Catholic doctrine that a person infected with the AIDS virus cannot morally engage in sexual intercourse."[41]

But not all canonists and theologians are in agreement on this matter. Some canonists continue to question whether this kind of sacramental union is valid since it cannot be consummated properly; while others would argue that it cannot be valid if couples enter into the marital commitment without the intention to procreate. While some would assume that one could counsel such couples to use a condom during marital sexual intercourse, T. J. O'Donnell opposes such a claim by interpreting this sexual intercourse as "a seriously sinful simulation of a marital act."[42] O'Donnell explains that condom use prevents total self-giving between spouses, which is essential for authentic marital sexuality.[43]

But while canon law permits marriage for infertile and postmenopausal couples and permits sexual intercourse for married couples who face similar obstacles,[44] so too the church should be able to acknowledge the sacramental character of a faithful marriage for HIV-positive or sero-discordant couples for whom procreation is not a goal of marriage.[45] Canonist Ladislas Orsy explains:

> A query often raised today is whether or not canonically impotent persons should (or could) be permitted to marry on the ground that they are able to achieve one of the joint ends of marriage, which is companionship. . . . The traditional answer is clearly stated in the Code, old and new: impotence is a diriment impediment. Still, the problem is not fully solved; the questioning continues. If nature has deprived some persons from pursuing both ends of the marriage, must our law deprive them from pursuing the one they can? Is there no room for doctrinal development?[46]

Orsy explains the confusing limitations of canon law by demonstrating that even couples who can experience mutual love and companionship are deprived of sacramental marriage if one partner is impotent. Orsy concludes, "ultimately the answer should come rather from the field of theology than from that of canon law."[47] What would happen if one brings together the stories of the women in this study and Orsy's analysis? The women in this study experienced the church's official teaching on procreation in marriage as an unrealizable ideal and believed that condom use for HIV prevention was consistent with mutual love and companionship in Christian marriage. Perhaps their reflection can signal a way forward for theologians and canon lawyers who might argue that canon law should not prevent couples affected by HIV from pursuing Christian marriage if they can achieve the purpose of mutual love in marriage.

A second aspect of *marriage for life* in the US bishops' treatment of Christian marriage is indissolubility, and this theme surfaced as a source of pain for some of the women in this study. The bishops argue that their teaching on marital permanence derives from the teaching of Jesus, citing the Gospel of Matthew:

> When Jesus had finished saying these things, he left Galilee and went to the region of Judea beyond the Jordan. Large crowds followed him, and he cured them there. Some Pharisees came to him, and to test him they asked, "Is it lawful for a man to divorce his wife for any cause?" He answered, "Have you not read that the one who made them at the beginning 'made them male and female,' and said, 'For this reason a man shall leave his father and mother and be joined to his wife, and the two shall become one flesh?' So they are no longer two, but one flesh. Therefore what God has joined together, let no one separate." They said to him, "Why then did Moses command us to give a certificate of dismissal and to divorce her?" He said to them, "It was because you were so hard-hearted that Moses allowed you to divorce your wives, but from the beginning it was not so. And I say to you, whoever divorces his wife, except for *porneia*, and marries another commits adultery."[48]

But the bishops' interpretation of this passage—that "Jesus himself teaches that divorce does not accord with the binding nature of marriage as intended by the Creator"—is overly simplistic. In commenting on the corollary passage in Mark's gospel, Pheme Perkins proposes a feminist interpretation of the text: "To the Pharisees' focus on divorce as a male prerogative, Jesus insists upon the equality of marriage intended in the creation stories."[49] The Torah allowed for divorce (Deut 24:1) at the initiative of the husband, but the grounds of divorce are not specified. In a feminist reading, the rule against divorce could have been intended by Jesus to protect women who would have been made more vulnerable if divorced by their husbands; thus Jesus creatively draws upon Jewish creation narratives to counter the Pharisees' interpretation of the Law of Moses. In this reading, Jesus values the well-being of married women and invokes the prohibition of divorce for this purpose; one could imagine, then, that were the well-being of women to be in jeopardy in our own age, Jesus would continue to value the well-being of women, perhaps even over the institution of marriage itself. But one notices further a difference between the Marcan Jesus and the Matthean Jesus. In Mark's Gospel, Jesus does not offer any exception to the teaching on divorce, but in Matthew's Gospel, "whoever divorces his wife, except for *porneia*, and marries another commits adultery" (19:9). The meaning of *porneia*, sometimes translated as "immorality" or "unchastity," remains contested.[50] Paul provides still another exception, in the case of a marriage between a believer and a nonbeliever (1 Cor 7:15); for Paul, the preservation of peace is greater than the preservation of an unpeaceful marriage. In canon law, this is called the Pauline Privilege (canon 1143). Given the differences in the treatment of divorce in Mark, Matthew, and 1 Corinthians, Michael Lawler argues, contrary to the US bishops' interpretation: "It is incorrect to speak of the New Testament *teaching* on divorce and remarriage, as if there was only one. There are several *teachings* and they do not all agree."[51]

While their selective reading of the New Testament provides evidence for their claim that divorce is contrary to God's plan, the bishops propose indissolubility in marriage as an absolute good. Even when faced with the case of spousal abuse, the bishops argue that marital separation would be licit and that the spouses might be able to obtain a declaration of nullity.[52] Spousal abuse is not grounds for arguing the legitimacy of divorce.

Here, again, is where the experiences of some of the women in this study highlight the potential inadequacies of official teachings on marriage. If marriage is supposed to enable a graced encounter with God—a symbol of Christ's love for the church—experiences of spousal abuse expose the flawed nature of a legalistic paradigm. The commitment of "support and assistance" offered by the bishops to women "caught in the tragedy of an abusive marriage" does not go far enough if the marriage itself is still theologically and canonically considered indissoluble.[53] It is not clear how allowing marital separation without divorce in such situations promotes the sanctity of marriage, unless by sanctity of marriage one means the unchanging nature of Catholic teaching on marriage. Prohibiting remarriage by divorced persons further punishes divorced persons rather than providing a compassionate response to tragedy. Some theologians have begun to challenge the magisterium's definition of indissolubility in light of the reality of marriage as a *human* reality. For example, Bernard Cooke explains:

> Men and women are gradually initiated into marriage as a human relationship and a Christian sacrament; the initiation is never completed in this life—no more than is a person's lifelong initiation into Christianity, for becoming married is for most Christians a major element in the broader initiation into the Christ. It would seem, then, that one should not talk about marriage as being completely or absolutely indissoluble but as becoming increasingly indissoluble as it becomes increasingly Christian . . . A Christian marriage is indissoluble, but short of the eschaton it is *incompletely indissoluble*.[54]

In my research, I found that violence in intimate relationships is far from uncommon in the United States. And pressure to remain in an abusive relationship contributes to the emotional pain and mental anguish suffered by battered women. Unfortunately, the church's teaching on indissolubility contributes to the disempowerment of women in abusive relationships. For example, Lettie told me that her first marriage lasted sixteen years, in part because of the pressure from her devout Catholic grandmother.

> I don't even know why I lasted that long. I should have just made up my mind and said goodbye before. But I respected my grandmother a lot. I didn't want her to die feeling that I was going to be alone. She was Catholic and didn't believe in divorce. She was living with us, and she had herself suffered in an abusive relationship and she survived it. But my first husband, he was so mean. He beat me, he said terrible things to me. He said degrading things to the children, he ignored them, he said he would be better off without them, hurtful things. He still hurts them. Even though they are adults now, he doesn't want to see them, he doesn't want to talk to them. He just turns away from everyone. That's the way he was with them when they were little. Resentment, neglect, anger. And it was so much worse when he was drinking. You would not believe it. I don't even know why I lasted that long.

For Lettie, as for the two collaborators who were rape survivors (Keesha and Crystal), abuse in sexual relationships was experienced as dehumanizing; their suffering prevented them from recognizing their self-worth and from recognizing God's loving care for them. In Lettie's case, it was the dissolution of her first marriage that provided her with a sense of dignity and control over her life again, an experience she described as "freedom." Catholic teachings on the indissolubility of marriage—enforced by her grandmother, herself a survivor of domestic violence—made Lettie's first marriage seem more like a prison than a sacrament.[55] Lettie's experience raises the question, posed here by Cooke: "How can we say that a relationship that in its human and existential aspects, and therefore in its sacramentality, has dissolved is indissoluble?"[56] If a Christian marriage is "a partnership of the whole of life" and is ordered to the "good of the spouses" as well as children, then what should we do when faced with a broken relationship that fails to live up to these descriptions? In the case of Lettie's first marriage, the church's teaching on indissolubility was not perceived as *good news*.

If we instead consider the meaning of *marriage for life* as marriage at the service of human flourishing we can creatively sketch a new course for theological reflection on the important, though not absolute, value of indissolubility. For indissolubility remains a valuable ideal. But marriage must be life-affirming for both partners. In the confusing context of marital disharmony, it might be difficult for married couples to discern how much conflict is to be tolerated in order to live up to one's promises of permanent commitment. I am certainly not proposing easy, no-fault divorce as a simple solution to the problem of wife abuse in US culture.[57] For most of the women interviewed in this study, the promise of permanence was experienced as life-giving and a source of grace in their marriages. Sue, Cheryl, and Diva expressed gratitude and joy at the ways their partners remained faithful and committed to them, even in times of great hardship. Crystal was committed to working through her ongoing difficulties with her spouse because she respected this value of permanence. But church teaching can and should simultaneously promote the value of committed love while also responding compassionately to persons for whom attempts at committed love became impossible. Within the Catholic canonical tradition, the declaration of nullity provides the opportunity for couples to remarry after a failed marriage; technically, the "annulment" is the official recognition that "some key element was missing from the very beginning which rendered the marriage invalid."[58] These can include a lack of maturity or a situation of constraint that limits the freedom of the person to consent to marriage.[59] Margaret Farley explains that a more difficult question to answer is whether or not a truly valid marriage (even one that was sacramental and consummated) may no longer bind. She begins her response by explaining:

> My own position is that a marriage commitment is subject to release on the same ultimate grounds that any extremely serious, nearly unconditional, permanent commitment may cease to bind. That is, an obligation to sustain a marriage ceases when (1) it truly becomes impossible to sustain it; (2) the marriage no longer serves the purposes, or has the *raison d'être*, it was meant to have; (3) another obligation comes into conflict with, and takes priority over, the marriage commitment . . . It is possible for a fundamental obligation to one's own self to justify ending a marriage (not because love of self takes

> priority over love of another, but because no relationship should be sustained that entails, for example, the complete physical or psychological destruction of a person—including oneself).[60]

Farley's analysis upholds the value of permanence even while describing legitimate limits; this signals a compassionate way forward for women struggling in dehumanizing marriage relationships. Similarly, Melissa Browning argues: "Christian churches should not only permit divorce but, in cases where one partner is in danger, divorce should be encouraged as the best option in a complex, tragic situation. Divorce can offer a liberative possibility for a woman whose partner endangers her life through infidelity or abuse."[61]

What emerges from these reflections and the pastoral encounters that necessitate our thinking on these matters, is that the church's consistent teaching on the primacy of conscience must be reaffirmed.[62] Yet conscience is strikingly absent from the US bishops marriage document. Resources for discernment in the midst of difficult and confusing relationships would be of great service to married couples today and may also serve to illumine for their pastors the complexities and messiness of marriage in real life. The Catholic moral tradition has always valued practical reason, and yet this virtue is often downplayed in a canonical or legalistic approach to marriage. Richard Gula explains the virtue of prudence:

> Prudence listens to experience, one's own and others, it seeks counsel, it looks into the future to anticipate difficulties and to size up consequences. It sifts through all these to come to a decision which fits the particular configuration of circumstances at hand. It chooses the best way to do the right action for now. The teaching of St. Thomas on prudence shows a particular respect for subjective sensing and grasping the invitation of God in a particular instance when material norms do not adequately take into account the complexity of the particular situation.[63]

How would Lettie's life have been different had her grandmother pressured her to see herself as loved by God and affirmed her obligation to discern God's will in her particular circumstances? Would it have made a difference if Lettie had been encouraged to consider church teachings on conscience and prudence, together with church teachings on marital indissolubility?

Perhaps one way to conceive of the value of indissolubility is to say that a marriage is indissoluble *as long as it* continues to affirm the equal dignity of both partners and their mutual love characterized by loving care. In this way, we place the conditions of the Vatican II definition of marriage on the canonical framework of Catholic theology of marriage, thus privileging the personalist over the legalist approach. We would thus promote the value of permanence for marriage commitments, concluding that it is good for couples to envision a shared future and to shape their personal identity according to that expressed commitment which can foster trust and love in the present. And yet, at the same time, we can recognize that commitments to permanence are still experienced in human, finite, limited, and sinful circumstances. Sexism and violence against women are part of the cultural landscape in which Christian marriage commitments are made, and even Christian women experience dehumanizing violence in intimate relationships. With their experiences in mind, then, the church must recognize that dissolution of a marriage can, in limited cases, be experienced as life-affirming.

Two main critiques of the bishops' pastoral letter surface from analysis of the stories of married women living with HIV. The first is that the bishops' focus on the inseparable connection between unitive and procreative love is not born out by the women's experiences of unitive love in condomistic intercourse. The second is that the pastoral letter's emphasis on the indissolubility of marriage, together with the raising up of the cross of Christ as a symbol for marriage, fails to protect women in abusive marriages because it implies that suffering in marriage should be accepted without qualification, and that self-giving love *to the end* is more valuable than a married woman's care of self. In general, then, one finds that the legalistic and romanticized descriptions of marital love yield confusing results for married women in marriages that seemingly fail to live up to the fundamental purposes of marriage described by the bishops.

BUILDING BLOCKS OF A HEALTHY CHRISTIAN MARRIAGE

In the Catholic moral tradition, since genital activity is only licit in heterosexual married relationships, questions of sexual morality are usually framed as questions of marital morality. These are often presented in a classicist natural law methodology.[64] In the past two decades, scholars of Christian sexual ethics have recovered principles from the Bible and Catholic social teachings to reframe and reform conversations around sexuality towards the goal of constructing a more person-centered and justice-oriented sexual ethics. In her groundbreaking work *Sex, Gender, and Christian Ethics*, published in 1996, Catholic theologian Lisa Sowle Cahill proposed that Christian sexual ethics engage in the task "more important than defining moral and immoral forms of sexual conduct," which she described as "the fundamental New Testament concern to transform all human relations toward greater equality, compassion, and solidarity."[65] She continues: "The task of a Christian social ethic of sex is to imbue sexual and reproductive behavior with the qualities of respect, empathy, reciprocity, and mutual fidelity which would allow sexual and parental love to be transforming agents in society in general."[66] Cahill's research developed a critical realist and feminist approach that blended scriptural and natural law justifications. By emphasizing respect, empathy, reciprocity, and mutual fidelity, Cahill brought to life the human dimensions of sexual acts highlighting the methodological problem of attempting to analyze sexual acts-in-themselves detached from the contextual analysis of the agent acting.

In his 1998 text *New Directions for Sexual Ethics*, Catholic theologian Kevin T. Kelly proposed a revision of Catholic sexual norms in order to dismantle patriarchy and formulate a satisfactory person-respecting sexual ethic that would address the HIV/AIDS crisis.[67] He proposed that a revised sexual ethic be built on the following foundational beliefs:

1. Belief in the full and equal dignity of women as human persons as a major touchstone in our age for judging the credibility of the Church's commitment to the dignity of the human person;
2. Belief in human freedom;
3. Belief in friendship, intimacy, and love;
4. Belief in the goodness of the human body, sexuality, and sensual joy;
5. Belief in the giftedness of human life;
6. Belief in the uniqueness of the human person and respect for personal conscience.[68]

Kelly grounded each of these foundational principles in scripture and the moral tradition, and yet framed them broadly enough that he hoped they would not become tools of domination or oppression. For example, Kelly affirmed the value of commitment without requiring marriage; Kelly affirmed the value of the giftedness of human life without reducing every act to its procreative potential.[69]

From these six foundational beliefs, Kelly developed norms that promoted social well-being while simultaneously acknowledging the influence of structural injustices. He phrased this as the "Yes, but . . ." answer in sexual ethics: "The 'Yes' or 'No' part of the answer enables us to be clear as to whether or not, as a general rule, this particular form of behavior is conducive to the good of the human person, integrally and adequately considered."[70] The second part of the answer—the "but . . ."—nuances the teaching because it allows "for the fact that individual moral agents are not all proceeding from the same starting-point."[71] Kelly's analysis coheres with Pope Benedict's application of the law of gradualism as applied to HIV prevention; there, Pope Benedict upheld both the objective and subjective dimensions of the moral act while encouraging the harm reduction strategy of condom use as a step in the proper direction, a way of gradually humanizing the sexual act.[72]

Kelly drew on the parable of the wheat and the weeds (Mt 13:24–30)[73] to illustrate the importance of subjective analysis in sexual ethics. In his interpretation, the owner of the field had faith in the healthy growth of his wheat, despite all of the weeds mixed in with it. The owner wanted to protect his crop from the misguided zeal of the servants who were intent on purifying the crop by pulling the weeds. But they did not seem to realize that pulling the weeds would harm the wheat. Kelly then applies this caution to sexual ethics: "Sometimes moral zealots can act very destructively because they are oblivious to the fact that what might look like a puny and undeveloped plant might, in fact, be a miracle of growth, given the adverse conditions under which it has had to struggle."[74] Kelly suggests that moralists begin by listening to the messiness of people's lived experiences and try to understand their struggles in the context of social injustices. Doing so may help moralists develop answers to complex sexual questions that are sensitive to the needs and struggles of people who may be doing their best in difficult situations. For Kelly, the attempt to have a single "Yes" or "No" answer that applies in every situation is too simplistic and fails to recognize the diverse ways that people experience the desire for wholeness and holiness even in complex and difficult situations. But an answer of "Yes, but . . ." may open up conversation and encourage discernment and moral growth instead of bringing judgment and shame.

Todd Salzman and Michael Lawler employ similar methods, describing their work as "revisionist" and "personalist."[75] Realizing the patriarchal and heterosexist assumptions embedded in much of the marriage and sexual ethics of the Christian moral tradition, they formulate a reconstructed understanding of "complementarity" as multifaceted—"orientational, physical, affective, personal, and spiritual."[76] As they move to their prescriptive analysis, they coin the phrase "just and loving truly human sexual acts" as a reformulated principle for sexual ethics.[77] Their sexual ethic thus opens up the possibility of affirming nonmarital and/or homosexual acts that are just, loving, and truly human. Theirs is not an "anything goes" approach to sexual ethics but it is rather an attempt to offer guidelines that facilitate human flourishing. They draw on Thomas Aquinas in their definitions of love and justice: "To love is to will the good of another;"[78] justice is "the virtue according to which, with constant and perpetual will, someone renders to someone else her or his due rights."[79] Salzman and Lawler further qualify that a just and loving truly human sexual act will have the following characteristics: equality of partners, free consent, mutual, long-term commitment, and fruitfulness.[80] They suggest that in order to evaluate a particular relationship or sexual act, one must engage in a careful hermeneutical analysis of how the foundational principle of "just and truly loving human sexual acts" can be applied in real, concrete, particular human relationships.[81]

Margaret Farley continues this trajectory within Catholic sexual ethics in her book, *Just Love: A Framework for Christian Sexual Ethics*. Farley argues that communities should attend not simply to the evaluation of particular sexual acts but more broadly to questions of appropriate sexual relationships:

> The most difficult question to be asked in developing a sexual ethic is not whether this or that sexual act in the abstract is morally good, but rather, when is sexual expression appropriate, morally good, and just, in a relationship of any kind. With what kinds of motives, under what sorts of circumstances, in what forms of relationships, do we render our sexual selves to one another in ways that are good, true, right, and just?[82]

Farley then proposes the following norms for sexual justice:

1. Do no unjust harm
2. Free consent of partners
3. Mutuality
4. Equality
5. Commitment
6. Fruitfulness
7. Social Justice[83]

One of the benefits of the approach offered by these moralists is that these norms provide a new lens through which we can analyze the definitions of Christian marriage within the Christian tradition. Certainly there is much overlap. The value of Farley's proposal is that the person evaluating his or her relationship will have more to consider besides the overly simplistic litmus test of procreation and indissolubility. Farley does not necessarily make the discernment easy for couples; for example, couples living with HIV will need to hold in tension both the norm of "do no unjust harm" and "fruitfulness." But Farley's guidelines provide a wider range of data in evaluating the health of a relationship. Farley offers this summary:

> Even more specifically, we may in terms of this framework say things like: sex should not be used in ways that exploit, objectify, or dominate; rape, violence, and harmful uses of power in sexual relationships are ruled out; freedom, wholeness, intimacy, pleasure are values to be affirmed in relationships marked by mutuality, equality, and some form of commitment; sexual relations like other profound interpersonal relations can and ought to be fruitful both within and beyond the relationship; the affections of desire and love that bring about and sustain sexual relationships are all in all genuinely to affirm both lover and beloved.[84]

The principles and norms suggested by Cahill, Kelly, Salzman, Lawler, and Farley do not represent consensus among Catholic moral theologians, but they do demonstrate a pattern among revisionist thinkers for rethinking the basic building blocks of a healthy marriage and for reconceiving what *marriage for life* might entail. No longer are procreation and indissolubility held up as absolute goods, untethered by attention to the quality of intimate relationships. Instead, these thinkers provide an alternate way of conceiving of guidelines for discussing responsible sexual loving that is sensitive to the problem of patriarchy in church teachings and inequality in human relationships. Theirs is an ethic that holds together personal responsibility and social justice, an ethic that communicates the value of the person, and an ethic that holds together an appreciation of the joys but also the dangers of sexual loving. In order for the church to adopt these revisionist norms for intimate relationships, the church would need to begin to trust that Christians are capable of discerning God's law for intimate relationships in complex circumstances. Pastoral documents could then encourage couples to discern and apply these principles in their everyday lives as a guide for thinking about what practices and forms of sexual loving are life-giving for the couple and for the wider world.

MARRIAGE *FOR LIFE*: A CHRISTIAN THEOLOGY OF MARRIAGE THAT TAKES SERIOUSLY THE EXPERIENCES OF COUPLES AFFECTED BY HIV AND AIDS

Christian marriage *for life* will have the following essential characteristics, each of which yields important norms for married life.

1. Affirmation of the inherent dignity of each spouse
2. Affirmation of spousal equality and marriage as mutual partnership
3. Promise of fidelity and commitment to a shared future
4. Openness to discernment of God's grace and respect for personal conscience
5. Life-affirming sexual ethics
6. Acceptance of finitude and recognition of marriage as human process of striving
7. Appreciation of social stability and active commitment to the common good

The first and perhaps most important element of any theology of marriage is that marriage should enable both partners to understand that their dignity resides in who they are as beloved of God.[85] Marriage *for life* will foster self-knowledge and self-acceptance. In accepting God's love for them, married persons should be empowered to speak honestly with their partners so they may name their own needs and desires. They will need to respect themselves, care for their bodies, and resist dangerous threats to their physical or emotional well-being. Marital violence is clearly an offense against the sacrament of marriage. For married people to resist such violence, they must be formed to think of themselves as beloved of God, worthy of love and affection, and empowered to care for themselves. A theology of marriage that promotes the full flourishing of both spouses will recognize that self-giving love has appropriate limits and will not tolerate abuse or expect sacrificial love that requires the destruction of the person; sacrificial love for the other, *if freely chosen and life-affirming* can be good and moral. Marriage should not separate us from the love of God (Rom 8:38) but instead should affirm each spouse as a beloved child of God worthy of love.

Secondly, marriage is an equal partnership.[86] Christian theology of marriage should be grounded in an egalitarian and relational anthropology. A healthy marriage depends on the self-giving love of both spouses, always aimed towards mutuality. The spouses are companions, journeying together on the road of life, a journey in which they offer one another support, love, comfort, and friendship. Within a true friendship, each desires the good of the other, but one also recognizes that the good of the other is deeply attached to one's own good; the couple experiences radical interdependency because of the value of their friendship-love. Each partner should recognize the other as his or her equal: *equal in dignity*, to be sure, but also *equal in voice*; that is, each partner contributes to their mutual discernment about the decisions that impact their relationship and family life. The power dynamics within the relationship are not hierarchical but instead should resemble a constant and messy back-and-forth exchange through which each spouse both gives and receives. The relationship's reciprocity is experienced not as a one-for-one exchange but as a communal sharing of the whole of life. *Humanae vitae* provides resources for just this sort of thinking, as when Pope Paul VI states: "Whoever really loves his partner loves not only for what he receives, but loves that partner for the partner's own sake, content to be able to enrich the other with the gift of himself."[87] To love one's partner for her own sake means that one must recognize one's spouse as an end in herself, not as a means to attain another value (such as procreation of children without concern for the health of one's spouse). Relationships built on injustice or exploitation cannot be said to illumine the love of God;[88] a renewed theology of marriage must consistently and emphatically empower spouses to understand their equality.

A third essential element in Christian marriage *for life* is the promise of fidelity and commitment to a shared future. The pledge of faithfulness that a couple makes—in a gradual process from courting through betrothal and then a public wedding and shared home life—communicates to each other and to their wider network of relationships that they see their future together, "in good times and in bad, in sickness and in health."[89] That a couple makes such a commitment does not guarantee that the couple will be able to live out this commitment, but it does signal the desire to live out such a commitment, which is itself a radical departure from trends in hookup culture.[90] Commitments demonstrate Christian hope, the virtue by which we rely on God with trust.[91] Hope reminds us that we are imperfect creatures with no sure knowledge of what the future holds, and yet Christians believe that our lives have a direction, a sense of purpose because of our ultimate end in God. Our commitments structure our life towards this ultimate end. The commitment of marriage means that we walk into that future with a partner who promises to be with us in the joys and the sorrows. To receive this commitment is itself empowering because it communicates that you are loved by someone who wants to share life's journey with you. Together, you look into the future as a "we" instead of simply two individuals. While the couple remains embedded in a network of relationships, the marriage partnership is privileged above other friendships and can become a symbol of God's love when it demonstrates to the world that covenants can be made and kept, that love can be steadfast and empowering, and that love is a dynamic and powerful force for good.

A fourth feature of marriage *for life* is the couple's attunement to the specific circumstances of their own situation and their willingness to discern together how God is calling them to respond to God's love in the uniqueness of their own circumstances. There is not a "one size fits all" code for every question a Christian married couple will face; instead, each couple must be discern together how they will subjectively live out their commitments. This openness to discernment and respect for conscience is life-affirming because they trust they will be given the tools to understand how God is inviting them to act. The couple has an obligation to discern the voice of God in conscience; this duty is an opportunity to encounter the living God. To claim that marriage is a sacrament means to affirm that marriage is "a symbol of the presence of God in the world."[92] In the Christian tradition, marriage is a vehicle for experiencing grace, and a couple's future life together will require many different discernments. While the church certainly lifts up some key values about married living, at each juncture the couple must discern how best to practice that value in their own context. The Catholic moral tradition values practical reason as a gift from God, and one way to think about the sacramentality of marriage is to consider how God is present in the large and small moments of a couple's life together.

A fifth feature of Christian marriage *for life* is a life-affirming sexual ethic that affirms self-care for both spouses. Sexual loving should promote the full and integral flourishing of both spouses. In other words, sex should be safe. Sex should always be consensual, mutually pleasurable, and loving; when practiced in this way, sexual loving fosters intimacy and trust. Each spouse can also experience self-acceptance through sexual lovemaking; one can become more comfortable in one's own body through the pleasures of sexual loving. This sexual ethic should be pro-life and pro-family in the broad sense: that is, it should give an account of sexual love that is life-giving and life-affirming for husband and wife and for the wider world. Catholic theologian Kevin Kelly explains, "The pro-life dimension of our being sexual beings should not be reduced to the procreational potentiality of human sexuality, even though that is an important aspect of it."[93] For HIV-affected couples this will require that special precautions are taken so that a spouse does not become infected through sexual loving or more ill by exposing one another to different strains of the virus.[94] Most fundamentally, this ethic requires all married persons to see their sexuality not as an uncontrollable urge or locus of shame but as a good gift of God; the proper response to this gift is to accept responsibility to make life-affirming choices about one's fertility.

A sixth feature of marriage *for life* is that marriage entails a human process of striving even while spouses simultaneously experience finitude. When marriage commitments are lived out in mutual love the marital relationship becomes an occasion of grace, an encounter with the living God. Church teachings must continue to encourage couples to do the best they can in their specific circumstances. But we must also remember that marriage is practiced in the "between times," between the "already" of Christ's victory over sin and the "not yet" of Christ's return in glory at the end of days.[95] Marriage is lived and experienced by fallible human beings in particular times and places. No marriage has escaped the problem of human sin. Patterns of this sinfulness are readily apparent in assumptions of gender inequality deemed "natural" in the Catholic Church's sacramental history and in the toleration of sexual violence that resulted.[96] But women are not only victims of sin; women are also sinners and women have failed to live up to marriage commitments just as men have failed. Theology of marriage must be sensitive to the *human* dimensions of marital love, even as theologians lift up the guiding ideals of our faith tradition. But it is always the case that some marriages will fail to live up to these ideals. A realistic theology of marriage will promote monogamy, fidelity, fruitfulness, and indissolubility in such a way as to raise these up as prophetic ideals for which all couples should strive, even as we recognize with pain and sensitivity that some married couples will be unable to realize these completely; the faith of the church requires not that these couples be abandoned but that they be supported, nurtured, and reassured of God's love for them.

Finally, the seventh feature of marriage *for life* is that marriage promotes social stability as the couple's love spills beyond themselves into the wider world. Concern for social stability is a wise component of the traditional theology of marriage. Healthy marriage is the foundation of a healthy society. Ideally, family life is the context in which one learns how to be kind, how to express empathy for a suffering person, how to practice reconciliation, how to have the courage to speak for oneself, how to negotiate conflict, how to be oneself and experience vulnerability in a safe place. In an ideal context, family life socializes children to respect other people's bodies, to learn about differences, and to begin to care for oneself. Family life provides occasions for both celebration and grief. So ideally the practice of Christian marriage should promote social stability and self-care simultaneously. To be *for life* in this broad sense also means that married couples should think of the sacramentality of their relationship as an invitation not just to experience the love of God within their marriages, but also as an invitation to be God's love for the world. Their love can bear fruit, whether or not they have children, if they cooperate with God by responding to the call to care for others and contribute to the common good. The US bishops provide helpful analysis when they write of the *life affirming* love of marriage for infertile or elderly couples:

> The marital union of a man and a woman is a distinctive communion of persons. An infertile couple continues to manifest this attribute. Even when their child-bearing years have passed, a couple should continue to be life-affirming. They can do this by staying involved in the lives of young people, and especially their grandchildren, as spiritual mentors, teachers, and wisdom figures. They can also continue to be nurturing through the exercise of care for those who are needy, disabled, or pushed to the margins of society, and by their support for or participation in works of charity and justice.[97]

Presumably, the wider understanding of the *life-affirming* nature of Christian marriage holds true not only for infertile or postmenopausal couples but for all Christian married couples. The bishops here document a broader interpretation of what it means to be pro-life without reducing the *life-affirming* aspect of marriage to procreation. A married couple affected by HIV and AIDS is also a "distinctive communion of persons" called to be life-affirming by mentoring young people, being good role models, or caring for the needy and marginalized. In her analysis of the Christian family, Lisa Sowle Cahill explains that "Christians must always be aware of neighbors and strangers who suffer as making real claims on them."[98] Christian marital love is never limited to the love between spouses. Spouses can contribute to the common good in their work outside the home, as well as through their participation in political and social movements, or by offering hospitality to loved ones and strangers alike. Evelyn Eaton Whitehead and James D. Whitehead explain that "love is creative beyond itself and it must be so if it is to endure."[99] As married couples balance the tensions between marital intimacy and the larger responsibilities of their lives, they must move from a focus on "we are" to "we care."[100] Evelyn and James Whitehead explain of their own marriage: "We feel the impetus to move beyond ourselves, to share this wealth, to bring others into the power of what our love has given us. This movement of expansion is itself an expectable dynamic of love as it matures."[101]

CONCLUSION

What is the purpose of Christian marriage? What is marriage *for*? When asked to describe the purposes of their own marriages, the women in this study described the need to privilege mutual love over procreative ends, particularly at different ages and life stages. For Diva, Lettie, Sue, Crystal, Keesha, Carmen, Cheryl, and Grace, simple acts of companionship were often described as touchstones of what the marital relationship is all about—accompanying one's spouse to doctor appointments, going to church together, reminding each other to take medicines, caring for the home together. Marriage did not shield these women from fear, stress, or suffering. Indeed, these women tell stories of financial troubles, violence, fear of infecting their spouses, loss of intimacy in sexual loving, greater vulnerability with each other, and fear that they cannot protect their children from grief and harm in the future. By emphasizing companionship and mutual love and by redefining procreative aims, as it implicitly does in the case of infertile couples, the church can promote a theology of marriage that responds to these women's struggles.

A new wave of scholarship in Catholic sexual ethics provides compelling arguments for rethinking the best way to conceive of the *purposes* of marriage and the goals of sexual loving. Drawing on this scholarship, I have proposed seven essential characteristics of what I call *marriage for life*: affirmation of human dignity, affirmation of spousal equality, promise of fidelity and commitment to a shared future, mutual discernment and respect for conscience, life-affirming sexual ethic, recognition of marriage as a human process marked by finitude, and appreciation of social stability and active commitment to the common good. These features of married love are not exhaustive but are offered as a proposal that is sensitive to the needs and special circumstances of couples affected by HIV and AIDS while also drawing on the best of the Christian tradition.

When couples promise to love, honor, and cherish one another, they do so without knowing what struggles they will have to endure as a married couple. For married persons living with HIV or AIDS, marriage can provide a loving relationship in which two people can support and care for each other and for their children (if any) through the stresses that come from HIV-related illness and stigma. When we take seriously the experiences of married women living with HIV we see that traditional accounts of the purposes of marriage, and especially the privileging of procreation, do not reflect fully these couples' experiences of the sacramental natures of their own marriages. What emerges instead is the need for the marriage relationship to affirm for married women their inherent dignity, their equality with their husbands, and their obligation to care for themselves, including the responsible use of their fertility.

NOTES

1. Here I mean that there is too often attention to the physical structure of the act apart from the relational context of the agent. See Richard M. Gula, S. S., *Reason Informed by Faith: Foundations of Catholic Morality* (New York: Paulist, 1989), 233–235.

2. Leo XIII, *Rerun novarum*, no. 9. Available online: http://www.vatican.va/holy_father/leo_xiii/encyclicals/documents/hf_l-xiii_enc_15051891_rerum-novarum_en.html (Accessed August 2, 2014). See also Michael J. Schuck, *That They Be One: The Social Teaching of the Papal Encyclicals 1740–1989* (Washington, DC: Georgetown University Press, 1991), 1–115, esp. 28, 79–80.

3. Edward N. Peters, ed. *The 1917 or Pio-Benedictine Code of Canon Law* (San Francisco, CA: Ignatius Press, 2001), Canon 1013. For an analysis of the theological development on the ends of marriage, see Theodore Mackin, S. J., *What is Marriage?* (New York: Paulist, 1982).

4. Christine E. Gudorf, "Encountering the Other: The Modern Papacy on Women," in *Feminist Ethics and the Catholic Moral Tradition: Readings in Moral Theology, No. 9*, eds., Charles E. Curran, Margaret A. Farley, and Richard A. McCormick, S. J. (New York: Paulist Press, 1996), 66–89. Gudorf decries the papal teachings on functional complementarity, the collapsing of womanhood with motherhood, and the romantic pedestalization of women.

5. Piux XI, *Casti connubii*, no. 26. Available online: http://www.vatican.va/holy_father/pius_xi/encyclicals/documents/hf_p-xi_enc_31121930_casti-connubii_en.html (Accessed July 9, 2014).

6. Ibid., no. 75. For analysis of this encyclical, see Bernard Cooke, "*Casti Connubii* to *Gaudium et Spes*: The Shifting Views of Christian Marriage," in *Marriage in the Catholic Tradition: Scripture, Tradition, and Experience*, ed. Todd A. Salzman, Thomas M. Kelly, and John J. O'Keefe (New York: Crossroad, 2004): 109–114.

7. Ibid., no. 76.

8. Indissolubility of the marriage bond was justified on the basis of scriptural and traditional warrants as well as the welfare of children (no. 16) and the welfare of women (no. 90). While marital separation was permitted, divorce was not. The language was absolutist in tone: "Let that solemn pronouncement of the Council of Trent be recalled to mind in which, under the stigma of anathema, it condemned these errors: 'If anyone should say that on account of heresy or the hardships of cohabitation or a deliberate abuse of one party by the other the marriage tie may be loosened, let him be anathema'; and again: 'If anyone should say that the Church errs in having taught or in teaching that, according to the teaching of the Gospel and the Apostles, the bond of marriage cannot be loosed because of the sin of adultery of either party; or that neither party, even though he be innocent, having given no cause for the sin of adultery, can contract another marriage during the lifetime of the other; and that he commits adultery who marries another after putting away his adulterous wife, and likewise that she commits adultery who puts away her husband and marries another: let him be anathemae. If therefore the Church has not erred and does not err in teaching this, and consequently it is certain that the bond of marriage cannot be loosed even on account of the sin of adultery, it is evident that all the other weaker excuses that can be, and are usually brought forward, are of no value whatsoever.'" *Casti Connubii*, nos. 88–89.

9. Theologian Michael Lawler names this shift in the primary understanding of marriage over time in the following way: (1) procreative institution => (2) procreative union => (3) interpersonal union. Michael G. Lawler, *Marriage and the Catholic Church: Disputed Questions* (Collegeville, MN: Liturgical Press, 2002), viii–ix.

10. As in this quotation: "By its very nature the institution of marriage and married love are ordered to the procreation and education of the offspring and it is in them that it finds its crowning glory." Vatican Council II, *Gaudium et spes (Pastoral Constitution on the Church in the Modern World)* in Austin Flannery, O.P., ed., *Vatican Council II: The Basic Sixteen Documents* (Northport, NY: Costello, 1996), 163–282, nos. 48–49.

11. Interdicasterial Commission for the Catechism, *Catechism of the Catholic Church* (CCC), (New York: Doubleday, 1995), 1601.

12. Todd Salzman and Michael Lawler argue that this emphasis on marital love as mutual does emerge in *Casti Connubii* although it is not developed there. Todd A. Salzman and Michael G. Lawler, *Sexual Ethics: A Theological Introduction* (Washington, DC: Georgetown University Press, 2012), 29–20.

13. Salzman and Lawler, *Sexual Ethics*, 34.

14. USCCB, *Marriage*, 11.

15. Ibid., citing *Catechism of the Catholic Church* (CCC), no. 2363.

16. Ibid., 15, citing CCC, no. 2363.

17. Ibid. No citation is given to substantiate this claim, either from sociological data, the literature on marriage and family, or church teaching.

18. Ibid., 14–15. For further reflection on the experiences of infertility and the need for theo-ethical reflection on the experiences of infertile couples, see Kathryn Lilla Cox, "Toward a Theology of Infertility and the Role of *Donum Vitae*," *Horizons* 40:1 (2013): 28–52.

19. The pastoral letter cites Pope Paul VI, *Humanae vitae*, no. 9: "Finally, this love is fecund. It is not confined wholly to the loving interchange of husband and wife; it also contrives to go beyond this to bring new life into being." Pope Paul VI, *Humanae Vitae*, Available online: http://www.vatican.va/holy_father/paul_vi/encyclicals/documents/hf_p-vi_enc_25071968_humanae-vitae_en.html (Accessed August 2, 2014).

20. USCCB, *Marriage*, 16–17. The document further elaborates on the importance of procreation in its comparison of married life to the Trinity: "Just as the Trinity of persons is a life-giving communion of love both in relationship to one another and to the whole of creation, so a married couple shares in this life-giving communion of love by together procreating children in the conjugal act of love." *Marriage*, 37. This seems to imply that infertile couples or couples who deliberately use contraception (even after careful discernment in conscience) fail to symbolize the life-giving communion of the Trinity in their married love.

21. Ibid., 17–18.

22. Ibid., 18.

23. Ibid., 18–19, drawing on Pope John Paul II, General Audiences, January 5 and 26, 1983, and *Familiaris consortio*, no. 32; see also CCC, no. 2370. John Paul II, *Familiaris Consortio* (1981), Available online: http://www.vatican.va/holy_father/john_paul_ii/apost_exhortations/documents/hf_jp-ii_exh_19811122_familiaris-consortio_en.html (Accessed August 2, 2014).

24. USCCB, *Marriage*, 19.

25. Ibid., 24, citing CCC, no. 2384. Emphasis is mine.

26. Ibid.

27. "God's plan for marriage persists," the bishops say, "despite the impact of original sin." Ibid., 25.

28. Ibid., 32.

29. "A man and a woman united in marriage as husband and wife serve as a symbol of both life and love in a way that no other relationship of human persons can." USCCB, *Marriage*, 11.

30. Ibid., 10–11.

31. Ibid., 33. Emphasis in the original text.

32. Richard Gula explains that moral freedom is an important aspect of our deliberation, as when he writes: "no one is morally obligated to do what he or she is incapable of doing." *Reason Informed by Faith*, 84.

33. Joel Gallant, MD, MPH, *100 Questions and Answers about HIV and AIDS*, 2ed. (Burlington, MA: Jones and Bartlett, 2012), 118. Gallant encourages HIV-positive women to achieve pregnancy via artificial insemination to avoid infecting the male partner, but this method is forbidden by official Catholic teachings.

34. Margaret Farley, *Just Love: A Framework for Christian Sexual Ethics* (New York: Continuum, 2006), 271.

35. The US Bishops write: "The procreative meaning of marriage involves not only the conception of children, but also their upbringing and education, including spiritual formation in the life of love. This formation can take place only within a human community formed in love." *Marriage*, 16.

36. Ibid., 4.

37. Canon 1058: "All can contract marriage who are not prohibited by law." *1983 Code of Canon Law*, English Trans. (Grand Rapids, MI: Eerdmans, 1983).

38. Canon 1084: "Antecedent and perpetual impotence to have sexual intercourse, whether on the part of the man or on that of the woman, whether absolute or relative, by its very nature invalidates marriage." Canon 1096: "For matrimonial consent to exist, it is necessary that the contracting parties be at least not ignorant of the fact that marriage is a permanent partnership between a man and a woman, ordered to the procreation of children through some form of sexual cooperation." Some theologians would argue against a literalist interpretation of consummation, explaining that marital consummation should refer not simply to sexual intercourse (as assumed in a contractual model of marriage) but rather to the everyday mutual and self-giving partnership of husband and wife (as assumed in a covenant model of marriage). See Mackin, *What is Marriage?*, 29–33. Much depends on one's interpretation of truly human acts, or consummation "in a human manner," (*humano modo*, canon 1061).

39. Canon 1055.

40. John McAreavey, *The Canon Law of Marriage and the Family* (Dublin, Ireland: Four Courts Press, 1997), 73.

41. W. A. Varvaro, "Prohibition against Marriage of AIDS Victims," in *Roman Replies and CLSA Advisory Opinions* (1987), 121.

42. T. J. O'Donnell, *Medicine and Christian Morality*, 2nd ed. (New York: Alba House, 1991), 226. O'Donnell claims that "condomistic intercourse in marriage is simply not marital intercourse."

43. See also Germain Grisez, "Moral Questions on Condoms and Disease Prevention." *National Catholic Bioethics Quarterly* 8:3 (Autumn 2008): 471–76.

44. Canon 1084.

45. See Lisa Fullam, "Same Sex Marriage: A Catholic Affirmation." Bondings 2.0: The Blog of New Ways Ministry, http://newwaysministryblog.wordpress.com/civil-same-sex-marriage-a-catholic-affirmation/ (Accessed June 30, 2014); Stephen J. Pope, "The Magisterium's Arguments against Same-Sex Marriage: An Ethical Analysis and Critique," in *Readings in Moral Theology, No. 15: Marriage*, eds. Charles E. Curran and Julie Hanlon Rubio (New York: Paulist, 2009), 300–329.

46. Ladislas Orsy, S.J., *Marriage in Canon Law: Texts and Comments, Reflections and Questions* (Wilmington, DE: Michael Glazier, 1986), 109–110.

47. Ibid., 110.

48. Mt 19:1–9. See also Mk 10:1–12.

49. Pheme Perkins, *Commentary on the Gospels, The New Oxford Annotated Bible* (Oxford: Oxford University Press, 2007).

50. Raymond Collins, *Divorce in the New Testament* (Collegeville: Liturgical Press, 1992), 205. See also Raymond E. Brown, *An Introduction to the New Testament* (New York: Doubleday, 1997), 194.

51. Lawler, *Marriage*, 96.

52. USCCB, *Marriage*, 25–6.

53. Ibid.

54. Bernard Cooke, "What God Has Joined Together . . ." in Kieran Scott and Michael Warren, eds., *Perspectives on Marriage: A Reader*, 2ed. (New York: Oxford University Press, 2001), 346–354, at 351.

55. It is also important to remember cases like Keesha's. Keesha explained that her substance abuse was a key factor in the breakdown of her marriage to Shawn. Not all cases of marriage failure are related to wife abuse.

56. Cooke, "What God Has Joined," 352.

57. Many studies have documented the negative effects of divorce on children. The US Census reports that children of divorced parents are more likely to live in poverty, for example. See US Census Bureau, *Marital Events of Americans (*August 2011): http://www.census.gov/prod/2011pubs/acs-13.pdf (Accessed June 20,2014). See also Judith Wallerstein, Julia M. Lewis, and Sandra Blakeslee, *The Unexpected Legacy of Divorce: A Twenty-Five Year Landmark Study* (New York: Hyperion, 2000). Olga Khazan reports on recent trends in marriage and childbearing in "The Luxury of Waiting for Marriage to Have Kids," *The Atlantic* (June 17, 2014): http://www.theatlantic.com/business/archive/2014/06/why-poor-women-dont-wait-for-marriage-to-give-birth/372890/ (Accessed June 20, 2014). While sustained attention to divorce is beyond the scope of this project, I do believe that, no matter the family structure, children deserve a loving, nurturing, stable, economically secure environment for their optimal growth and development; adults bear responsibility for protecting children from harm.

58. Patrick Lagges, "Annulment: The Process and Its Meaning," *Marriage and Family* 73:4 (April 1991): 18–24.

59. Ibid., See also Lawler, *Marriage*, 103–113.

60. Margaret Farley, "Divorce, Remarriage, and Pastoral Practice." In *Readings in Moral Theology, No. 15: Marriage*, eds. Charles E. Curran and Julie Hanlon Rubio (New York: Paulist, 2009), 426–455, at 444–445.

61. Melissa Browning, *Risky Marriage: HIV and Intimate Relationships in Tanzania* (Lanham: Lexington, 2014), 180.

62. For an excellent treatment on conscience in the Catholic tradition, see Linda Hogan: *Confronting the Truth: Conscience in the Catholic Tradition* (New York: Paulist, 2001).

63. Gula, *Reason Informed by Faith*, 316.

64. As an example, see Congregation for the Doctrine of the Faith, *Persona Humana* (1975), available online: http://www.vatican.va/roman_curia/congregations/cfaith/documents/rc_con_cfaith_doc_19751229_persona-humana_en.html (Accessed August 5, 2014).

65. Lisa Sowle Cahill, *Sex, Gender, and Christian Ethics*, 117.

66. Ibid., 119.

67. Kevin T. Kelly, *New Directions in Sexual Ethics: Moral Theology and the Challenge of AIDS* (London: Geoffrey Chapman, 1998), 11.

68. Ibid., 139.

69. Ibid., 145, 162.

70. Ibid., 187.

71. Ibid.

72. Cf. chapter 5.

73. He put before them another parable: "The kingdom of heaven may be compared to someone who sowed good seed in his field; but while everybody was asleep, an enemy came and sowed weeds among the wheat, and then went away. So when the plants came up and bore grain, then the weeds appeared as well. And the slaves of the householder came and said to him, 'Master, did you not sow good seed in your field? Where, then, did these weeds come from?' He answered, 'An enemy has done this.' The slaves said to him, 'Then do you want us to go and gather them?' But he replied, 'No; for in gathering the weeds you would uproot the wheat along with them. Let both of them grow together until the harvest; and at harvest time I will tell the reapers, Collect the weeds first and bind them in bundles to be burned, but gather the wheat into my barn.'"

74. Kelly, *New Directions*, 187.

75. Salzman and Lawler, *Sexual Ethics*, xix, xxiii. See also Salzman and Lawler, *The Sexual Person: Toward a Renewed Catholic Anthropology* (Washington DC: Georgetown University Press, 2008).

76. Ibid., 81.

77. Ibid., 82.

78. Thomas Aquinas, *Summa Theologica*, Trans. Fathers of the English Dominican Province (New York: Benziger, 1948), Ia–IIae, Q. 28, 1C.

79. Ibid., IIa—Iae, Q. 58, 1.

80. Salzman and Lawler, *Sexual Ethics*, 82–83.

81. "Whether any given sexual act, heterosexual or homosexual, is truly human is determined, not by the naked application of abstract moral principles, but by a careful, hermeneutical analysis of how those principles apply in real, concrete, particular human relationships." Ibid., 87.

82. Farley, *Just Love*, 207.

83. Ibid., 207–244.

84. Ibid., 231.

85. The dignity of men and women is explicitly affirmed in the *Catechism*, no. 369.

86. CCC, nos. 372, 1605. It should be noted that while many modern theologians appeal to Genesis 1–2 as scriptural evidence of the "equality" of women and men, these texts were not always interpreted so positively. Within Christian tradition, theologians have interpreted women as inferior because man was created first, because woman was created as man's "helpmate," and because Eve was blamed for the first disobedience, making women responsible for sin. See also Timothy 2:9–15, 1 Peter 3:1–7, 1 Corinthians 11:3–12.

87. Pope Paul VI, *Humanae vitae* (1968), no. 9.

88. As an example, Pope John Paul II lamented the discrimination women have experienced and explicitly denounced gender-based violence in his "Letter to Women," (1995), available online: http://www.vatican.va/holy_father/john_paul_ii/letters/documents/hf_jp-ii_let_290619 95_women_en.html (Accessed June 4, 2014), nos. 3–5. See also the 1994 pastoral letter by the Committee on Women in Society and in the Church, United States Conference of Catholic Bishops, *Strengthening the Bonds of Peace: A Pastoral Reflection on Women in Society and in the Church,* which teaches that discrimination against women "contradicts the will of God" and which explicitly rejects sexism. Available online: http://www.usccb.org/about/laity-marriage-family-life-and-youth/womens-issues/strengthening-the-bonds-of-peace.cfm (Accessed June 4, 2014), nos 6–8.

89. Sacred Congregation of Rites, *Rite of Marriage*, 1969, in *The Rites of the Catholic Church* (New York: Pueblo, 1982), no. 60.

90. Donna Freitas, *Sex and the Soul: Juggling Sexuality, Spirituality, Romance, and Religion on America's College Campuses* (New York: Oxford University Press, 2008) and Kathleen Bogle, *Hooking Up: Sex, Dating, and Relationships on Campus* (New York: New York University Press, 2008).

91. See Thomas Aquinas, *Summa Theologica*, IaIIae, Q. 17–18.

92. Lawler, *Marriage,* 10. The *Catechism* concurs: "[Their] mutual love becomes an image of the absolute and unfailing love with which God loves man [sic]." CCC, no. 1604.

93. Kelly, *New Directions*, 162–168, at 162.

94. A correlative concern is the responsibility that these couples have to prevent the spread of HIV to their children. Mother-to-child transmission of HIV can be reduced if the pregnant woman is on anti-retroviral therapy, if she undergoes a Caesarian delivery instead of a vaginal delivery, and if the infant is given anti-retroviral medications at birth.

95. For scriptural justifications of this "already and not yet" vision of human life in the Reign of God, consider Mt 25:31–46; Rv 22:12–13; Lk 11:20; 1 Cor 10:11; Mk 13; Lk 11:2; 1 Cor 15:20–28.

96. Christine E. Gudorf, "Western Religion and the Patriarchal Family," in Kieran Scott and Michael Warren, eds., *Perspectives on Marriage: A Reader* (New York: Oxford University Press, 2001), 285–304. For an overview of some of the key developments in the theology of Christian marriage see Peter Jeffery, *The Mystery of Christian Marriage* (New York: Paulist, 2006), 194–226.

97. USCCB, *Marriage*, 15.

98. Lisa Sowle Cahill, *Family: A Christian Social Perspective* (Minneapolis: Fortress Press, 2000), 131.

99. Evelyn Eaton Whitehead and James D. Whitehead, ""Marriage Becomes a Journey," in *Perspectives on Marriage: A Reader,* 2ed., ed. Kieran Scott and Michael Warren (New York: Oxford University Press, 2001): 116–126, at 125.

100. Ibid., 125.

101. Ibid., 126.

Chapter Seven

Implications for Parish Life: Survival, Sex, and Prayer in Everyday Pastoral Contexts

> I give you a new commandment, that you love one another. Just as I have loved you, you also should love one another. By this everyone will know that you are my disciples, if you have love for one another.
> Jn 13:34–35.

Most Catholic married couples come to understand the church's theology of marriage through pastoral moments in their own marriage journey—their first meeting with their pastor when preparing for marriage, or the planning of their wedding liturgy, or a retreat for engaged couples. These moments of pastoral evangelization might introduce theological themes that are later reinforced during weekly parish liturgies, adult education programs within their parish, or articles in their diocesan newspaper. In these pastoral encounters, what messages do women hear about their vocations as wives, their roles within marriage, and the church's expectations for their living and loving?

In at least three of such pastoral moments women often hear mixed messages about the church's expectations for them in the vocation of marriage. In some contexts this consists of explicit teachings about female fertility, expected roles within the home, or the demands of parenting. In other contexts, these expectations are implied in subtle ways, by associating women with home life or by failing to unpack the practical implications of women's equal dignity when describing the unique contributions women can make to both private and public life.

For Catholic women to flourish in marriage, they must hear affirming and empowering messages in ordinary church settings. It should be plainly obvious to all women who participate in Catholic liturgies and who benefit from parish ministries that God loves them and that the church is a place of support and encouragement. In everyday contexts, church teachings and practices must explicitly affirm women as beloved of God, respect wives as equal partners with their husbands, and offer a coherent and compelling sexual ethic that affirms self-care and self-concern. Yet in at least three pastoral moments the Catholic Church offers confusing messages about expectations for women in married and family life. Drawing on the stories of the women interviewed, I note the persistence of confusing messages and put forward some of their suggestions for transforming church life at local levels. In particular, I focus on the possibility for rethinking family ministries, marriage preparation, and the wedding liturgy so that in these everyday contexts of faith formation women hear of God's loving care for them and of their obligation to care for themselves as part of what it means to be a disciple of Jesus and member of the Body of Christ.

RETHINKING FAMILY MINISTRIES: A MISSION TO COMFORT THE AFFLICTED AND AFFLICT THE COMFORTABLE

While Carmen criticized the Catholic Church for not welcoming people affected by AIDS, her story can help us reflect on the opportunities to develop church ministries that would be more effective in reaching struggling women like Carmen. Carmen was convinced that were it not for her support group, and especially her first contact there, whom she calls her sponsor, she would be dead. In 2006, Carmen told me:

> Evelyn—she is my sponsor—I can't think of a way in which she didn't help me! Sometimes you don't die of the diseases but of the thoughts. Do you understand me? The thoughts. When you know that you have this disease, that you are eventually going to die of it, and sometimes I was so depressed. She gave me her number, and Evelyn said "I am here for you 24/7." Can you believe that? And you know what, she was. Sometimes I called her at one o'clock in the morning, two o'clock in the morning, and she would tell me that everything was going to be fine, that I should let myself rest. When I look back at that, I think, wow, she really did that for me. She really cared. No one ever treated me like that before, no one ever seemed to care about me. And it wasn't sexual, just a friend. She did it for everyone in that group. So supportive. And others in that group, well, I can tell you, it is so terrible to hear the new person say "I can't tell my family. I will die of this disease and I can't tell my family because they will reject me." The newest member of our group, he said that, that his family would reject him. And it just makes me think, that why can't we treat each other better, you know?

Carmen felt no support from her local Catholic parish, but the AIDS support group where she met Evelyn and attended regular meetings was her life line. What can the church learn from Carmen's story? Carmen was grateful that she had found supportive networks, but worried that other Catholic men and women would not get the support they needed. When we further reflect on Carmen's story, we can ask: Who is more like Jesus in Carmen's experiences? Who is living up to the commandment to love your neighbor as yourself? What would it mean for church members to be more like Evelyn than the parents of the newly diagnosed young man in Carmen's support group?

If Catholic offices of family ministries at the diocesan and parish levels could take up this challenge and strategize to better affirm and support women struggling to get by in difficult circumstances, they could serve the needs of HIV-affected families in their midst. One of the themes that emerged in my collaborators' stories was the theme of survival. They reported patterns of medical, emotional, psychological, spiritual, and financial stress. In the framework of Catholic diocesan ministries, family ministries are charged with supporting and strengthening families by offering continuing education and programs for spiritual enrichment, and by advocating for family-friendly social policies. At root, Christians must ask, how can the church community encourage the empowerment of women and self care of women amidst complex social threats and everyday struggles of family life?

Some publications from family ministries offices name gay marriage, legal abortion, and contraceptive use as the dominant threats to marriage today. But for most married couples in the United States, it would seem that the threats to their marriages arise from the more immediate struggles to have stable employment, affordable child care and educational opportunities for their children, safe neighborhoods, stable community institutions and support networks, and places of employment that offer family-friendly policies including parental leave plans, medical benefits, and flexible work hours.[1] These are the kinds of struggles named by the women in this study. None of the women felt their marriages were threatened by same-sex marriage, abortion, or contraception. Marriage programming that focuses on natural family planning education, anti-abortion advocacy, or anti-homosexuality campaigns fails to address the complex threats that challenge the flourishing of married couples. Instead, family ministries should develop programs that focus on communication skills, conflict resolution, budgeting and financial planning, home buying, establishment of cooperative child care networks, and family support networks.

Catholic leaders recognize the importance of programming that helps parents to appreciate and celebrate the holiness of ordinary family life.[2] In the US bishops' statement, "Putting Children and Families First," the bishops advocate for parish programs that would help parishes to serve the parents and children of the community.[3] Such examples include welcoming the participation of children within liturgy, establishing religious education programs for children and teens, and offering workshops for parents on topics such as loving discipline, sexual education of their children, and shared chores within the home. Summer camps like Vacation Bible School and other youth programs can offer assistance to families with school-age children, especially families that might not otherwise be able to afford summer camps or enrichment activities because of the prohibitive cost.

In addition to promoting family-specific workshops, the agenda of parish-based family ministries should help parents understand that they are called to do more than simply love their spouse and children. Church participation should provide an opportunity to learn about the challenges faced by people of different economic classes and to foster mutual relationships. Julie Hanlon Rubio has convincingly argued this point for some time now, drawing on both theology of marriage and Catholic social teachings. Rubio explains that family life is not meant to be exclusive, fostering only the good of family members, but inclusive, obligated to take seriously the welfare of local, national, and even international communities. The family must situate its own good in the context of the common good, and it must make a commitment to serve the poor.[4] In Catholic teachings, the family is described as the primary place of faith formation, the "domestic church," where children are schooled in virtue.[5] Family ministries can help give parents the resources to teach their children about these important social commitments. By helping parents to become aware of advocacy opportunities, anti-racism efforts, anti-poverty reforms, and other opportunities for political action, family ministries can help parents to stay informed about the social issues to which they should give their attention as Christian parents. Family ministries at the parish level could walk together in the AIDS Walk, create a food pantry for families in need, or provide meeting space for Al-Anon[6] or support groups for AIDS affected families. In addition, family ministries can assist parents in discerning the values they hope to promote in the ways they spend their money. Sally Purvis explains, "Our relationships, behaviors, and choices about earning, saving, and spending—as well as our political choices—have implications far beyond the narrow scope of our daily lives, and those implications must become part of our daily choices."[7] Members of a family could be encouraged to spend more time together, to eat family meals together, and to engage in community service together outside the home. In these daily interactions family members learn about their obligations to one another and to the wider world.

There are many opportunities for family ministries to promote educational programs that explicitly affirm married women as beloved of God and equal partners with their spouses. These ministry offices could develop programs that support the stewardship of girls' gifts for service and work outside the home. In addition, the church can better promote civil institutions that would enable the flourishing of family life. Much more could be spent to advocate for family-friendly policies that would reduce pressure on working adults, ensure the safety of children in schools, and create opportunities for parents to educate their children about their obligations to contribute to the common good. In this way, family ministries can model a comprehensive pro-life agenda that assists spouses in integrating their personal commitments with the church's social commitments. Church attendance should both nurture and challenge. Surely this is a difficult balance, but as Dorothy Day reportedly named her vocation to "comfort the afflicted and afflict the comfortable,"[8] so too this is a task that can be undertaken by parish ministries today. Family ministries must hold together both the need to support vulnerable people and to challenge comfortable families.

RETHINKING MARRIAGE PREPARATION: SEX, INTIMACY, AND FREEDOM FROM VIOLENCE

In the United States, all engaged couples who wish to be married in the Roman Catholic Church must participate in a marriage preparation program. Most are organized at the parish level in collaboration with a diocesan office of family ministry. Many programs rely on the leadership of married couples together with clergy who assist the couples in their paperwork and planning of their wedding liturgy. In most cases, couples who are preparing for marriage within the church must meet with a priest or deacon within their parish, attend a series of classes or a retreat (covering issues such as communication, intimacy, sexuality, and financial planning), explore their relationship and expectations of marriage by filling out a marital inventory, and discuss these findings with a married couple, family counselor, or priest.

In 1988, the NCCB Committee on Pastoral Practices published *Faithful to Each Other Forever: A Catholic Handbook of Pastoral Help for Marriage Preparation*[9] as a resource for those involved in marriage preparation work. It remains a very useful and comprehensive pastoral tool.[10] The Family Ministries Office of the Archdiocese of Chicago has also published its own document entitled *In the Spirit of Cana: Guidelines for Pastoral Outreach to Christian Marriage*[11] as a resource for those involved in marriage preparation programs within the church. Other pastoral resources are intended for use by the couple preparing for marriage.[12]

There is much to praise within these publications. Each offers descriptions of marriage as a faithful and loving partnership. Drawing on canon law, papal encyclicals, the documents of Vatican II, the Bible, and data from the social sciences, the authors emphasize fidelity, mutual love, and children as gifts from God. These publications refer to this time of preparation as a special opportunity for engaged couples to explore their own hopes, fears, and expectations about married life, while also offering the pastoral minister an opportunity to evangelize the couple. All of these marriage preparation resources are meant to help the couple prepare not only for the day of their wedding but also, and more importantly, for their future life together afterwards. They provide an important opportunity to socialize men to respect women and to better understand church teachings on egalitarian marriage partnerships. While acknowledging that this is sometimes difficult for couples who are busy preparing for the celebration, the literature takes an important future-oriented view.

The authors take special care in helping the engaged persons to reflect on their own experiences of family life in order to analyze their own expectations about the family they hope to create with their partner. Special emphasis is given to communication, conflict resolution, and trust. Some utilize a case studies approach,[13] while other publications ask questions for the couple to consider individually and discuss together.[14] These materials and sacramental preparation programs invite the couple to reflect with honesty on their own needs and desires, their faith commitments, and their hopes for the future with their partner. They invite the couple to engage in the process of marital preparation with maturity and to take the time to consider responsibly the promise and commitment they are going to make in marriage.

In a study conducted by the Creighton University Center for Marriage and Family, interviews with married individuals who completed marriage preparation in the Catholic Church indicated that sacramental preparation programs are beneficial for a majority of couples. Two-thirds of the respondents perceived marriage preparation as a valuable experience, with the following aspects rated as most helpful: providing time for couples to learn about each other, collaboration among clergy and lay leaders in the marriage preparation program, and addressing the "five Cs" (communication, commitment, conflict resolution, children, and church).[15] Thus, these programs fill important needs among engaged couples. All of the publications invite the couple to think about the ups and downs, and the highs and lows of married life, in order to prepare realistically for moments of frustration, pain, or tragedy that might challenge their relationship in the future. Each discusses illness, grief, and financial instability.

For couples directly affected by HIV and AIDS, marriage preparation brings unique challenges. In the eight publications I read that were aimed towards the married couple, not a single one mentioned HIV or AIDS. Only the Chicago Family Ministries *Guidelines* mention HIV and AIDS explicitly, and this publication is written for pastoral ministers (and therefore would not be normally available to the engaged couple). There, in the section entitled "Health Concerns," the *Guidelines* explain that persons living with a debilitating disease are not prohibited from entering into Christian marriage. The authors explain: "While some of the demands of married life may be a bit more stressful for them *and for their partners*, if one has the mental capacity to make a solemn (i.e., covenant) commitment, physical disabilities are not a *de facto* impediment."[16] Regarding persons living with HIV, the document continues:

> There are questions concerning sexual intimacy and procreation which need to be dealt with honestly, tactfully, and on a case-by-case basis. Again, be careful of oversimplified or presumptive moral, canonical, or pastoral responses. Whether through canonical exceptions, permanent abstinence, or some discussible moral interpretations of family planning techniques, these issues need not automatically preclude marriage for a given couple.[17]

These guidelines, which do not explicitly mention condom use, do suggest that there may be permissible alternatives to permanent abstinence for HIV-affected couples. The *Guidelines* suggest that pastoral ministers refer the couple to counselors who could help them discuss "the physical, psychological, social, and spiritual implications that HIV/AIDS will have on their relationship" with sensitivity and confidentiality.[18] Yet there is no way of verifying that this information is communicated to the couple, or of assessing the minister's sensitivity, especially since the engaged couple is not given this information in print.

While these guidelines remain vague, the publication's explicit mention of HIV and AIDS is admirable. Overall, the resources of the Archdiocese of Chicago are valuable for pastoral ministers and for couples preparing for the sacrament of marriage. But they have limitations. In light of the concerns that arose in the experiences of the women I interviewed, these publications could be supplemented by other resources that focus greater attention on self-care of married persons before and within marriage. Too often pre-marriage books characterize marital love as self-sacrifice and romanticize sexual lovemaking without also helping couples to understand the complex and messy challenges of love for God and of mutual love.[19] Couples preparing for marriage should be taught not only about the need to give of themselves to their spouses, but also about how to name their own needs and desires, accept their spouse's love and sacrifice, and care for themselves physically, emotionally, and psychologically.

Specifically, these pastoral publications could make improvements in four distinct areas: first, by addressing the unique emotional and health concerns of couples who are sexually experienced; second, by explicitly affirming the dual vocation of both spouses to work in the public and private spheres; third, by expanding the sexual education guidelines beyond natural family planning; and fourth, by including more information regarding domestic violence as an affront to human dignity and an offense against the sacrament of marriage.

Realistic Approach to Premarital Sex

The Catholic Church teaches that sexual activity is acceptable only within heterosexual monogamous marriage and that sexual loving between married spouses should remain open to the possibility of procreation. Yet many engaged couples who are preparing for marriage are already sexually active, or have engaged in sexual activity in previous relationships.[20] Seven of the eight women in my study had engaged in sex prior to marriage. To ignore this reality is willful blindness on the part of church ministers. The Centers for Disease Control and Prevention estimates that in the United States, 250,000 persons are HIV-positive and do not know they are infected.[21] Since engaged persons preparing for marriage within the church may have participated in unsafe sex, and may not have been tested for HIV, they might be among this group.[22] In light of the HIV epidemic within the United States, and the rise in heterosexual transmission rates, marriage preparation programs must encourage couples to discuss their past sexual histories with honesty and openness; these programs should explicitly encourage voluntary HIV testing and disclosure to one's partner for all persons who have been or are sexually active, as well as their engaged partners.[23] This information should be straightforward in the literature given to every couple; such information could protect the partners and also the possible children of such unions. The tone of sensitive material should be encouraging and hopeful, not stigmatizing or fear-based.[24] Three of the women in this study provided advice for pastoral ministers. Grace explained:

> For couples who are preparing for marriage, here's my advice. The first thing is don't assume you're marrying a virgin, and that's okay, but you should take responsibility to get tested. And you can learn from my story. If you do test positive, I hope not, but if so, life's not over. You can live with it. There are lots of married people who are positive; you can be in a serodiscordant relationship; there are lots of people out there like that. And I think the church just needs to be like Father Karl. Because without him, I don't know how things would have turned out for me. It probably would have been much different, without knowing I was supported, right from the beginning. That meant a lot to me.

When asked what advice she would give to a newly engaged couple, Cheryl explained: "Become friends first. Communicate. Try not to go to bed angry. If he's having a bad day, listen to him." Diva offered the following advice for pastoral ministers: "The church should meet people where they're at. That's what the church should do. They can have an open mind."

While couples who are sexually experienced are not disqualified from reception of the sacrament of marriage, marriage preparation programs that neglect to discuss these concerns with engaged couples will miss the opportunity to help them think about the consequences of past relationships on the commitment they are preparing to make. In addition, engaged couples who are sexually active may benefit from a discussion of how they intend to prepare for their relationship's transition into faithful married love. In discussing their sexual history with each other the couple can discuss their own levels of satisfaction and their hopes for increased intimacy and better communication with each other about the sexual expression of their love. By including this component within marriage preparation programs, pastoral ministers have an opportunity to minister to the couple in an important time of transition in their life and to emphasize that sexuality is a good gift from God. It would be appropriate to suggest to the couple that as married persons they will have the responsibility to care for themselves and for each other. It is not enough to leave this to the discretion of the individual minister who prepares the couple.

Dual Vocation for Husbands and Wives[25]

Another flaw of these marital preparation programs is their affirmation of gender roles that discourage wives from working outside the home. Scripts found in this literature can be confusing and even damaging for women like Sue, Lettie, Diva, and Grace, all of whom worked outside the home in jobs that enabled them to provide for their families and to experience their worth and dignity through their gift of self in the world. Recall that Sue worked as an AIDS educator, Grace as a social worker, Lettie in personnel management, and Diva as a health care aide. Grace described her work as her "prayer." Women preparing for marriage in the Catholic Church may, after reading these publications, feel subtle pressure to give up their employment, either immediately or in the future, so that they can focus their time and attention on caring for the home and for their children (if any).[26] This is problematic for several reasons. First, for many couples it may not be financially feasible for only one spouse to work.[27] But whether or not one is compelled to work by financial necessity, women's work outside the home should not be simplistically denounced as harmful to the family. Instead, the energy that animates each person to contribute to the common good through work outside the home should be seen as a sign of God's invitation to renew the community. Rather than being regarded as selfish, for both husbands and wives this vocation to work can be seen as a Christian duty.

These assumptions about appropriate roles for women also arise within these publications in both discussions of expectations about household chores and child rearing. *A Marriage in the Lord* informs couples that discussions of these expectations are likely to create conflict, and explains that a 2006 study by Neil Chethik, found a "direct link to men being more satisfied with their sex life when the woman perceived the division of household duties to be fair."[28] The author continues:

> Even if the housework was not divided equally, the perception of fairness was what mattered. The problem remains getting men to do more around the house. The survey found that nagging, criticism, and accusations did not motivate men to do more housework, but creating a master plan, giving notice as to when things should be done, and changing expectations (usually lowering them) did.[29]

This marriage manual's treatment of this very real concern could have been recast in a framework of justice, communication, or mutual responsibility. Instead it repeats, in subtle ways, the assumption that work within the home is the responsibility of the woman and that women should lower their expectations for assistance from their partners.

Discussion regarding care of children frequently falls into the same trap. Parenting is described as a mother's natural gift and vocation, while fathers receive little encouragement in their roles as parents.[30] Some texts describe husbands as providers and protectors without also naming ways that as fathers they can be nurturing caregivers.[31]

While these publications treat neither topic well, expectations surrounding housework and parenting remain important topics for engaged couples to consider. It turns out that couples are hungry for realistic strategies to navigate these thorny issues; one study reports that couples married five years or less identified three particularly difficult areas of concern in their marriages: balancing job and family; frequency of sexual relations; and financial issues.[32] The authors of the study suggest that premarital programs continue to develop resources for engaged couples to prepare them for marital stresses stemming from time, sex, and money. Many couples in the US context hope and expect that both spouses will work outside the home. When both husband and wife share the responsibilities of earning the family income, raising children, caring for the home, and contributing to the common good, then both partners must struggle to balance public and private life, work and home life. While it is important for couples to communicate about their hopes for balancing work and home life, and about any fears they have, it is not helpful to imply that work outside the home is inappropriate for women or necessarily harmful for children.

Julie Hanlon Rubio, in her exploration of the "dual vocation" of Christian parents, explains that Christian discipleship "presumes a public vocation."[33] To follow Jesus means that one's life cannot be focused only on one's family. Work outside the home, for men as well as women, can constitute an important aspect of one's public vocation.[34] Both parents can work outside the home while also maintaining a healthy home environment; in this way both spouses can contribute to the common good of the wider community.

For Rubio, "the notion of public vocation implies that the full self-realization of a Christian requires involvement in public life."[35]

For couples with children, this dual vocation may require that the family depend on childcare outside the home. But Rubio attempts to dismiss the public stigma from such a decision by situating childcare in a social context. For Rubio, childcare outside the home is "care of children by members of a community"; furthermore, "care of children by non-relatives can be beneficial to children."[36] In response to the objection that having a high number of children in childcare outside the home is harmful to society, Rubio claims that "if community responsibility for children is a worthy ideal, community care for and influence on children should not be threatening; it should be exciting."[37]

Bonnie J. Miller-McLemore, also a working mother herself, reflects theologically upon the reality of life for working mothers in the contemporary US context. She notes that the number of married women in employed positions is more than five times what it was in 1940; half of all women with children under one work outside the home.[38] Miller-McLemore wonders, do these women "have it all?" She concludes that the phrase "having it all" is a romanticized, distorted, and even oppressive concept because women do not have equity with men in either the workplace or the family. For example, women make only about seventy cents for every dollar earned by men, and report that their household chores have only grown, not diminished, over the years.[39] She continues:

> When "having it all" really means "doing it all," it is a dubious honor at best. The idea arose within an economic and social system that viewed child-rearing, homemaking, and community life as "non-work," and which naively viewed market labor as almost completely independent of the labors of family and community. The dilemmas of work and family simply reveal the distortions of these views. Childrearing, housework, and community service are hard—and socially essential—work.[40]

In analyzing how this dilemma affects women, Miller-McLemore contends that one cannot ignore the realities of class and race and the effects of these factors on women's opportunities and struggles.[41] Upper-class mothers often secure labor from those in lower economic brackets—housekeepers, live-in nannies, gardeners, caterers, decorators, and so on—and in doing so approximate the illusion of "having it all" while depending on the labors of less well-situated women. Miller-McLemore's vision of gender justice instead requires more evenly distributed family responsibilities among men, women, children, and community institutions. She writes:

> A corrected interpretation of "having it all" must restore appropriate responsibility to men, local community institutions, the workplace, government, and

> public policymakers. . . . Women should not be blamed for their unrealistic expectations or their failure to work it all out, not seen as fools or guilty of wanting too much when their problems are quite relative to a particular moment in history that has forced both a false separation between paid work and family care, and an unnatural divorce between work and love, which belong together.[42]

The marriage preparation publications I surveyed fail to assist engaged couples in discerning the best approach to overcoming these hurdles within their marriage and instead rely on either romanticized notions of "having it all" or traditional accounts of gender role differentiations that prevent women from seeing work outside the home as a valuable contribution to the common good.[43]

Natural Family Planning

A third element of these publications is the promotion of Natural Family Planning (hereafter NFP) for all married couples. Marriage preparation programs within the Catholic Church aim to evangelize engaged couples on the church's theology of marriage and sexuality.[44] The programs teach that through their sexual loving married couples are invited to cooperate with God as co-creators, and that welcoming children and caring responsibly for children is a unique gift to be celebrated.[45]

While the church promotes responsible use of marital fertility and cooperation between husband and wife, official Catholic teaching rejects the "artificial" separation of the unitive and procreative dimensions of marital sexuality.[46] Catholic theology of marriage teaches that couples should desire to welcome children.[47] The church endorses NFP for all married couples, both couples who wish to postpone pregnancy, and couples who desire to achieve pregnancy. Marriage preparation programs in the United States offer couples information about NFP techniques and classes, and instruction books are widely available.[48]

While these publications inform readers about the scientific basis for natural methods of controlling fertility, they frequently do so within a framework that reinforces essentialist[49] views of men and women and promotes fear of and confusion about "unnatural" methods of birth control.[50] Consequently, these educational materials could confuse women preparing for marriage in the Catholic Church. Additionally, because of the moralistic tone of some of the publications, couples who choose other methods of fertility control may feel guilty, even if their decision was arrived at after careful discernment in good conscience.

For some highly motivated couples, natural family planning might be the best method of sexual planning. In learning the techniques of fertility monitoring, a woman will become more in tune with her body by becoming aware of the days in her monthly cycle in which conception is a possibility if she and her husband engage in sexual intercourse. But a variety of circumstances, including irregular menstrual cycles, irregular sleeping patterns, lactation, taking medications, and emotional stress, make it difficult—and sometimes impossible—for a woman to successfully interpret her signs of fertility.[51] If the couple does not intend to conceive, long periods of sexual abstinence may be required.[52]

For couples who, after careful discernment, have concluded in good conscience that God is not calling them to begin a family or to have another child, NFP can be difficult to follow, emotionally stressful, and ineffective. While NFP literature frequently describes the increased cooperation and communication between couples using NFP, the more realistic expectation is that the woman takes on much greater responsibility in monitoring her signs of fertility and communicating with her husband about how they can schedule their love-making to avoid pregnancy.[53]

NFP manuals, especially those texts authored by Catholics, are prone to emphasize procreation as "God's will" and as an expectation of married couples. One book explains to newlyweds: "We emphasize here as we do elsewhere in this manual: you need a sufficiently serious reason to avoid pregnancy. If you don't have a really good reason to postpone pregnancy, your honeymoon is a wonderful time to start your family. In God's plan, marriage is for family."[54] But is the honeymoon *really* the best time to start a family? The first year of marriage is widely known to be a difficult year of adjustments and transition for both husband and wife.[55] When NFP publications tell couples that they need a "sufficiently serious" and "really good" reason to postpone pregnancy, engaged couples might become confused as they wonder if their own reasons are reasonable and serious or if their reasons are selfish and sinful. A consequence of this depiction of marriage is that women, who accept greater physical burdens and responsibilities to fulfill the duty of procreation, are pressured to consider motherhood as an obligation instead of a calling to discern in conscience. The pressure of these considerations could cause serious anxiety for an already overwhelmed bride and groom.

In addition, NFP literature promotes breastfeeding and discourages women from working outside the home and thereby neglecting her "responsibilities" as mother. One pamphlet explains that "God's plan" of "natural mothering" entails "mother-baby inseparability" described thus: "When mother goes to church, so does baby. When mother goes shopping, attends a meeting, or visits a friend, so does baby. And when baby indicates a need to nurse, mother obliges. When a mother goes to bed at night or for a nap, baby is usually in the same bed, nursing as needed while his mother sleeps."[56] Another pamphlet distributed by Couple to Couple League explains that "leading authorities" and "experts" agree that "every child needs one person as a full-time caretaker for the first three years, a person who has time day and night to devote *herself* to the needs of the child."[57] This depiction belies the fact that for most of human history children were not raised by a single person within a nuclear family structure as these "experts" imply.[58] For engaged couples preparing for marriage, the not so subtle pressures within such publications imply that the vocation to marriage requires openness to procreation, welcoming of children, a husband/father whose work can support the financial needs of the family, and a wife/mother willing and able to stay home full-time to nurse and care for the children and maintain the home. While early childhood development and the need for parents to responsibly care for their children is important, such restrictions for women fail to accept that some women could have vocations other than nursing and child-rearing. The implicit assumptions about the roles of husband and wife are not egalitarian; the husband is not assumed to have a nurturing role in the caretaking of his children, while the mother's exclusive devotion to her children overshadows her own self-care or her contribution beyond the household.

If the theology of marriage depends on an affirmation of the dignity of women, their equality with men, and the overarching affirmation that they are beloved of God and called to care for themselves in relationship, then a woman's preparation for the sacrament of marriage should not require that she relinquish any personal vocation to work outside the home. The tone of these publications can make readers feel guilty for responding to God's call to contribute to the common good through their work. They refuse to acknowledge that balancing of work and family life remains not just a struggle for women but also a much neglected responsibility of men. Furthermore, by recommending the "self-sacrifice"[59] and "self-gift" of women, who must "take up their cross" in order to practice NFP, these publications reinforce scripts from the Christian tradition that fail to affirm women and fail to take seriously their own need for self-care.[60]

Engaged and married couples should instead be encouraged to communicate about their hopes and/or fears about parenthood and should be encouraged to think about parenthood as a vocation to which some, but perhaps not all, married couples are called. Marriage preparation programs should honor the experiences of women who, after careful discernment, have decided they are not ready to begin a family. Some young women fear pregnancy, are not ready for the sacrifices that it would entail, or feel ill-equipped to become parents. For these women, self-care and responsible use of fertility demand that they prevent procreation, at least temporarily. To see a woman in her totality is to see her as she is embedded in social relationships, including her commitments within and outside the home, her love for her spouse, and her hopes for her own personal growth. She is a person with multiple roles and responsibilities, all of which must be discerned and balanced in her own unique circumstances. To reduce her to her procreative potential or potential role as mother fails to fully honor her many God-given gifts and dignity. It is equally unfair, then, for anyone to characterize a married woman's reluctance to conceive as self-evidently an "unnatural resistance to motherhood."[61] Rather, in her unique, messy, and complex context, a married woman must discern together with her husband the vocation to parenthood.

For couples who have discerned in conscience that they are not called (at least at this time) to procreate, NFP would require periodic abstinence. Theologians who challenge this method point to the other benefits of sexual intercourse, including shared mutual pleasure and emotional bonding.[62] In such an interpretation, contraceptive marital sex can be life-affirming because of the mutual love shared between the spouses. Theologian Cristina Traina has argued from her personal experience, "for me contraception does not impede self-gift but, like pregnancy, allows it the freedom to proceed unworried by consequences."[63] Many theologians have argued that one could look to the totality of a marriage and not a single isolated sex act to determine the procreative dimension of marital sexuality. Still others argue that the contraceptive ban relies on a physicalist interpretation of human nature that ignores the psychological, sociological, and spiritual dimensions of human beings that support sex without fertility.[64] In one way or another, the vast majority of Catholic moral theologians note that the teachings of *Humanae vitae* have not been "received" by the faithful, the evidence of which is found in surveys of reported Catholic couples who rely on contraception within their marriages.[65]

Thus, couples preparing for marriage in the Catholic Church today could be invited to reflect on a wider range of sources of moral wisdom than simply the 1968 birth control encyclical. Couples could be invited to consider as well their own experience and the unique context of their own marriage commitment. Marriage preparation could include a description of the church's teaching on the obligations and rights of conscience and the moral imperative to follow one's conscience after due deliberation. While these publications can help the couple to form their consciences, they could do so without implying that holiness depends upon practicing NFP or neglecting one's obligations to the common good.

Finally, for couples living with HIV, practicing NFP would require permanent abstinence, since NFP forbids barrier methods of birth control (such as the male condom). But the women in this study rejected the claim that God was calling them to abstain from sexual activity. Instead, in conscience, they came to a different conclusion. While previous chapters have detailed their stories and the compelling arguments from a variety of moral theologians on this question, it is important here to simply say that at the everyday pastoral level women should be encouraged to discern God's invitation to love God, self, and neighbor in the complex circumstances in which each woman finds herself. If NFP were offered as one acceptable method but not the only method, perhaps women in irregular situations would still feel affirmed and validated in their choices instead of feeling that the church's ideal position is out of reach, and that they are unable to thus be "good Catholics."[66]

Silence About Domestic Violence

A fourth theme, domestic violence, receives little attention in the marriage preparation publications that I surveyed. In 85 percent of cases in the United States, domestic violence is in fact wife abuse.[67] Therefore a theology of marriage that explicitly affirms the dignity and equality of married women must clearly denounce intimate partner violence. Anthony Garascia's *Before "I Do"* includes "respect" and "communication" as "Foundational Factors That Form a Healthy Marriage," in which he writes: "there is no place for physical violence and/or speech that belittles and intimidates," and, further, couples must commit "to resolving disputes in a nonviolent manner."[68] *A Marriage in the Lord* also briefly addresses this theme,[69] encouraging couples who are dealing with issues of abuse to seek help from their local Catholic Charities office or from a mental health organization, and informing couples that "no one must stay in an abusive marriage."[70] These explicit condemnations of domestic violence are important. However, given national statistics and the evidence that abuse is often a part of pre-marital relations, and in light of the treatment of the empowerment of women in other areas of these texts, survivors of abuse may find that overall these texts provide confusing messages about their dignity and equality.

For example, on the page following the treatment of domestic violence in *A Marriage in the Lord*, the authors begin the section on "Sexual Intimacy" by claiming that "God expects us to give ourselves totally, body and soul, to our spouse in marriage."[71] To reinforce this claim, the author quotes three passages from the Bible (in full):

> For this reason a man shall leave his father and his mother, and be joined to his wife; and they shall become one flesh (Genesis 2:24).
> The husband must fulfill his duty to his wife, and likewise also the wife to her husband. The wife does not have authority over her own body, but the husband does; and likewise also the husband does not have authority over his own body, but the wife does (1 Corinthians 7:3–4).
> And rejoice in the wife of your youth. As a loving hind and a graceful doe, Let her breasts satisfy you at all times; Be exhilarated always with her love (Proverbs 5:18–9).[72]

These passages can be misinterpreted in ways that are problematic. Traditional interpretations of these passages have often blessed and legitimated the power of men/husbands over women/wives. This legacy of patriarchal marriages could be sincerely discussed within Catholic marriage preparation programs so that engaged couples can be informed about how the institution of marriage has changed over time. The meaning of biblical texts is not self-evident, but rather must be interpreted. The second text above, from 1 Corinthians, has been used within the Christian tradition to sanction marital rape, since the "marital duty" implied that the wife's body belonged to her husband. That this text follows the editor's claim that "God expects" total spousal self-gift in marriage could be particularly confusing to a woman who feels pressure to give herself sexually to her husband even if she has other more pressing personal concerns. While the quotations from Genesis and Proverbs are likely intended to affirm the goodness and playfulness of sexual intimacy, their effect, when given as evidence of God's expectations for marital love, instead gives the impression that women are created for the delight of their husbands—a delight which is not described in mutual terms but in terms of the husband's pleasure in his wife.

Anthony Garascia quotes from Ephesians 5:25-32 in *Before "I Do"*:

> Husbands, love your wives, as Christ loved the church. He gave himself up for her to make her holy, purifying her in the bath of water by the power of the word, to present to himself a glorious church, holy and immaculate, without stain or wrinkle or anything of that sort. Husbands should love their wives as they do their own bodies. He who loves his wife loves himself. Observe that no one ever hates his own flesh; no, he nourishes it and takes care of it as Christ cares for the Church—for we are members of his body.
>
> For this reason a man shall leave his father and mother, and shall cling to his wife, and the two shall be made into one. This is a great foreshadowing; I mean that it refers to Christ and the church. In any case, each one should love his wife as he loves himself, the wife for her part showing respect for her husband.[73]

While Garascia does not explicitly quote the most problematic passage from Ephesians 5—"wives should submit to their husbands as to the Lord"—still, the conclusion of the passage which he selects does not affirm equal power between spouses. These texts have been interpreted in the Christian tradition as conferring power on the husband, as "head," who then had the right to discipline his wife and children, legitimizing his control over them.[74]

In light of the patriarchal teachings embedded in much of the Christian scriptures, it is decidedly risky to quote these passages in texts that are meant to prepare contemporary couples for a lifetime of mutual love in marriage. Special care should be taken to re-interpret biblical references to the authority or headship of men and submission of women in traditional accounts of patriarchal marriages, which have little to say to couples today who seek instead egalitarian and mutually loving marriages. If marriage preparation texts use scriptural passages as sources for authoritative teachings, the authors must demonstrate how the interpretation of such texts can be "Word of

God" for contemporary couples. Marriage preparation texts could claim that wifely submission is not required for couples today, or could re-interpret the meaning of submission. Without this kind of textual analysis, readers who are preparing for marriage might become confused, since the marriage manual would seem to imply that patriarchal messages of the Bible still hold true when in fact church teaching has developed.[75]

Domestic violence is contrary to the dignity and flourishing of married women.[76] What might seem less obvious are the ways that an emphasis on procreation as a "duty" of Christian couples and the lack of attention to patriarchal assumptions about marriage in the Bible create expectations for unequal power relationships between men and women because of implicit understandings about what is "natural" for women, or about what God intends for marital women's self-sacrifice or self-gift within marriage. Violence against women is deeply rooted in cultural traditions of patriarchy sanctified by Christianity that have denied women equal power with their husbands. Wife battering, while now explicitly condemned by the church,[77] is rooted in beliefs of women's inferiority, views sustained by the church in previous eras.[78] Violence against women remains a threat to the stability of marriage. Marriage preparation programs could explicitly denounce violence against women and invite readers to carefully study Scriptural texts whose traditional interpretations do not affirm women as equal partners within marriage. A pastorally sensitive approach is necessary—one that socializes men to respect women as equals but that also empowers women in abusive relationships to recognize and name that abuse. Women in abusive relationships must be given the tools—including the tools of theological analysis—to counter the claim that their experience of abuse is "natural" or "part of God's will" for them. Including the stories of survivors could provide an eye-opening and practical method by which marriage preparation materials could educate couples and empower women. For example, Karen Leslie Hernandez explains that writing about her experience of domestic violence was empowering, and her story can help pastoral ministers name abuse as contrary to God's will. For years, Hernandez asked, in the midst of broken marriage, "Where is God?" She concludes:

> God is not in the uttering of unkind things. God is not present in the action of instilling fear in your partner. God is not present in degradation. God is not present in the threat of violence against your partner. God is not present in lies and deceit. God is not present in the demeaning of anyone. God is not present in infidelity. God is simply not present in abusive behavior—ever.
> God is in the hope you hold as partners in a relationship. God is in the respect you show in a relationship. God is in the kindness and effort you show in a relationship… If you are in an abusive relationship, please seek help.[79]

Marriage preparation programs in the Catholic Church should explicitly denounce intimate partner violence and encourage persons in abusive relationships to seek help, as Hernandez advocates.

These four flaws within existing Catholic marriage preparation texts—inadequate attention to sexually experienced couples, inattention to the dual vocation of Christian couples, exclusive focus on NFP, and silence about domestic violence—are significant and merit further attention. To prepare for the commitment of marriage, engaged couples need to discuss these important issues. Couples cannot know what their future married life will bring, but a realistic, welcoming, and affirming marriage preparation program can help couples think about areas of their relationship that need greater attention, and the significance of the vows they are preparing to take. For couples affected by HIV and AIDS, the current manuals for marriage preparation contain significant gaps. This is most evident in the treatment of sexual norms that discourage "unnatural" methods of family planning, including barrier methods of birth control (such as the male condom). Within marital preparation programs in the United States, the experiences of couples living with HIV are largely ignored.

RECLAIMING THE WEDDING LITURGY

In addition to these marriage preparation resources, the Catholic wedding liturgy contains messages that associate women exclusively with unilateral submission, household chores, procreation, and motherhood.[80] These claims emerge in three specific areas of the liturgy: first, in the scriptural texts proclaimed in the Liturgy of the Word; second, in the prayers of blessing for the married couple; and third, in the rubrics of the *Rite* that govern posture and liturgical action.[81] Nevertheless the *Rite* could be revised so that it explicitly affirms spousal equality without perpetuating gender essentialism; a focus on the vows within the 1969 ICEL liturgy are a helpful and hopeful first step in such a transformation.

The scriptural passages proclaimed in the wedding liturgy are selected by the bride and groom from among a list of suggested texts in the *Rite*.[82] In the introduction to the *Rite*, this aspect of the liturgy is said to show the gathered community "the importance of Christian marriage in the history of salvation and the duties and responsibility of the couple in caring for the holiness of their children."[83] One can assume, therefore, that in such a framework, the chosen texts are expected to be heard and accepted by the gathered community as a reflection of God's will for the couple. In the liturgy, these texts are proclaimed as "Word of the Lord" or as "Gospel of the Lord."[84] Unlike the marriage preparation manuals, which have the opportunity to assist couples in textual analysis and interpretation of the texts in the Bible that refer to marriage, the couple's wedding liturgy is not the appropriate place for textual analysis and a lesson on biblical hermeneutics. Instead, these texts are proclaimed; such proclamation implies assent to their literal or assumed meanings.

There are significant limitations in the selected texts for the *Rite of Marriage*; the texts portray women as peripheral to the story of salvation, as subordinate to their male partners, and as valuable only through their procreative potential. If the couple chooses as the First Reading the *Rite's* suggested passage from the Book of Sirach, we hear proclaimed: "Happy the husband of a good wife."[85] The brief reading describes a good wife as a woman who brings joy to her husband, is thoughtful, possesses governed speech and firm virtue, is modest and chaste, and keeps a radiant home.[86] This is problematic because it can be interpreted to mean that the primary duty of a married woman is to please her husband and care for the family home; one is hard pressed to find examples of mutual love in such a text. Other readings describe how women were given away as though property of their fathers, and not as equal partners making a free choice of a marital partner.[87] Traditional interpretations of these texts imply that a wife's role is characterized by service to her husband.

The fertility of women remains a key theme among these texts in the *Rite*, as when the Psalmist proclaims: "Your wife shall be like a fruitful vine in the recesses of your home; Your children like olive plants around your table. Blessed are those who fear the Lord."[88] Traditional interpretations of these texts imply that infertility is a curse, and that a woman's role should be limited to child-bearing and maintaining the family home.

Modern interpretations of the "mutual affection" and "equal regard" lauded in Romans 12:10 and 12:16 seem to contradict more traditional interpretations of wifely submission proclaimed in Ephesians 5:22 and 1 Peter 3:1, the latter reading only six verses later describing women as "the weaker female sex."[89] While some couples will choose not to select these particular readings, favoring instead a proclamation of the goodness of creation,[90] or of the covenant between God and Israel,[91] the fact that the *Rite of Marriage* recommends selection from among this wider list creates the impression that these texts are considered to be a reflection of God's will for women and of the church's theology of marriage. Such an assumption is problematic for women who expect their marriages to be equal partnerships in which they are affirmed in their inherent dignity prior to their proven fertility in the experience of motherhood.

In light of this ambiguity, it is problematic when theologians overlook the oppressive texts within the *Rite* and characterize the Biblical texts as conferring a "rich portrait of marriage."[92] If these texts are "fruitful sources of theological insight into the sacrament,"[93] even while they retain an emphasis on the headship of husbands and duty of wives to bear children, submit to their husbands, and lay down their lives for others, then it is not surprising when women become confused by contemporary affirmations of the "equal dignity" of spouses which seemingly contradicts the depiction of God's will in the texts of their wedding liturgy. Couples who desire to find liberating scriptural passages commanding mutual respect and faithful love will be disappointed. As Julie Hanlon Rubio concludes, "those who are searching for an inspiring passage about the joys of love between husband and wife and the delights of parenting should look elsewhere."[94]

These problems are true also of the blessings within the *Rite of Marriage*, though perhaps to a lesser extent. The blessings of the *Rite*, like the biblical texts, focus on the two-fold obligation of the couple to fidelity and fecundity. For example, in the Opening Prayer, the presider asks of God, "Increase their faith in you and in each other, and through them bless your Church with Christian children."[95] This theme continues as the presider asks the couple in Question 3 of the Statement of Intentions, "Will you accept children lovingly from God, and bring them up according to the law of Christ and his Church?" The couple must respond affirmatively, "We will."[96] While the *Rite* does give the presider the power to omit the references to procreation and children "if, for example, the couple is advanced in years," nevertheless the standard liturgy offers an interpretation of marriage that has as a primary focus the expectation that the couple will have children.[97]

The Nuptial Blessing also implies expectations for the wife that are different than those for her husband. Most of these blessings offer a longer blessing specifically for the woman. One Nuptial Blessing reads, in part:

> You gave man the constant help of woman so that man and woman should no longer be two, but one flesh, and you teach us that what you have united may never be divided. Father, by your plan man and woman are united, and married life has been established as the one blessing that was not forfeited by original sin or washed away in the flood.
> Look with love upon this woman, your daughter, now joined to her husband in marriage. She asks your blessing. Give her the grace of love and peace. May she always follow the example of the holy women whose praises are sung in the Scriptures. May her husband put his trust in her and recognize that she is his equal and the heir with him to the life of grace. May he always honor her and love her as Christ loves his bride, the Church . . . Bless them with children and help them to be good parents. May they live to see their children's children.

The prayer's focus on the woman is interesting because the congregation prays that she will be given the graces of "love" and "peace," so that she may follow the examples of unnamed "holy women" in the Bible. Do these unnamed holy women possess skills of leadership, assertiveness, intelligence? Or were these unnamed women praised for their fulfillment of "feminine" roles, or for their obedience or submission? Such distinctions are not made within the prayer. While the equality of the spouses is affirmed, the affirmation comes within a prayer for the husband. The congregation prays that he will honor his wife and love his wife.

Another Nuptial Blessing reads, in part:

> Help them to create a home together (and give them children to be formed by the gospel and to have a place in your family). Give your blessings to N., your daughter, so that she may be a good wife (and mother), caring for the home, faithful in love for her husband, generous and kind. Give your blessings to N., your son, so that he may be a faithful husband (and a good father).[98]

In this second blessing, one can see that the expectations for the wife include caring for the home, while such an obligation is not mentioned for the husband.

In order to understand the way these prayers offer a synthesis of the Roman Catholic vision of marriage, we must note the historical background of these texts. In the ninth century, the Roman tradition included only the blessing of the bride in its ritual of marriage, while the Spanish and Frankish traditions included a blessing of both the bride and the bridegroom. Most prayers for the bride focused on her fertility. Kenneth Stevenson tells us that this conflict in traditions was preserved for many more years, and that it became a central point of argument after the Second Vatican Council when the *Rite of Marriage* was being revised.[99] The set themes have remained constant: creation of man, creation of woman, commandment to multiply, prayer for the bride (and outside the Roman tradition, for the bridegroom), for the couple's future, for marital virtues of fidelity and love, for grace to follow the esteemed characters of the Old Testament, for the gift of children, and for life in eternity.[100]

During the revision of the *Rites* in 1969, some parties hoped to preserve the prayers of the "tradition," both in language and emphasis; however, among other parties there was a desire to reject those aspects of the tradition that were patriarchal and instead enliven and renew the living tradition by attending with greater emphasis to descriptions of marriage as an egalitarian relationship. The Nuptial Blessings in the 1969 *Rite* represent a compromise position, since portions are taken from prayers of the "tradition" while the opening interrogatories added a more inclusive language. Still, the blessings reveal, quite explicitly, the distinctive expectations for wives within the sacrament of marriage. These expectations include caring for the home, following the example of holy women, and living a discipleship characterized by grace, peace, love, kindness, faithfulness, and generosity. While in itself the obligation to care for the home or to follow the example of holy women is not problematic, what remains troubling is the expectation that these are more fitting for women than men, and that husbands are not also called, like wives are, to live a discipleship characterized by grace, peace, love, and generosity. No description is available for what constitutes the husband's role as "good husband and father." Thus, even though official church teaching asserts that marriage is an equal partnership and that this partnership should be shaped by the mutual love between spouses, what comes across in the blessings of the liturgy is instead the assumption that women should assume a role characterized by humility and service, and that their fertility in some way reveals God's special plan for them.

With regard to the rubrics of the liturgy, Paul Covino asks: "Are the messages and the values conveyed in our liturgies consistent with what we believe about what is taking place?"[101] Covino believes that the rubrics and prayers of the wedding liturgy offer a "primary theology" of the sacrament of marriage.[102] While this theology of marriage has helpful elements, we must also attend to the potential problems.

Julie Hanlon Rubio explains that if we read the fundamental gestures of the Catholic wedding as a "text," we will discover some of the basics of Catholic theological thinking on marriage.[103] For Rubio, the wedding is significant in that it situates the couple's relationship within the broader context of the church community, inviting the couple to think about their relationship not as a private and romantic commitment but as a partnership that finds its deepest expression in shared passion for public service.[104] This countercultural message from the wedding liturgy has special significance for Catholics in the United States, for whom a criticism of consumerism, materialism, and extravagant spending may be especially warranted. Rubio especially emphasizes the difference between "popular" weddings, which focus on the bride and give special attention to the bridal party and procession, and the Catholic *Rite*, which officially suggests that the bride and groom enter together, accompanied by their parents, following the priest in the entrance procession.[105] Covino explains:

> The wedding liturgy marks not only the new union between husband and wife, but in a very real way their taking leave of their parents and family of origin. The entrance procession as outlined in the Rite of Marriage gives ritual expression to our Catholic reverence for our families of origin and to the need for leave-taking.[106]

For Covino, this entrance procession symbolically represents the church's belief that the bride and groom enter marriage mutually and as equal, complementary partners.[107] American Catholics should be instructed, according to Covino, that the more common practice of the father of the bride accompanying the bride to the altar, which gives the impression that the father is "giving away" his daughter, does not reflect the faith of the church community.[108]

Covino and Rubio also point to other aspects of the church's *Rite* that are not reflected in typical American Catholic celebrations of marriage: the expectation that the couple would greet guests at the door of the church; the expectation that all parishioners are invited to the wedding liturgy; the positioning of the couple during the vows so that those in attendance can see and hear the couple exchange their vows; and the gathering of a special collection so that the generosity of those in attendance on this special day may reach beyond the couple to serve some social good.[109] Both authors similarly decry the consumerism that is reflected in many Catholic weddings today and claim that such elaborate and expensive plans do not reflect the "authentically Christian understanding of marriage."[110] Unless the texts of the Scriptures proclaimed and of the blessings invoked actually reflect spousal equality, then those in attendance will continue to be confused by the mixed messages about the expectations for women and men in the sacrament of marriage.

These ambiguities point instead to the need for a liturgical renewal that would explicitly express the equality of women and men within marriage. This renewal would require either omitting some traditional prayers, or making them optional. Since liturgy has great power in shaping our dispositions and in shaping our self-perceptions, the renewal of the *Rite of Marriage* should be a priority for the church. It is not enough that the Nuptial Blessing pray that the husband will recognize his wife as his equal, especially when the prayer itself alludes to the text of Ephesians 5 by invoking the metaphorical relationship of Christ and the church. If the church intends to affirm the dignity of women and their equal power with men, such claims must be explicit in the liturgical expression of the sacrament of marriage.

There are hopeful seeds of this kind of renewal already embedded within the *Rite*. First, the church sees the bride and groom as ministers of the sacrament of marriage.[111] In their free consent and in their promises to love and care for one another, they confer upon each other the sacrament. The presider and the congregation are present to publicly witness the couple's exchange of vows and to offer their love and support, but the bride and groom are ministers of the sacrament for each other.

In addition, the exchange of vows within the *Rite of Marriage* offers a succinct vision of marriage with honesty, love, stability, and fidelity at the center. The vows exchanged between the couple proclaim, "I promise to be true to you in good times and in bad, in sickness and in health. I will love you and honor you all the days of my life."[112] The 1969 *Rite* revised the language of these vows so that women no longer vow to "obey" their husbands.[113] This is an important shift that should not be taken lightly. The vows, in their profession of fidelity through hard times and commitment throughout life, provide an ideal vision of the Christian understanding of marital commitment. In the language of the vows, procreation is strikingly absent. Wives do not promise to bear children, but rather promise to be companions in life's journey and to be honest and loving partners. While some would interpret the duty to procreate as part of "honoring" one's spouse, this is not at all self-evident. For these reasons, these vows can still be considered liberating for women and men. The vows call the couple to mutual fidelity, mutual love, and mutual commitment. That they are reciprocated within the liturgy points to some understanding of the equal partnership envisioned by this part of the *Rite of Marriage*. While the wedding liturgy continues to offer confusing messages with regard to the dignity and equality of women within the sacrament of marriage, there have been important shifts of emphasis since Vatican II, and seeds of a more egalitarian vision are already present within the current *Rite*.

CONCLUSION

Family ministries, marriage preparation programs, and the prayers of the wedding liturgy provide opportunities for the church to evangelize couples and the wider church about the heart of the Christian vocation to marriage. These moments provide an opportunity for the church to proclaim its public theology of Christian marriage. Unfortunately, the legacy of patriarchal marriage traditions and the lingering effects of this sexism in Christian theology and practice continue to obfuscate the church's claim that Christian marriage is a *partnership* and that this partnership is ordered towards the *good of spouses*.[114] Church teaching promotes the full flourishing of both spouses in marriage, but in at least three pastoral moments women hear confusing messages about what is expected of them in marriage and family life. Now, more than ever, it is important that men and women hear, in everyday faith formation, that men and women are equal and that marriage should be life-affirming for both spouses. In these pastoral moments, couples should be invited to consider how God is calling them—in their unique circumstances—to embrace the call to love one another and by so doing, to experience the grace of God who is Love (1 Jn 4:8).

NOTES

1. Michael G. Lawler and Fail S. Risch, "Time, Sex, and Money: The First Five Years of Marriage," *America* (May 14, 2001): 20–22. See also David Popenoe and Barbara Whitehead, *The State of Our Unions* (National Marriage Project, Rutgers University, 2006).

2. The United States Conference of Catholic Bishops' *For Your Marriage* website offers information about Catholic theology of marriage as well as "person on the street" interviews in which couples speak in their own words about the ways they show love and commitment for their spouses every day. The website encourages increased communication between spouses and focuses on everyday acts of marital love as the key to understanding the challenges of

marriage in our culture. The site also includes information about family counseling, marriage therapy, and resources for persons with special concerns related to alcoholism, domestic violence, or infertility. United States Conference of Catholic Bishops, http://www.foryourmarriage.org (accessed January 25, 2008).

3. Ad Hoc Committee on Marriage and Family Life, National Conference of Catholic Bishops, *A Family Perspective in Church and Society: A Manual for All Pastoral Leaders*, 10th Anniversary Ed. (Washington, DC: USCCB Office for Publishing, 1998).

4. Julie Hanlon Rubio, "Does Family Conflict with Community?" *Theological Studies* 58 (December 1997): 597–617; *A Christian Theology of Marriage and Family* (New York: Paulist, 2003) and *Family Ethics: Practices for Christians* (Washington DC: Georgetown University Press, 2010), 190–213.

5. John Paul II, *Familiaris Consortio*, (1981), Available online: http://www.vatican.va/holy_father/john_paul_ii/apost_exhortations/documents/hf_jp-ii_exh_19811122_familiaris-consortio_en.html (Accessed August 2, 2014), no. 21.

6. Al-Anon is a network of support groups who provide support for friends and family of problem drinkers. See the website of Al-Anon Family Groups: http://www.al-anon.alateen.org/ (Accessed August 2, 2014).

7. Sally Purvis, "A Common Love: Christian Feminist Ethics and the Family," in *Religion, Feminism, and the Family*, ed. Anne Carr and Mary Stewart Van Leeuwen (Louisville, KY: Westminster John Knox Press, 1996), 121. See also Lisa Sowle Cahill, *Family*, 130–137.

8. "Dorothy Day," Website of the Catholic Worker Movement: http://www.catholicworker.org/dorothyday/ddbiographytext.cfm?Number=72 (Accessed August 2, 2014).

9. National Conference of Catholic Bishops Committee on Pastoral Practices, *Faithful to Each Other Forever: A Catholic Handbook of Pastoral Help for Marriage Preparation* (Washington, DC: United States Conference of Catholic Bishops, 1988).

10. Except for the fact that it is out of print and not widely available.

11. Cana Conference of Chicago, Family Ministries Office of the Archdiocese of Chicago, *In the Spirit of Cana: Guidelines for Pastoral Outreach to Christian Marriage: Formation, Celebration, and Continuing Education* (Chicago, IL: Archdiocese of Chicago, 2005, Rev. 2011). See also Austin Flemming, *Parish Weddings* (Chicago, IL: Archdiocese of Chicago Liturgy Training Publications, 1987).

12. Archdiocese of Chicago Family Ministries Office, *A Marriage in the Lord*, 5th ed. (Chicago, IL: Archdiocese of Chicago, 2007). The companion book for pastoral ministers is *A Ministry to Marriage: Leader's Guide to A Marriage in the Lord* (Chicago, IL: Archdiocese of Chicago, 2007); Paul Covino, Ed., *Celebrating Marriage: Preparing the Wedding Liturgy*, Rev. Ed. (Portland, OR: Pastoral Press, 1994); Anthony Garascia, *Before "I Do": Preparing for the Sacrament of Marriage* (Notre Dame, IN: Ave Maria Press, 1999); Joseph M. Champlin, *Together for Life: A Preparation for Marriage and for the Ceremony* (Notre Dame, IN: Ave Maria Press, 2000).

13. Anthony Garascia, *Before "I Do,"* 50–51.

14. Family Ministries Office, *A Marriage in the Lord*, 58–59.

15. Lee M. Williams, Lisa A. Riley, Gail S. Risch, and David T. van Dyke, "An Empirical Approach to Designing Marriage Preparation Programs," *American Journal of Family Therapy* 27 (1999): 271–283.

16. Family Ministries Office, *In the Spirit of Cana*, 2–30. Italics in original.

17. Ibid., 2–31.

18. Ibid.

19. *A Marriage in the Lord* explicitly quotes 1 Corinthians 7:3–4 and Proverbs 5:18–19. See Family Ministries Office, *A Marriage*, 46. See also David M. Thomas' explanation of how marital love should be thought of as gift: "Christian marriage enriches each spouse because the love at its heart is fundamentally altruistic. Each person in marriage offers himself or herself to the other in a somewhat paradoxical move that exemplifies the New Testament notion that it is in giving that we receive and in dying that we gain life. When we give of ourselves, we don't lose anything. . . . Success in marriage is more about giving than getting. . . . Agapaic love is love written large. It is that kind of love that enables us to give ourselves, our attention, our time, our energy, our thoughts, our entire being to another as a gift. And we don't ask for

anything in return." David M. Thomas, *Christian Marriage: The New Challenge* (Collegeville, MN: Liturgical Press, 2007), 28–31.

20. Data from the Guttmacher Institute, a non-profit institution that studies reproductive health, indicates that 95 percent of survey respondents reported they had had premarital sex; 93 percent said they did so by age thirty. 2005 data show median age at first marriage is just over twenty-five for women and twenty-seven for men. Sharon Jayson, "Most Americans have had premarital sex, study finds," *USA Today* (December 19, 2006) Section 1A; Within the Diocese of Denver, 91 percent of engaged couples surveyed in 2000 reported that they were sexually active and 66 percent were cohabiting, in a study done in preparation for their diocesan document *What God Has Joined*, See *AD2000* 14:5 (June 2001), 8; While the proportion of adolescents who are sexually experienced has decreased in recent years, 34 percent of ninth graders and 61 percent of twelfth graders report having had sexual intercourse; 7 percent of high school students say they first had intercourse before age 13. See Grunbaum et al., "Youth Risk Behavior Surveillance, United States, 2001," *Morbidity and Mortality Weekly Report*, 51(SS-04) (2002) 1–62. See also Lawrence B. Finer, "Trends in Premarital Sex in the United States, 1954–2003," *Public Health Reports* 122 (January–February 2007): 73–78.

21. Centers for Disease Control and Prevention, *Revised Recommendations for HIV Testing of Adults, Adolescents, and Pregnant Women in Health Care Settings* (Atlanta, GA: CDC, September 2006). These data are part of the reason why the CDC now recommends routine HIV testing, so that more people will know that they are HIV positive and can then both access care and treatment for themselves and also reduce risk behaviors to prevent spreading the virus to others.

22. Recall, for example, the story of Grace, who was exposed to HIV through sexual intercourse with her boyfriend, whom she later married (chapter 2). Grace explained, "It can happen to anyone."

23. Engaged persons who are drug users or former drug users, or who are members of any other HIV "risk" group, should also be encouraged to take the HIV test and to discuss these risk behaviors with their engaged partners.

24. Unfortunately, one text currently used in diocesan marital preparation programs increases stigma of HIV-affected persons by treating AIDS as an example of "societal evils." See Christopher West, *Good News about Sex and Marriage* (Cincinnati: Servant Books, 2004), 43.

25. I credit Julie Hanlon Rubio with the phrase "dual vocation." See Rubio, *A Christian Theology of Marriage and Family* (New York: Paulist, 2003): 89–110.

26. For Gina Messina-Dysert, the pressure was explicit. The Catholic priest with whom she met for pre-Cana counseling told her "Now that you are going to be married your role is to be a wife and mother. Working outside the home will no longer fit into your life. Your duty is to have children and care for your family." Gina Messina-Dysert, "Selfish Working Mothers Destroying the Natural Order?" (June 5, 2013): http://feminismandreligion.com/2013/06/05/selfish-working-mothers-destroying-the-natural-order-by-gina-messina-dysert/ (Accessed June 6, 2013).

27. Arlie Hothschild with Anne Machung, *The Second Shift: Working Parents and the Revolution at Home* (New York: Viking, 1989); Christine Firer Hinze, "Bridge Discourse on Wage Justice: Roman Catholic and Feminist Perspectives on the Family Living Wage," in *Feminist Ethics and the Catholic Moral Tradition*, ed. Charles E. Curran, Margaret Farley, and Richard A. McCormick, S.J. (Mahwah, NJ: Paulist, 1996), 511–540.

28. Family Ministries Office, *A Marriage*, 34.

29. Ibid.

30. Ibid., 60, 71; Garascia, *Before "I Do,"* 89.

31. Family Ministries Office, *A Marriage*, 56–61; Garascia, *Before "I Do,"* 40, 84.

32. Gail S. Risch, Lisa A. Riley, and Michael G. Lawler, "Problematic Issues in the Early Years of Marriage: Content for Premarital Education," *Journal of Psychology and Theology* 31 (2003): 253–269; Michael G. Lawler and Gail S. Risch, "Time, Sex, and Money: The First Five Years of Marriage," *America* 184 (2001): 20–21.

33. Rubio, *A Christian Theology of Marriage*, 99.

34. Ibid., 99.

35. Ibid., 109.

36. Rubio, "Does Family Conflict with Community?"
37. Ibid.
38. Bonnie J. Miller-McLemore, "Family and Work: Can Anyone 'Have It All'?" in Anne Carr and Mary Stewart Van Leeuwen, eds., *Religion, Feminism, and the Family* (Louisville, KY: Westminster John Knox Press, 1996), 279.
39. Ibid., 279. Gender inequality and income inequality in the US even received the attention of President Barack Obama in his 2014 State of the Union Address, when he said, "Today, women make up about half our workforce. But they still make 77 cents for every dollar a man earns. That is wrong, and in 2014, it's an embarrassment. A woman deserves equal pay for equal work. She deserves to have a baby without sacrificing her job. A mother deserves a day off to care for a sick child or sick parent without running into hardship—and you know what, a father does, too. It's time to do away with workplace policies that belong in a "Mad Men" episode. This year, let's all come together—Congress, the White House, and businesses from Wall Street to Main Street—to give every woman the opportunity she deserves. Because I firmly believe when women succeed, America succeeds. . . . Inequality has deepened. Upward mobility has stalled. The cold, hard fact is that even in the midst of recovery, too many Americans are working more than ever just to get by—let alone get ahead. And too many still aren't working at all." The full text of the State of the Union Address can be found here: http://www.whitehouse.gov/the-press-office/2014/01/28/president-barack-obamas-state-union-address (accessed June 30, 2014). Further analysis can be found at "State of the Union 2014" at http://www.whitehouse.gov/sotu (Accessed June 30, 2014); Jordan Weissmann, "U.S. Income Inequality: It's Worse Today Than It Was in 1774," http://www.theatlantic.com/business/archive/2012/09/us-income-inequality-its-worse-today-than-it-was-in-1774/262537/ (Accessed June 30, 2014). For global perspective on this problem, see United Nations Development Programme, *Humanity Divided: Confronting Inequality in Developing Countries* (Geneva: UNDP, 2014), available online: http://www.theatlantic.com/business/archive/2012/09/us-income-inequality-its-worse-today-than-it-was-in-1774/262537/ (accessed June 30, 2014). President Obama has tried to rectify this injustice. See The White House, Office of the Press Secretary, "Expanding Opportunity for All" (April 8, 2014): http://www.whitehouse.gov/the-press-office/2014/04/08/fact-sheet-expanding-opportunity-all-ensuring-equal-pay-women-and-promot (Accessed August 2, 2014).
40. Ibid.
41. Ibid., 281.
42. Ibid., 291. See also Margaret A. Farley, "New Patterns of Relationships: Beginnings of a Moral Revolution," *Theological Studies* 36 (December 1975): 627–646, and *Just Love: A Framework for Christian Sexual Ethics* (New York: Continuum, 2006).
43. Unfortunately the preparatory document for the Synod on the Family perpetuates this distortion by criticizing "pervasive gender ideology" and by upholding gender essentialism. See *Instrumentum Laboris: The Pastoral Challenges of the Family in the Context of Evangelization* (2014):http://www.vatican.va/roman_curia/synod/documents/rc_synod_doc_20140626_instrumentum-laboris-familia_en.html(Accessed August 2, 2014).
44. This aim is explicit in these publications. One reads, "The formal marriage preparation period is in most instances an opportunity for the Church to evangelize and catechize those who come to celebrate the Sacrament of Matrimony. . . . It is an opportunity for adult faith formation." Family Ministries Office, *In the Spirit of Cana,* xi.
45. John Paul II, *Familiaris consortio* (1981), 14.
46. Paul VI, *Humanae vitae* (1968), 12.
47. The *Catechism* explains that procreation is a duty: "Called to give life, spouses share in the creative power and fatherhood of God. Married couples should regard it as their proper mission to transmit human life and to educate their children; they should realize that they are thereby cooperating with the love of God the creator and are, in a certain sense, its interpreters. They will fulfill this duty with a sense of human and Christian responsibility." Interdicasterial Commission for the Catechism, *Catechism of the Catholic Church* (CCC), (New York: Doubleday, 1995), no. 2367.
48. Some widely used publications include Mary Shivanandan, *Catholic Update: The How and Why of Natural Family Planning* (Cincinnati, OH: St. Anthony Messenger Press, 1995);

Charles and Elizabeth Balsam, *Family Planning: A Guide for Exploring the Issues*, 3rd ed. (Liguori, MO: Liguori Publications, 1994); John F. Kippley and Sheila K. Kippley, *The Art of Natural Family Planning*, 4th ed. (Cincinnati, OH: Couple to Couple League, 2005); Lyn Billings and Ann Westinore, *The Billings Method: Controlling Fertility Without Drugs or Devices* (Lewiston, NY: Life Cycle Books, 2000). See also: Donald DeMarco, *New Perspectives on Contraception* (Dayton, OH: One More Soul, 1999), Mary R. Joyce, *Women and Choice: A New Beginning* (St. Cloud, MN: LifeCom, 1985), Hanna Klaus, *Natural Family Planning: A Review*, 2nd ed. (Bethseda, MD: Natural Family Planning Center, 1995), Janet E. Smith, ed., *Why Humanae Vitae Was Right: A Reader* (San Francisco, CA: Ignatius Press, 1993), United States Catholic Conference, *Human Sexuality: A Catholic Perspective for Education and Lifelong Learning* (Washington, DC: USCCB, 1990), Christopher West, *The Good News About Sex and Marriage: Answers to Your Honest Questions About Catholic Teaching* (Ann Arbor, MI: Servant Publications, 2000), Mercedes Arzu Wilson, *Love and Fertility: How to Avoid or Achieve Pregnancy . . . Naturally!* (Dunkirk, MD: Family of the Americas Foundation, 1992); Merryl Winstein, *Your Fertility Signals: Using them to Achieve or Avoid Pregnancy, Naturally* (St. Louis, MO: Smooth Stone Press, 1998). For a non-Catholic perspective, see Toni Weschler, *Taking Charge of Your Fertility: The Definitive Guide to Natural Birth Control, Pregnancy Achievement, and Reproductive Health* (New York: HarperCollins, 2006).

49. Gender essentialism asserts that biological differences between men and women prescribe role differentiations that demand unequal distributions of power within the family and limit the contributions women can make in the public sphere. Gender essentialism is harmful for men as well as for women. When we instead recognize the influence of socialization, it becomes far more difficult to name any natural qualities of women or men that are not dependent, in some way, on culture, history, family of origin, or social location. While sexual difference is a given aspect of human anthropology, this aspect of our embodied nature does not necessitate strict role differentiations. See Lisa Sowle Cahill, "The body-in context," in *Sex, Gender, and Christian Ethics* (Cambridge: Cambridge University Press, 1996), 73–107, esp 82–105, *Family: A Christian Social Perspective* (Minneapolis, MN: Fortress, 2000), 91; Margaret A. Farley, "The Church and the Family: An Ethical Task," *Horizons* 10:1 (1983) 50–71; Susan A. Ross, *Extravagant Affections*, 99; *Proceedings of the Catholic Theological Society of North America* 44 (1989), 199–205; Christine E. Gudorf, "Western Religion and the Patriarchal Family," in *Perspectives on Marriage: A Reader*, 2ed., ed., Kieran Scott and Michael Warren (New York: Oxford University Press, 2001): 285–304; Christine E. Gudorf, *Body, Sex, and Pleasure: Reconstructing Christian Sexual Ethics* (Cleveland, OH: Pilgrim, 1994) 29.

50. John and Sheila Kippley, *The Art of Natural Family Planning*, 279–294; Charles and Elizabeth Balsam, *Family Planning: A Guide*, 7–8, 15–21; "The Deadly After-Effect of Abortion: Breast Cancer," "The Pill," "Tubal Ligation," and "Vasectomy," (Cincinnati, OH: The Couple to Couple League).

51. The signs of fertility are basal temperature, taken upon waking in the morning, and changes in vaginal mucus monitored daily and recorded throughout the month. Irregular sleeping patterns can disrupt the woman's ability to monitor her basal temperature, and many medications, including over-the-counter cold medications, affect her mucus patterns. Emotional stress, athletic training, and lactation can delay ovulation, and prevent regular monthly patterns. For couples who hope to conceive, NFP can help the couple to time their love-making to optimize the potential for conception.

52. James Trussell and Laurence Grummer-Strawn, "Contraceptive Failure of the Ovulation Method of Periodic Abstinence," *Family Planning Perspectives* 22 (March/April 1990): 70.

53. The man does not need to take his daily temperature, monitor any sexual fluids, or record this information on a written chart or in a computer program. While many of the NFP training guides recommend that the husband assist the wife, this isn't always possible or preferable (when, for example, the woman checks her vaginal mucus before urination). While it is true that husband and wife need to communicate about whether sexual intercourse is advisable based on their willingness to conceive, one can imagine that this communication might not only include the "unity of their deeper purpose" (as *Humanae vitae* describes it) but also genuine frustration or conflict with regard to sexual abstinence or confusing patterns of fertility. If the woman is responsible for communicating to her husband about the timing of their

love-making, she is also in the position to reject her husband's sexual advances during imprudent times of her cycle. One can imagine that these conversations could lead to resentment over time.

54. *The Art,* 103. Later in the book the authors explain: "You and your spouse can look into each other's eyes only for so long. Then you start noticing the pimples—your mutual personality defects. In the natural order of things, a newly married couple soon direct their energies to their children, children who are the physical expressions of their love, their joint projects. Children are a great blessing and joy to their parents in more ways than one." Ibid., 238. The Kippleys' understanding of a childless marriage as incomplete and selfish might seem immature and even offensive to many married couples today. If a spouse feels compelled to have children because she can no longer accept the personality defects of her partner, this hardly seems virtuous.

55. Gail S. Risch, Lisa A. Riley, and Michael G. Lawler, "Problematic Issues in the Early Years of Marriage," *Journal of Psychology and Theology* 31 (2003): 253–269.

56. "Breastfeeding: Does it really space babies?" (Cincinnati, OH: Couple to Couple League, 1998).

57. "The First Three Years: They're Important," (Cincinnati, OH: Foundation for the Family, 1999). Emphasis mine.

58. Charles J. Reid, Jr., "The History of the Family," in *Concilium 1995/4: The Family* (Maryknoll, New York: Orbis, 1995), 10–17. See also Don S. Browning, *Marriage and Modernization: How Globalization Threatens Marriage and What to Do About It* (Grand Rapids, Michigan: Eerdmans, 2003); Don S. Browning, Bonnie J. Miller-McLemore, Pamela D. Couture, K. Brynolf Lyon, and Robert M. Franklin, eds., *From Culture Wars to Common Ground: Religion and the American Family Debate* (Louisville, KY: Westminster John Knox Press, 1997); David Matzko McCarthy, *Sex and Love in the Home: A Theology of the Household* (London: SCM Press, 2004); The *Good Life: Genuine Christianity for the Middle Class* (Grand Rapids, Michigan: Brazos, 2004).

59. After quoting Luke 9:23–25, one text explains, "Losing your life for his sake doesn't refer only to ultimate martyrdom. It also applies to those little martyrdoms of everyday life in which you 'die' to some expression of self-will and find yourself correspondingly enriched. . . . Don't feel sorry for yourself. Instead, give meaning to your sufferings. Join your difficulties with the suffering of the Lord Jesus." John and Sheila Kippley, *The Art of Natural Family Planning*, 252–253.

60. I find it particularly troubling that many pastoral references have begun to include recommendations that the couple explore Christopher West's interpretation of the "theology of the body," as expressed in Christopher West, *Theology of the Body Explained* (Boston, MA: Pauline Books & Media, 2003) or Christopher West, *Good News About Sex & Marriage* (Cincinnati, OH: Servant Publications, 2000). While time does not permit me to address the flaws of these texts, they fail at a basic level to affirm self-care as a moral virtue and central commandment of Christian discipleship.

61. As quoted in Cristina L. H. Traina, "Papal Ideals, Marital Realities: One View from the Ground," in Patricia Beattie Jung and Joseph Andrew Coray, eds., *Sexual Diversity and Catholicism* (Collegeville, MN: Liturgical Press, 2001), 269–288, at 277. Traina cites Karol Wojtyla (John Paul II), *Love and Responsibility*, trans. H. T. Willetts (New York: Farrar, Straus, and Giroux, 1981), 237–239.

62. Gudorf, *Body, Sex*; John T. Noonan, Jr., "Contraception: The Doctrine and the Context," in Paulinus Ikechukwu Odozor, C.S.Sp., ed., *Sexuality, Marriage, and Family: Readings in the Catholic Tradition* (Notre Dame, IN: University of Notre Dame Press, 2001) 423–463; Richard A. McCormick, S.J., "*Humanae vitae* 25 Years Later," in Odozor, *Sexuality, Marriage*, 478–485.

63. Traina, "Papal Ideals," 279.

64. Christine E. Gudorf, "Contraception and Abortion in Roman Catholicism," in Daniel C. Maguire, ed., *Sacred Rights: The Case for Contraception and Abortion in World Religions* (New York: Oxford University Press, 2003), 55–78, at 67.

65. Philip S. Kaufman, *Why You Can Disagree and Remain a Faithful Catholic* (New York: Crossroad, 2000), 52, 101, 199. Kaufman cites a 1993 NCR/Gallup poll in which 73 percent of

all American Catholics and 63 percent who attend Mass weekly agreed that "you can be a good Catholic without obeying Church teaching on birth control." More recently, the Pew Forum *U.S. Religious Landscape Survey* indicates that Catholics in the United States continue to be divided on issues such as abortion, birth control, and homosexuality. See the interactive analysis at Pew Forum on Religion and Public Life, *U.S. Religious Landscape Survey* (2008), http://religions.pewforum.org/portraits#.

66. One canonist explains: "It appears to be irrefutable according to Catholic doctrine that a person infected with the AIDS virus cannot morally engage in sexual intercourse." W. A. Varvaro, "Prohibition Against Marriage of AIDS Victims," in *Roman Replies and Canon Law Society of America Advisory Opinions* (Washington, DC: Canon Law Society of America, 1987), 121. See chapters 4 and 5 for further analysis of this complex issue.

67. Centers for Disease Control and Prevention, *National Crime Victimization Survey: 1992–1996* (Atlanta, Georgia: Centers for Disease Control and Prevention, 1998).

68. Garascia, *Before "I Do,"* 27, 29.

69. The treatment is only two paragraphs in length.

70. *A Marriage*, 44.

71. Ibid., 46.

72. Ibid.

73. *Before "I Do,"* 38.

74. This interpretation is found in Pius XI, *Casti Connubii* (1930), http://www.vatican.va/holy_father/pius_xi/encyclicals/documents/hf_p-xi_enc_31121930_casti-connubii_en.html (Accessed August 2, 2014), no. 26. For theo-ethical analysis of violence against women in marriage, see Don S. Browning, "Domestic Violence and the Ethic of Equal Regard," in *Equality and the Family: A Fundamental, Practical Theology of Children, Mothers, and Fathers in Modern Societies* (Grand Rapids, MI: Eerdmans, 2007) 374–387; Daniel C. Maguire and Sa'diyya Shaikh, eds., *Violence Against Women in Contemporary World Religions* (Cleveland, OH: Pilgrim Press, 2007); Linda A. Bell, *Rethinking Ethics in the Midst of Violence: A Feminist Approach to Freedom* (Lanham, MD: Rowman & Littlefield, 1993); Joanne Carlson Brown and Carole R. Bohn, eds., *Christianity, Patriarchy, and Abuse: A Feminist Critique* (Cleveland, OH: Pilgrim Press, 1989); Rita Nakashima Brock and Rebecca Ann Parker, *Proverbs of Ashes: Violence, Redemptive Suffering, and the Search for What Saves Us* (Boston, MA: Beacon Press, 2001); Beverly Wildung Harrison, *Making the Connections: Essays in Feminist Social Ethics*, ed. Carol S. Robb (Boston, MA: Beacon, 1985).

75. This is not the only possible method of analysis. Marriage preparation manuals could engage multiple methods of biblical interpretation. My point is simply that the texts should be analyzed; they cannot speak for themselves. Elisabeth Schussler Fiorenza distinguishes between four methods: hermeneutics of suspicion, hermeneutics of proclamation, herememeutics of remembrance, and hermeneutics of celebration. See *Bread Not Stone: The Challenge of Feminist Biblical Interpretation* (Boston: Beacon, 1995), 1–22.

76. For an overview of international statistics with analysis, see UNFPA, "Gender-Based Violence: A Price Too High," in *State of World Population 2005: The Promise of Equality* (New York: United Nations Population Fund, 2005), 65–73; "Combat Violence Against Women," in UN Millennium Project Task Force on Education and Gender Equity, *Taking Action: Achieving Gender Equality and Empowering Women* (Sterling, VA: United Nations Millennium Project, 2005), 110–121.

77. United States Conference of Catholic Bishops, *When I Call For Help* (Washington, DC: United States Conference of Catholic Bishops, 2002).

78. For centuries husbands were duty bound to "discipline" their wives. Rosemary Radford Ruether, "The Western Religious Tradition and Violence Against Women in the Home," in Joanne Carlson Brown and Carole R. Bohn, eds., *Christianity, Patriarchy, and Abuse: A Feminist Critique* (Cleveland: Pilgrim, 1989), 41–41, at 34–35. See also R. E. Dobash and R. Dobash, *Violence Against Wives: A Case Against the Patriarchy* (New York: Free Press, 1979), 137.

79. Karen Leslie Hernandez, "Where is God in Abusive Relationships?" (June 13, 2014): http://feminismandreligion.com/2014/06/13/where-is-god-in-abusive-relationships-by-karen-leslie-hernandez/ (Accessed July 8, 2014).

80. Sacred Congregation of Rites, *Rite of Marriage*, 1969, in *The Rites of the Catholic Church* (New York: Pueblo, 1982), 560.

81. Cf., chapter 5.

82. *Rite*, nos. 67–105. It is customary to have three readings and one sung Psalm. In most cases the first reading is selected from the Old Testament, followed by the sung Psalm, followed by a reading from the epistles of the New Testament, followed by a sung Alleluia, followed by a gospel reading from the New Testament. The couple can choose from the following selections: Gn 1:26–28, 31a; 2:18–24; 24:48–51, 58–67; Tb 7:9–10, 11–15; 8:5–10; Sg 2:8–10, 14, 16a; 8:6–7a; Sir 26:1–4, 16–21; Eccl 26:1–4, 16–21; Jer 31:31–32a, 33–34a; Rom 8:31b–35, 37–39; Rom 12:1–2, 9–18; 1 Cor 6:13c–15a, 17–20, 12:31; 13:8a; Eph 5:2a, 21–33; Col 3:12–17; 1 Pt 3:1–9; 1 Jn 3:18–24; 1 Jn 4:7–12; Rv 19:1, 5–9a; Ps 33:12, 18, 20–22; Ps 34: 2–9; Ps 103:1–2, 8, 13, 17–18a; Ps 112: 1–9; Ps 128: 1–5; Ps 145: 8–10, 15, 17–18; Ps 148: 1–4, 9–14; 1 Jn 4:7b, 8, 11, 12, 16; Mt 5:1–12; Mt 5:13–16; Mt 7:21, 24–29; Mt 19:3–6; Mt 22:35–40; Mk 10:6–9; Jn 2:1–11; Jn 15:9–12; Jn 15:12–16; Jn 17:20–26. The 1990 *Order for Celebrating Marriage* includes five additional texts: Prv 31: 10–13, 19–20, 30–31; Rom 15:1b–3a, 5–7, 13; Eph 4:1–6; Phil 4:4–9; Heb 13:1–4a; 5–6b. Currently this *Order* is available only in Latin; the English text is expected to be approved by the United States Conference of Catholic Bishops in the near future. For a brief commentary on these readings, see Paul Covino, *Celebrating Marriage*, 51–83; Joseph M. Champlin, *Together for Life*, or Robert Crotty and John Barry Ryan, *Commentary on the Ritual Readings* (New York: Pueblo, 1982).

83. Introduction to the *Rite of Marriage*, no. 6. in *Rites*, 555.

84. *Lectionary for Mass for Use in the Dioceses of the United States*, 2nd ed (Washington, DC: Confraternity of Christian Doctrine, 2002).

85. Sir 26:1–4;13–16.

86. One commentary notes that this description of a good wife is from the husband's point of view, which seems to place too great an emphasis on her function to provide him happiness. Paul Covino, ed., *Celebrating Marriage* (Portland, OR: Pastoral Press, 1994), 61.

87. Gn 24:48, 51, 67; Tb 7:10, 12; Prov 31:10.

88. Ps 128:3–5. See also the Genesis mandate to "be fruitful and multiply," Gn 1:28, and the blessing on Rebekah that her thousands of descendants may "gain possession of the gates of their enemies," Gn 24:60.

89. 1 Pt 3:7.

90. Gn 1 26-28, 31a, or Gn 2:18–24.

91. Jer 31:31-32a, 33–34a.

92. As Paul Covino claims in a recent publication, "Marriage Ministry and the Rite of Marriage," *Origins* 37:21 (November 2007): 333–339, at 336. See also Mark Searle, "Marriage Rites as Documents of Faith: Notes for a Theology of Marriage" in Mark Searle and Kenneth W. Stevenson, *Documents of the Marriage Liturgy* (Collegeville, MN: The Liturgical Press, 1992).

93. Covino, "Marriage," 336.

94. Rubio, *A Christian Theology*, 45.

95. *Rite of Marriage*, no. 108.

96. Ibid., no. 59.

97. *Rite*, no 24. Couples affected by HIV/AIDS could presumably request that these references be omitted, as is possible for couples who marry late in life.

98. Ibid., no. 120.

99. Kenneth Stevenson, *Nuptial Blessing: A Study of Christian Marriage Rites* (London: Alcuin SPCK, 1982), 46, 188.

100. Ibid., 46.

101. Covino, "Marriage Ministry," 335.

102. Ibid., 334.

103. Rubio, *A Christian Theology*, 25.

104. Ibid., 37–43.

105. Ibid. See *Rite of Marriage*, no. 20; Covino, *Celebrating Marriage*, 13–27.

106. Covino, "Marriage Ministry," 337.

107. Ibid.

108. Ibid.
109. Ibid., 337–338; Rubio, *A Theology of Marriage,* 25–43. See also Austin Flemming, *Parish Weddings* (Chicago, IL: Liturgy Training Publications, 1987).
110. Covino, "Marriage Ministry," 339.
111. CCC, no. 1623. For a description of theological trends since Vatican II, see Joseph Martos, *Doors to the Sacred* (Garden City, NY: Doubleday, 1981), 379–387.
112. *Rite,* no. 60.
113. Stevenson, *Nuptial*, 188.
114. CCC, no. 1601.

Conclusion

> So when he had washed their feet, and taken his garments and reclined at the table again, he said to them, "Do you know what I have done to you? You call me Teacher and Lord; and you are right, for so I am. If I, then, the Lord and the Teacher, washed your feet, you also ought to wash one another's feet."
> Jn13:12–14

HIV/AIDS is one of the most pressing public health, economic, and human rights crises of our time. But the response of Christians has too often been slowed by an inability to listen to the experiences of those most knowledgeable about HIV. This project is only able to tell a very small part of a very large story. While partial, contextual and limited, the study is no less valuable for church members. In these concluding remarks I point to ongoing ecclesial investigations that could benefit from attention to these women's stories, I describe the limitations of this study, and I reflect upon the need for storytelling and listening as part of what it means to be church. Storytelling and listening together reflect the starting point of solidarity that is necessary more than ever in this time of HIV/AIDS. The hope of this project is that it not only helps my readers to better understand this particular problem, but that we are motivated to respond, to let it challenge us, that we may understand in a new way the demands of Christian discipleship.

A SHIFTING LANDSCAPE

This project has sought to listen to the experiences of a cohort of eight Catholic, married, HIV-positive women to better understand what thwarts their flourishing. My recommendations for church communities are aimed at preventing HIV infection, naming and eliminating stigma to create an inclusive church community, and crafting a theology of marriage that recognizes the lingering impacts of sexism in Christian marriage traditions and works to empower women to be equal partners who experience marriage as graced encounter with God. The project is thus at the intersection of many different but related fields: health care ethics, sexual ethics, social ethics, and feminist ethics, to name a few. Much has changed in these fields since the research began.

The papacy of Pope Francis has marked a major shift in how the Catholic Church is perceived in the world. The pope's focus on social justice and the way he presents himself as a humble pastor have refocused attention to themes of mercy and solidarity. Within Catholicism, ongoing ecclesial conversations on marriage and the family have raised the hopes among some that Pope Francis will initiate a substantive revision of canon law and theology of marriage. The Extraordinary General Assembly of the Synod of Bishops, held in the Vatican during October 2014, met to investigate "The Pastoral Challenges of the Family in the Context of Evangelization."[1] In the preparatory document, *Instrumentum Laboris*, there was a genuine attempt to solicit the views of a wide range of Catholic faithful including the voices of both clergy and lay people.[2] The *Instrumentum* focused on three areas in advance of the 2014 Extraordinary General Assembly: first, how the Gospel of the Family can be preached in the present-day; second, how the Church's pastoral care program for the family might better respond to new challenges today; and third, how to assist parents in developing a mentality of openness to life and in upbringing their children.[3]

Does this document address the concerns that surfaced in the stories of my collaborators? To some degree, yes. The *Instrumentum* acknowledged the importance of listening, of responding with mercy, and of speaking a word of hope in difficult pastoral moments. Consider the following:

- The primary task of the Church is to proclaim the beauty of the vocation to love which holds great potential for society and the Church. To meet this urgency, the episcopate throughout the world is being called, *cum et sub Petro*, to listen humbly to the Holy Spirit and reflect on today's pastoral challenges (preface).
- The Church needs to provide care for families living in critical and stressful situations, ensuring that the family be attended in its entirety. The quality of the relationships within the family must be of utmost concern for the Church. Initial support originates in a parish, which is the "family of families." It is the principal center of a renewed pastoral care which receives and guides people and is animated by sentiments of mercy and tenderness. In this regard, parish organizations have a significant role in sustaining the family (no. 46).

- Other difficulties affecting the family, in additional to physical illnesses, including AIDS, are: mental illness, depression and the death of a child or spouse, all of which call for a pastoral approach which takes into account the unique family situation. . . . The power and urgency of proclaiming the Gospel of mercy is crucial for a Christian community in the course of providing for and receiving persons in these difficulties, especially when a family is particularly in need (no. 79).

The tone of the *Instrumentum* is pastoral and sensitive to the realities of suffering. A major motif of the document is that the church should be a place of mercy and assistance, not a place of shame or disregard. And the women in this study would be pleased to see that the difficulties of their lives are acknowledged as the plight of families affected by AIDS receives explicit mention when discussing "critical situations" worldwide.

Nevertheless, there are some peculiar elements and discouraging developments. The document begins by proclaiming the "Gospel of the Family" and ends with a prayer to the Holy Family of Nazareth, "the sure point of reference and comfort for every family."[4] Drew Christiansen finds the scriptural foundations, especially the focus on Jesus's family, to be a curious beginning: "A biblical theology of the family that focuses on the Holy Family and thinks of the (nuclear) family as uniform through history is faithful neither to the text, nor to history of the church's pastoral experience."[5] Christiansen notes that the gospels provide difficult sayings on the family, and that the Synod risks over-sacralizing and hyper-inflating the importance of the family.

Another curious element is the revisionist history implicit in the claim: "Throughout the centuries the Church has maintained her constant teaching on marriage and family,"[6] which seems to say that marriage teachings are unchanging and have not developed over time. The document then cites *Gaudium et spes*, helpfully emphasizing marriage as a "community of life and love," but does not attend to the significance of this theology as a shift away from previous magisterial teachings that focused on hierarchical ends of marriage.[7] The *Instrumentum* reports a widespread lack of understanding of church teaching, and seems to imply that one answer would be increased catechetical efforts,[8] especially efforts to explain church teaching in fresh language.[9] Julie Hanlon Rubio remarks: "The working document sometimes gives the impression that the Synod's response will be to condemn the culture and repeat old teachings dressed up in language that sounds new to very few."[10]

Given that the role of the woman in the family is a particularly important question, it is troubling that the document is dismissive of the so-called "ideology of gender theory," which is reported as a problem that must be addressed by restating Christian anthropology,[11] even while the "theology of the body" series is lifted up as a possible resource in this construction of Christian anthropology.[12]

Finally, even while there is evidence of a lack of reception of some teachings, many of those same teachings are simply restated. Archbishop Joseph Kurtz of Louisville, Kentucky, the President of the United States Conference of Catholic Bishops, explained in an interview for *National Catholic Reporter* that the emerging conversations on marriage and family are an opportunity to re-evangelize the faithful. "We know there is a need for greater, effective teaching on key tenets of the faith, such as the indissolubility of marriage, the importance of sexual difference for marriage, the natural law, and the married couple's call to be open to life."[13] Cardinal Vincent Nichols of Westminster explained that the Synod's goal was not to change church teachings, as when he argued: "You may have heard or read that this Synod has been about changing the teaching of the Church on marriage, family life or sexual morality. This is not true. It was about the pastoral care that we try to offer each other, the 'motherly love of the Church,' especially when facing difficult moments and experiences in family life."[14]

The 2014 Extraordinary General Assembly was widely covered by the media, and was undoubtedly an opportunity for deep reflection on the theology of marriage and contemporary challenges to family life. The final report of the 2014 Synod, *Relatio Synodi*, was released on October 18, 2014, and functions as the working document for the 2015 Ordinary General Assembly.[15] The final report contains many of the same elements as the preparatory document, including an invitation to "look to the reality of the family today in all its complexity, with both its lights and shadows,"[16] the recognition that "the dignity of women still needs to be defended and promoted,"[17] the importance of "building relationships of self-giving and creative reciprocity, which are empowering and supportive,"[18] and a call to accompany families "in such a way that the real-life experience of the entire ecclesial community can be added to the teaching of the contents of the faith."[19] Whether the ongoing attempts to listen to the experiences of the faithful around the world will lead to different conclusions in the 2015 Synod remains an open question. There could be genuine listening and a willingness on the part of the bishops to reconsider church teachings and even change some teachings. It is also possible that the lack of reception of some teachings could be interpreted as the result of confusion, sin, or failure of communication on the part of the magisterium. A third middle way might yield an attempt to restate the same teachings in a more compelling and pastoral language, a change in tone but not substance. At this point it is too early to know what the bishops' deliberations will yield, and how Pope Francis will frame the Synod's work when he issues his own post-synodal apostolic exhortation.

Two additional groundswells of social change are worth mentioning explicitly. Implementation of the Patient Protection and Affordable Care Act is underway, even while resistance to the law continues, mostly along predictable partisan lines. But public dialogue about the law has forced US citizens to think anew about the promise of health care as a human right, and the implications of such an ideal for civil society. Similarly, when the US Supreme Court ruled that the Defense of Marriage Act was unconstitutional, supporters of same-sex marriage across the country were jubilant. In the coverage of this debate, it has become clear that the definition of marriage remains contested both legally and theologically; there is not yet consensus in the United States regarding the purposes of marriage and whether marriage is a human right. As Christians engage in these complex debates about health care and marriage, much is at stake. My hope is that the analysis of this book will contribute positively to these ongoing deliberations among US Catholics. We live in a country with deep divides, including economic inequalities, racial disparities in health care access, and persistent misogyny and heterosexism in mainstream culture. If we are to heed Pope Francis's call to be *a church in the streets*, Catholics must be more attentive to the everyday experiences of people wounded by generational poverty, racism, sexism, homophobia, and other kinds of structural injustices. A theo-ethical method that incorporates ethnography or participatory action research[20] can provide one way of fostering this much needed discussion within academic and ecclesial contexts; my hope is that this project provides one example of the merits of this kind of work.

LIMITATIONS OF THE STUDY

The methodology of the project is grounded in the belief that attention to human experience (which is integral to Catholic ethics) requires listening to the everyday experiences of Catholics, and especially to those who are marginalized and whose voices are not typically heard in academic or pastoral/theological circles. While this project provided a descriptive account of some women's experiences, their particular experiences arise out of unique familial, geographical, and personal contexts which may be radically dissimilar from my readers' contexts. That they are unique and specific does not invalidate their potential contribution to normative ethics. But neither do their stories invalidate the important contributions of other sources of Christian ethics, including the Bible and Christian traditions. My aim was to bring their life experience into dialogue with the teachings of the church.

Still, this study has real limitations. I interviewed only eight women. These women were not selected from a random sample but rather were recruited through a convenience sampling methodology. Since they were recruited through social service agencies within Chicago, the participants might be more likely to be poor than women selected from a random sample.

Because each woman had known her HIV-positive status for some time, their descriptions of coping with HIV infection might be very different from those by women who are newly diagnosed. The sample of women I interviewed did not include any women younger than thirty-seven years of age at the time of our first meeting, even though HIV infection rates are highest among women between ages twenty-five and thirty-four. In addition, the study entailed a single in-person interview followed by multiple telephone conversations. While I did establish a good rapport with participants, it would have been impossible for a woman to share her whole story within the time constraints. Indeed, even the data from the interviews I conducted included more information than I could bring to the reader. Thus, I have inevitably left out many powerful stories in the attempt to create space for the ones to which I do attend. Further, while the interviews did include discussion of the women's experiences of marriage, I did not interview their spouses. While the majority of participants are involved in support groups that meet regularly, I did not observe their support group meetings. In the future the research could be expanded to include a comparative study of women from other faith traditions, women from other geographical contexts, or an expanded study that would include both spouses in a study on marriage; however, these were beyond the scope of this project.

STORYTELLING AS AN ASPECT OF SELF-CARE

The eight women who shared their stories with me were forthright about their struggles, fears, questions, and hopes. In describing their past struggles—including, for some, failures to love and care for themselves—they had to honestly and openly admit to themselves and to me that they share some responsibility for their situations. This process of sharing their stories was itself an aspect of self-care because in the process of sharing their stories they wanted their experiences to matter for a wider audience. Feminist theologian Denise Ackerman explains that storytelling lies at the very heart of feminist theological praxis because "telling and listening to the stories of those who are suffering, discriminated against, or oppressed is an essential starting point for counteracting silence, denial, and stigma."[21] Indeed, the very act of telling one's story counters silence and denial.

The process of storytelling also invites self-reflection. It offers the opportunity to reflect on one's past, make some sense of one's suffering, and think about goals for one's future. In the process of describing their personal journeys some women wrestled with feelings of shame and of anger. But this was also an opportunity for honesty and self-acceptance, a way for each woman to admit to herself that she can move forward with trust in herself and with some sense of hope.

Ackerman explains the sense-making function of storytelling and of the need for churches to listen to the stories of the marginalized:

> Telling stories is intrinsic to claiming our identity and, in the process, finding impulses for hope. For those living with HIV/AIDS there is a need to claim and to name their identities in order to move away from the victim status often thrust upon them. Telling our stories also has a sense-making function. The act of telling the story assists the narrator in making sense of her or his experiences in an often chaotic world. Whether stories are revealing in shaping identities or whether they are making sense of situations that call for understanding, they should be heard in churches.[22]

The women interviewed in this study felt ignored and silenced within their church. They encountered silence within their parishes, fear among co-workers, and reluctance in church publications to deal with the complex and messy questions that arise for HIV-positive persons who are married. Until their experiences are acknowledged by the wider church community such ignorance, distrust, and silence may continue.

Physician and ethicist Margaret E. Mohrmann explains that persons who are sick often attempt to make sense of their illness through storytelling. For Mohrmann, active listening is essential for physicians, nurses, social workers, and pastoral caregivers. She explains, "There is much to be learned from the way patients tell their own tales of suffering: what they emphasize, the chronology as they have experienced it, the side events that sound unrelated to us but clearly are not to them, what they fear it all means."[23]

Life with HIV is about more than CD4 counts and opportunistic infections. In Mohrmann's descriptions we see that the medical terminology is but one description of the experience of illness and disease. She recalls, as an example, the letters of Flannery O'Connor when she was dying of lupus. Morhmann explains that O'Connor's letters do not mention anemia, bone marrow suppression, or renal failure. Instead, O'Connor wrote of her condition, "The wolf, I'm afraid, is inside tearing up the place."[24] Morhmann concludes:

> It is important to get diagnoses right: to recognize psoriasis and lupus, cancer and schizophrenia, AIDS and alcoholism. . . . It is no less important to recognize that for the sufferer the name of the disease, spiritually speaking, is humiliation or fear or malaise or endless pain or loneliness or despair or the end of a career or the end of a life. It is no less important to recognize that this is a human being to whom a terrible thing is happening and, whatever other name this terrible thing bears, its name is tragedy.[25]

To listen, and to really hear, takes time, compassion, and a willingness to be, in Morhmann's words, "silently present." These experiences challenge the listener to see the one who suffers as a whole human person, a person with dignity, voice, courage, and integrity, even if also a person vulnerable, afraid, or angry. To be invited to tell one's story can be empowering in itself, for it confirms that one's experience is valuable.

But while storytelling can help women to lay claim to their voices, indeed, to their right to speak, such storytelling is not without risk. The storyteller is in a particularly vulnerable position because this self-disclosure can invite judgment, blame, or, in some cases, violent reprisal. We do well to remember the horrific death of Gugu Dlamini of South Africa who was beaten to death in her village when she publicly revealed her HIV-positive status.[26] Ms. Dlamini, mother of a thirteen-year-old daughter, was an AIDS activist who was trying to educate her neighbors about the virus. They did not respond by listening.

While HIV-positive women in the United States today might not fear the extreme violence that Gugu Dlamini suffered, they know all too well that storytelling involves risk. They are all too familiar with the ignorance and fear in their communities. Their storytelling takes courage. But the hope of my collaborators, in participating in this study, was that they could contribute, even in some small way, to the church's deeper understanding of their experiences.

LISTENING AS AN ACT OF SOLIDARITY

Empathetic listening is transformative not only for the one who is able to tell her story but for the listener as well. Such listening does not alleviate suffering, but active listening can honor the person who suffers by communicating that her story is important. The one who listens is a witness to the storyteller's struggle and can honor the storyteller by being present with her and by standing in solidarity with her. To listen to another's suffering, even with the greatest of empathy, is *not* to experience it oneself. To listen might relieve some anxiety, but generally speaking will not eliminate the suffering. It is instead to honor that person's suffering, to admit that it is tragic, to witness its difficulty and to be present with the suffering person in her pain.

To really listen means that one must begin by not speaking. The listener must resist the urge to interrupt, to speak one's own words of sense or explanation, and instead must let the stories of others unsettle us, challenge us, and even change us. This posture can be transformative on both personal and social levels. First, it can be transformative because it upsets power dynamics of hierarchy and privilege. The listener accepts the speaker's authority to speak from experience. This stance is grounded in recognition that no one can have full and complete knowledge, but the work of understanding is a communal process, a coming to know together. Secondly, this posture of listening values all as teachers and requires that the listener adopt a posture of learning. We do not know it all. We must invite guides with personal experiences to tell us how it is for them. Finally, this posture requires that we resist simplistic answers. Answers do come, but after mutual deliberation, after an unsettling process of listening and thinking, and after one's willingness to be transformed.

As public discourse is becoming increasingly polarized, the practice of empathetic listening can enable Christians to wrestle with the messy complex moral problems facing our neighbors. The vocation to solidarity, to which all Christians are called, invites Christians to think of our responsibilities not only to ourselves and our family members but also of our need to be responsible for, and to be accountable to, the common good. Empathetic listening can transform the church's attention to the questions of HIV and AIDS, which are not just abstract questions of canon law or bioethics but concerns about real people and the injustices and sufferings that prevent their flourishing. Now is the time for the church to hear these voices, and to take them into account when thinking theologically about these concerns.

In 2014, in the Holy Thursday ritual that Catholics know so well as the institution of the Eucharist, Pope Francis emphasized not only the presence of Christ in the bread and wine broken and shared, but also in the face of the suffering person. By washing the feet of incarcerated persons, Pope Francis signaled to Christians everywhere that we are called to recognize the human dignity of even those most marginalized and to meet the face of Christ in our neighbor. In 2001, when he was Jorge Bergoglio, he washed and kissed the feet of twelve AIDS patients at a hospice in the Argentinian capital.[27] This model of service, first lived by Jesus and now modeled by the pope, is a model for all Christians to emulate.

It is true that HIV/AIDS is only one pressing moral concern among many others in our world, but it affects real people who suffer every day. We are invited today to be a listening church, a church on the streets, to wash one another's feet, to meet people where they are and witness the love of God in the brokenness and messiness of everyday life. The church can more effectively preach the saving message of Jesus when the church itself is a place where people experience healing, encouragement, compassion, mercy, and love.

NOTES

1. General Secretariat of the Synod of Bishops, *Instrumentum Laboris* (June 2014): http://www.vatican.va/roman_curia/synod/documents/rc_synod_doc_20140626_instrumentum-laboris-familia_en.html (Accessed July 10, 2014).
2. Ibid. The Introduction of the *Instrumentum* explains the timeline and process by which people contributed responses to the questionnaire.
3. Ibid., no. 158.
4. Ibid., 159.

5. Drew Christiansen, "The Gospel of the Family." *America Magazine* (June 26, 2014). http://americamagazine.org/issue/family-context (Accessed July 10, 2014).
6. *Instrumentum*, 4.
7. Ibid., 4.
8. Ibid., 17–18.
9. Ibid., 30.
10. Christiansen, "Gospel of the Family." *America.*
11. *Instrumentum*, 23, 126–127.
12. Ibid., 18.
13. Brian Roewe and Joshua J. McElwee, "US Bishops Vote to Stay the Course." *National Catholic Reporter* (June 20–July 3, 2014), 15.
14. Doug Culp, "Follow Up on the Synod," *FAITH Magazine* (December 2014), 17.
15. Extraordinary General Assembly of the Synod of Bishops, *Relatio Synodi: The Pastoral Challenges of the Family in the Context of Evangelization* (October 18, 2014). http://www.vatican.va/roman_curia/synod/documents/rc_synod_doc_20141018_relatio-synodi-familia_en.html# (Accessed December 2, 2014).
16. Ibid., no. 5.
17. Ibid., no. 8.
18. Ibid., no. 9.
19. Ibid., no. 36. See also no. 46.
20. I have come to believe that Participatory Action Research (PAR) provides a helpful method that overcomes some of the deficiencies of the ethnographic approach I undertook in this research project. In particular, PAR requires a long-term partnership and expects that over time there is a natural breakdown between distinctions of "researcher" and "researched" since PAR is a community-based process of creating knowledge and mobilizing for political action. See A. McIntyre, *Participatory Action Research* (Los Angeles: Sage Publications, 2008); Meredith Minkler and Nina Wallerstein, *Community-Based Participatory Research for Health* (San Francisco: Jossey-Bass, 2003); and S.L. Kindon, et al., *Participatory Action Research Approaches and Methods: Connecting People, Participation, and Place* (London: Routledge, 2007).
21. Denise M. Ackermann, "From Mere Existence to Tenacious Endurance: Stigma, HIV/AIDS and a Feminist Theology of Praxis," in Isabel Apawo Phiri and Saronjini Nadar, eds., *African Women, Religion, and Health: Essays in Honor of Mercy Amba Ewudziwa Oduyoye* (Maryknoll, New York: Orbis, 2006) 221–242, 231.
22. Ibid.
23. Margaret E. Mohrmann, M.D., *Medicine as Ministry: Reflections on Suffering, Ethics, and Hope* (Cleveland, OH: Pilgrim Press, 1995), 67. See also Howard Brody, *Stories of Sickness* (New Haven, CT: Yale University Press, 1987), Arthur Kleinman, M.D., *The Illness Narratives: Suffering, Healing, and the Human Condition* (New York: Basic Books, 1988).
24. Mohrmann, *Medicine*, 68.
25. Ibid., 69.
26. Donald G. McNeil, Jr., "Neighbors Kill An HIV+ AIDS Activist in South Africa," *New York Times* (December 28, 1998), Health, 2.
27. Delia Gallagher, "Pope Francis Washes Feet of Disabled." CNN Online. (April 17, 2014). http://www.cnn.com/2014/04/17/world/europe/pope-francis-washes-feet-of-disabled-people/ (Accessed July 31, 2014).

Afterword

> I thank my God through Jesus Christ for all of you, because your faith is proclaimed throughout the world. For God, whom I serve with my spirit by announcing the gospel of his Son, is my witness that without ceasing I remember you always in my prayers.
> Rom 1: 8–9

During the summer of 2014 I initiated contact with each research participant. I had last spoken with each woman in the summer of 2007 or 2008, approximately one to two years after the first in-person interview. I was eager to learn about how each woman was feeling, and whether anything in her life had changed significantly since our last contact. Talking with the women again was humbling because I realized again how HIV is a part of their everyday lives; even though I have certainly learned a lot about HIV, I cannot speak about living with HIV from personal experience in the way that these women can. I felt a range of emotions during our conversations and realized the work yet to be done by my faith community in order to better address their needs and concerns.

SUE MELTON[1]

Sue is still happily married and while she has had an AIDS diagnosis, her viral load was low again during her last check up. Sue has been very proactive about seeking medical care and learning about her HIV medications. She has never taken a drug holiday. Sue takes fifty-six pills a day now, and is experiencing the long-term toxicity of her HIV medications. But she is still grateful that they have helped her live so long with HIV infection. She is hopeful that her family will benefit from the implementation of the Patient

Protection and Affordable Care Act, but is worried that some AIDS-specific benefits will be cut. Sue continues to work in AIDS education to combat stigma and to raise awareness about sexual health. Sue and her husband continue to struggle financially, and the recession made this worse. "We are basically in the working poor. We still have to eat oatmeal for dinner some nights. It's very difficult." Sue took a three-year break from her local Catholic parish when she could no longer bear to sit in the back of the church, as the priest insisted she must. Then, she had a moment she described as an awakening.

> I realized how clueless he was. I realized he is one man in one building and he does not speak for the whole church. I realized that I did not need his approval to have my faith. I know I would not be here today if I did not have faith. I still believe in Catholicism but that priest does not speak for the whole church. What I've learned is that priests are human. It sounds strange to say it like that because of course they are. But what I mean is that my years of suffering in the back of church are partly my fault. I should have educated him. He is human. We all make mistakes. I wish that I had had the courage to speak up for myself years ago. I carried around that fear and stigma like a boulder on my back for so many years. But now I don't feel it there anymore.

Sue is hopeful that Pope Francis will continue to emphasize love and mercy. "The church will keep the basics, but it needs to change. Sometimes growth is painful, but change can be good."

CHERYL KING[2]

The first thing Cheryl told me is that her HIV is undetectable, "Thanks be to God!" Cheryl thanks God every day for her sobriety and she relies on God to stay clean. Cheryl is still happily married and active in the same support group as when we last spoke, although she tells me about some of the women in that group who have passed away.

> The strangest thing is when you go to a funeral for a positive sister and nobody says the word HIV or AIDS at all, and the newspaper says she died after a long struggle with cancer, and you start to wonder how many of her family and friends even knew about what she had been struggling with for so many years. And I don't want to dishonor her in death, but what do I say when someone asks me how I knew her? Do I say how many times we cried together and told each other not to give up? Do I say we were sharing information about HIV drugs and helping each other cope for the past ten years? That's the truth, it is. But I haven't said that. I just say we were friends and I'm really going to miss her.

When I ask her about her medical care, Cheryl says "Obamacare screwed everything up at first. It is hard for us poor people. But maybe in the end it will get better." Her husband is unable to see the same medical provider that he has seen for the past ten years. His new doctor does not know him and his history and the doctor is not an HIV specialist so doesn't really understand his HIV drugs, according to Cheryl. She says it is funny when she and her husband feel they know more about HIV than the doctor. Cheryl is trying to get a referral to see an HIV specialist instead of a primary care doctor but when we talked she had just planned how she would get the form signed the next day. "I have to take four different buses to get out there but I mapped it out and I think I can figure it out tomorrow. I hope it is not too hard."

CARMEN RAMIREZ[3]

Carmen told me that she feels blessed in her life and that she never expected to live this long. When she remembers the day she was diagnosed with HIV, she thought her life was over. But now, she is fifty-two years old and has been living with HIV since 1996 and she feels that life is worth living. She has wonderful doctors and remains active in her support group. She is learning English and her daughter, who is bilingual, is helping her. But Carmen tells me that things have changed in her personal life since we spoke in 2008. First, she explains that she is no longer married. I asked if her husband passed away, but she said, "No, it was not that. He left. But it was a good thing, yes, it was good. We were not happy together." Carmen then goes on to explain the relationship further. I remembered that she had told me that she and her husband often argued. Carmen said that she "should have recognized that as a bad sign back then, but thought things would get better." But she says that he was the kind of person who just wanted a wife who would do everything for him. "He was very traditional, and at first I like that about him, but then I realized how unhappy I was just doing everything for him." It was her daughter who helped Carmen to recognize that her husband was mistreating her. "She said, 'he does not respect you. You deserve better.' And I saw that she was right." Carmen tells me that she will not marry again. "I plan to just focus on my daughters. I want to help them, to be there for them. Sometimes a man is a distraction." As we say goodbye, Carmen tells me not to worry about her. "I'm happy. I'm healthy. I'm fine. Don't worry."

DIVA JACKSON[4]

Diva is still happily married and her HIV is under control, but she was in pain from a broken foot when we talked. She told me that things were still "pretty much the same" since our last conversation. She has normal side effects from the medicines she takes, but has not faced drug resistance or problems accessing her medications. Her husband's status is similar, although at the time he was facing unpleasant side effects from new medications. But he has good care for his HIV and Hepatitis C infections. Both Diva and her husband have remained clean "by the grace of God," she says. Diva sings in the choir at her church and says that she feels the Spirit's presence when she can lift up her voice and belt out the lyrics of her favorite worship hymn. Diva remains active in two support groups, although she is now the oldest woman in each group. "I'm like a grandmother to these newly diagnosed girls. Anything they ask, I know the answer. Any issues they have, I've been there. So I help them a lot." Diva explains that her family remains very important to her. She has now disclosed her HIV status to all of her adult children, and they have accepted her and support her. The biggest joy in her life is her new granddaughter. The biggest source of stress in her life is how to help her son who is incarcerated. "I keep bringing him to prayer and I don't know what to do." Diva tells me that she knows she bears responsibility for her children, even her adult children, and that she regrets that she was not a better mother when they were younger. "My addictions prevented me from loving them in the way they deserved. And now, I need to be there for them. But it is hard to know how to help them, especially my son. He's my constant worry." Diva tells me that she relies on God and that she knows God will help her sort it out. "I got lots to be thankful for," she tells me. "Food on the table, roof over my head, a nice apartment with my husband and daughter and her five-year-old son. We're safe. Trust in the Lord and he will provide."

GRACE CEKIK[5]

Grace tells me that she has a lot to tell me. She moved away from Chicago. She still works in the medical field, but let go of her advocacy role so she does not have any HIV specific speaking engagements anymore. But she wanted to tell me about her relationship break-up and about her health. For starters, Paul, the man with whom she was in a serious relationship in 2006, became abusive. She said it began slowly. He became increasingly unkind, difficult to live with, and demanding. After a few years the hurtful comments became worse. He told her that no one else would want to be with her. "He would cut me down all the time—demeaning remarks, manipulative behavior. He made me feel like I was the crazy one, like I had unrealistic expectations because I didn't want my partner yelling at me all the time. I kept wanting to talk about it, work it out, but then one day we had this huge fight. He said horrible things, threw something at me, spit on me, and walked out. He made no contact for four years. In hindsight, I think it was good that it happened that way because I don't know if I ever would have left him. I put up with the abuse for so long. But now I see how awful it was and I wonder: How did I ever live that way?" Grace never had children, and says that she had to let go of that dream. "But I think I would have been a good mom." Three years ago Grace started to get sick. "My numbers weren't good." She had a scary experience when she took a new kind of HIV drug and had a severe allergic reaction. "I was hospitalized, and I thought it was the end." But when she was discharged her doctors told her they would try a different combination of medications. For some time she went on disability. "When you're on disability, taking meds is your full time job, ha ha. You'd think it would be easy but when you feel awful, it is actually hard!" Grace feels lucky that she has wonderful friends and family members who have cared for her through the messiness of her relationship break-up and through her battles with HIV virus. And she feels lucky for her job and for the excellent medical care she has received. Grace has continued to drift away from the institutional Catholic Church, but she meditates every day. "I guess I'm more spiritual than religious," she tells me. When I ask her what she would like church members to learn from her story, she says: "I'd like people to see HIV like any other disease. Treat people living with HIV like you treat people with diabetes or lung disease. Also, preach a message of love and acceptance. And finally, accept same-sex marriage. Recognize that marriage is about love, and lift that up. When two people love each other, that is good and beautiful. I had that with Sam." Grace told me that she still wonders what her life would have been like if Sam had not become infected with HIV.

LETTIE MENDOZA[6]

Lettie Mendoza died, somewhat unexpectedly, in 2007. Lettie's ovarian cancer had returned and she had other complications related to her underlying HIV diagnosis. Her husband said she was just too tired to fight anymore. The HIV finally won. A rosary, followed by a Mass of Christian Burial, was celebrated for Lettie in her local parish and was well attended by family and friends, including members of her support groups. Lettie's daughter expressed her feelings in this way: "My heart hurts. I know she is happy and she is not in pain anymore. But I miss her every day." One of Lettie's relatives memorialized Lettie in this way: "She was loving, caring, giving, compassionate, intelligent, and wise. She was like a mother to me, to all of us. She encouraged me and guided me through all the ups and downs of life." One of Lettie's co-workers said, "she was a sweet lady. We will miss her." Another of Lettie's friends from work explained: "It is so hard to understand how one day she is right there with you and another day she is gone. I will miss her on our break times. We used to laugh so much together." While the presider never mentioned Lettie's HIV status, he did refer to her "illness" and her "medical struggles over the years." One friend from her support group explained that she was glad that the funeral did not focus on Lettie's struggle with HIV/AIDS because HIV was only one part of Lettie's life. In the end, Lettie was not defined by her HIV status; instead, she was defined by her virtues and her loving relationships.

UNKNOWN: KEESHA WALKER AND CRYSTAL SMITH

My last contacts with Keesha Walker and Crystal Smith were in 2008, and I was not able to follow up with them in 2014. I found no evidence of their deaths, but their phone numbers and addresses had changed multiple times. My attempts to contact them through their former case managers and social workers were unsuccessful. I am thus unable to report whether Keesha and Shawn remain separated, or if Crystal and her husband found marriage counseling helpful. I do not know how their HIV infection has progressed, or what new struggles they face in their lives.

CONCLUDING REFLECTIONS

When I reflect upon my conversations with Sue, Cheryl, Carmen, Diva, and Grace, and with Lettie's loved ones, I realize how their stories have had such an impact on me during the last eight years, even without regular contact with them. Some parts of their updates were unsurprising to me: I knew that long-term drug toxicity would be a challenge and I expected to hear them say that the social injustices that thwarted their flourishing in 2006—issues such as poverty and domestic violence—would persist despite their strong wills. I was delighted to hear that Cheryl and Diva have continued to stay away from addictive substances and that they remain active in their support groups for women living with HIV. But I was troubled by the portraits of Carmen's and Grace's relationship troubles, especially since I had a positive impression of these two relationships in 2008. That both women were in relationships that became abusive indicates the ongoing need to socialize men to respect women and to continue to raise awareness about gender-based violence in church settings. My follow-up conversations with five of the eight women validated my study's conclusions, especially regarding the need to eradicate HIV-related stigma, the need to reframe sexual ethics in light of concerns of human dignity and social justice, and the importance of promoting a theology of marriage that is person-centered, not institution-centered. But learning of Lettie's death, and my inability to contact Keesha and Crystal, also reinforced for me the tragic thread in these women's stories and the fact that my study did very little, if anything, to improve their livelihoods.

I continue to believe that the theology of accompaniment provides an important corrective to traditional methodologies in Christian ethics, and I hope more of my colleagues will commit to research that is more explicitly grounded in the data of everyday people's experiences. But as Steve Reifenberg explains, the theology of accompaniment is a radical approach:

> Accompaniment is not simply walking together. It requires recognizing real-world complexities, acknowledging the asymmetries of power and privilege, and being willing to address these while walking together. There is something fundamentally but beautifully radical in this idea. In a society so focused on individual attributes and achievement, this simple concept of walking beside another, humbly and ever toward justice, could change the world.[7]

I hope, with Reifenberg, that this method becomes a force for good in the world, an impetus for social change. Reifenberg further comments on the theological anthropology that undergirds this approach: Each person is social by nature and we are held together by bonds of interdependence.

> Accompaniment flips the impulse of "how do we help them?" into an assertion—"we're in this together." We are connected, tied, and bound together. We need to walk together and learn together, and maybe, together, we can envision and create better, more equitable tomorrows, both for the big issues "over there" and also in our daily lives, loving our neighbors—that is, everyone—as we love ourselves.[8]

As I conclude this project, I realize anew the importance of learning together as one way of abiding by the commandment to love our neighbors as we love ourselves. My hope is that Christians can imagine a shared future in which all people experience God's love and are empowered to care for themselves in fulfilling interdependent relationships. My hope is that all women living with HIV will hear the church community say, in word and through social action:

> *God loves you.*
> *Your voice matters.*
> *You deserve respect.*
> *We care about you.*
> *We want you to live a deeply fulfilling life.*
> *We're in this together.*

NOTES

1. Melton, Sue [pseud.]. Interviewed by the author, July 3, 2014.
2. King, Cheryl [pseud.]. Interviewed by the author, July 15, 2014.
3. Ramirez, Carmen [pseud.]. Interviewed by the author, July 8, 2014.
4. Jackson, Diva [pseud.]. Interviewed by the author, July 9, 2014.
5. Cekik, Grace [pseud.]. Interviewed by the author, July 8, 2014.

6. Mendoza, Lettie [pseud.]. Interviewed by the author, September 9, 2007. Personal communication with loved ones occurred on November 1, 2007; July 6, 2014; July 8, 2014; and July 9, 2014; and December 26, 2014.

7. Steve Reifenberg, from *In the Company of the Poor: Conversations with Dr. Paul Farmer and Fr. Gustavo Gutierrez*, Eds. Michael Griffin and Jennie Weiss Block (Maryknoll: Orbis, 2013), 194.

8. Reifenberg, *In the Company of the Poor*, 196.

Appendix

COMMUNITY RESOURCES: ORGANIZATIONS THAT ASSIST PEOPLE LIVING WITH HIV/AIDS IN CHICAGO

The women in this study would like to thank the following organizations for offering them assistance since their HIV diagnosis. Please consider getting involved in their work or in the work of similar organizations where you live. Remember, *we are in this together*.

AIDS FOUNDATION OF CHICAGO

The mission of the AIDS Foundation of Chicago is to lead the fight against HIV/AIDS and to improve the lives of people affected by the epidemic. Founded in 1985 by community activists and physicians, the AIDS Foundation of Chicago is a local and national leader in the fight against HIV/AIDS. The AIDS Foundation of Chicago collaborates with community organizations to develop and improve HIV/AIDS services, fund and coordinate prevention, care, and advocacy projects, and champion effective, compassionate HIV/AIDS policy. Website: http://www.aidschicago.org/.

CAMP BENEDICT

Camp Benedict is an educational and recreational family camp serving the needs of AIDS affected families in the upper Midwest. People living with HIV/AIDS can come together for summer camp experience in this beautiful environment and experience community and empowerment. Camp Benedict is grounded in the belief that all people deserve honesty, respect, acceptance, empowerment, and unconditional love. Website: http://www.campbenedict.org/.

CATHOLIC CHARITIES HIV/AIDS SERVICES (COOK COUNTY AND LAKE COUNTY)

Catholic Charities, in its mission of charity to anyone in need, continues to live the Gospel message by working to strengthen and support individuals, families, and communities based on the value and dignity of human life. Catholic Charities provides professional counseling and case management services to families and individuals who are experiencing a wide range of social and personal problems, including homelessness, family violence, substance abuse and addiction, sexual abuse, illness such as HIV/AIDS, and other problems that affect the family's or individual's ability to cope. Services may be one or a combination of the following: responding to a crisis, referral to a needed service, help with accessing services and benefits, advocacy, help with developing a plan of action and following through, money management, professional counseling and family therapy. Spanish-speaking staff is available. Website: http://www.catholiccharities.net/GetHelp/OurServices/HIVAIDSServices.aspx.

HOWARD BROWN HEALTH CENTER

Howard Brown Health Center (HBHC) was founded in 1974 and is now one of the nation's largest lesbian, gay, bisexual, and transgender (LGBT) organizations. The agency serves more than 16,000 adults and youth each year in its diverse health and social service delivery system focused around seven major programmatic divisions: primary medical care, behavioral health, research, HIV/STD prevention, youth services, elder services, and community initiatives. HBHC serves men and women, infants, youth, and children. Services include HIV testing, research, medical care, support groups, mental health therapy, educational outreach, special programs for survivors of domestic violence, and case management. Website: http://www.howardbrown.org/.

POSITIVE WOMEN'S NETWORK USA

Positive Women's Network—United States of America (PWN-USA) is a national membership body of HIV-positive women, inclusive of transgender and cisgender women, working to achieve HIV policies and programs grounded in gender equity and human rights. Website: http://pwnusa.wordpress.com/.

PROJECT VIDA

Project VIDA is a culturally focused HIV/AIDS prevention and direct services community-based organization located on Chicago's West Side. Project VIDA was founded by a consortium of volunteers in 1992 to address the unique needs and concerns of Latino and African American individuals at risk for or currently living with HIV/AIDS. Project VIDA's mission is "to improve quality of life and reduce health disparities in underserved communities by promoting self-empowerment and providing holistic health education and direct services." Project VIDA has served more than 173,700 clients and community members, mostly in Chicago's heavily-populated Latino and African-American neighborhoods. Website: http://www.projectvida.org/home.

TEST POSITIVE AWARENESS NETWORK (TPAN)

Test Positive Awareness Network (TPAN) is a community-based organization providing comprehensive health and wellness programs to everyone impacted by HIV/AIDS. Their services include case management, support groups, needle exchange, HIV testing, and educational outreach. TPAN publishes Positively Aware (http://www.positivelyaware.com/) whose annual Drug Guide is a resource for persons living with HIV all over the world (http://www.positivelyaware.com/2014/14-03/drugguide.shtml). TPAN also publishes the HIV Services Directory, even though funding for that effort was dramatically cut in 2011 (http://www.tpan.com/services-directory). TPAN website: http://www.tpan.com/.

VITAL BRIDGES

Vital Bridges' mission is to help people throughout metropolitan Chicago impacted by HIV and AIDS to improve their health and build self-sufficiency by providing food, nutrition counseling, housing, care coordination, and prevention services. Website: http://www.heartlandalliance.org/vital/.

Bibliography

1983 Code of Canon Law, English Trans. Grand Rapids, MI: Eerdmans, 1983.

Abbott, Walter J. *Documents of Vatican II*. New York: Guild, 1966.

Ackermann, Denise M. "A Voice Was Heard in Ramah: A Feminist Theology of Praxis for Healing in South Africa." In *Liberating Faith Practices: Feminist Theologies in Context*, ed. Denise M. Ackermann and M. Bons-Storm. Leuven: Peeters, 1998.

Ad Hoc Committee on Marriage and Family Life, National Conference of Catholic Bishops, *A Family Perspective in Church and Society: A Manual for All Pastoral Leaders*, 10th Anniv. Ed. Washington, DC: USCCB Office for Publishing, 1998.

Adams, Carol J., and Marie M. Fortune. *Violence against Women and Children: A Christian Theological Sourcebook*. New York: Continuum, 1995.

AIDS Foundation of Chicago. "HIV/AIDS in Chicago 2010." Accessed June 24, 2014. http://aidschicago.org/pdf/chicago_factsheet_2010.pdf.

Ajayi, James Olaitan. *The HIV/AIDS Epidemic in Nigeria: Some Ethical Considerations*. Rome: Gregorian University Press, 2003.

Allen, John. "The Word from Rome: Vatican in Condom Debate." *National Catholic Reporter*. May 5, 2006.

Andolsen, Barbara Hilkert. "*Agape* in Feminist Ethics." *Journal of Religious Ethics* 9 (1981): 69–83.

________. "Elements of a Feminist Approach to Bioethics." In *Feminist Ethics and the Catholic Moral Tradition*, ed. Charles E. Curran, Margaret A. Farley, and Richard A. McCormick, 350–63. New York: Paulist Press, 1996.

Andolsen, Barbara Hilkert, Christine E. Gudorf, and Mary E. Pellauer, eds. *Women's Consciousness, Women's Conscience: A Reader in Feminist Ethics*. Minneapolis: Winston, 1985.

Arcel, Libby Tata. *Torture*. Copenhagen: International Rehabilitation Council for Torture Victims, Fall 2002.

Archdiocese of Chicago Family Ministries Office. *A Marriage in the Lord*, 5th ed. Chicago, IL: Archdiocese of Chicago, 2007.

Ashley, Benedict M., and Kevin D. O'Rourke. *Health Care Ethics: A Theological Analysis*. 4ed. Washington, DC: Georgetown University Press, 1997.

Baldovin, John. "Holy Sacrifice of the Mass." *Worship* 80:2 (March 2006).

Balsam, Charles and Elizabeth. *Family Planning: A Guide*.

Barnett, Tony, and Alan Whiteside. *AIDS in the Twenty-first Century: Disease and Globalization*. New York: Palgrave Macmillan, 2002.

Barr, Sarah. "Needle Exchange Programs Face New Federal Funding Ban." Kaiser Health News Online. December, 21, 2011. Accessed July 30, 2014. http://www.kaiserhealthnews.org/stories/2011/december/21/needle-exchange-federal-funding.aspx.

Bassett, William W., ed. *The Bond of Marriage*. Notre Dame: University of Notre Dame Press, 1968.

Bayer, R. *Private Acts, Social Consequences: AIDS and the Politics of Public Health*. New York: Free Press, 1989.

Beattie, Tina. *New Catholic Feminism: Theology and Theory*. New York: Routledge, 2006.

Berg, B. L. *Qualitative Research Methods*. Needham Heights, MA: Allyn & Bacon, 1989.

Berger, Michele Tracy. *Workable Sisterhood: The Political Journey of Stigmatized Women with HIV/AIDS*. Princeton, NJ: Princeton University Press, 2004.

Bernadin, Joseph Cardinal. *Consistent Ethic of Life*, ed. Thomas G. Fuechtmann. Kansas City, MO: Sheed & Ward, 1988.

Biederman, Joseph, et al., "Patterns of Alcohol and Drug Use in Adolescents Can Be Predicted by Parental Substance Use Disorders," *Pediatrics* 106. 2000.

Black, Peter, and James Keenan, "The Evolving Self-Understanding of the Moral Theologian: 1900–2000." *Studia Moralia* 39 (2001): 291–327.

Blodgett, Barbara J. *Constructing the Erotic: Sexual Ethics and Adolescent Girls*. Cleveland, OH: Pilgrim Press, 2002.

Boisclair, Regina A. "Amnesia in the Catholic Sunday Lectionary: Women—Silenced from the Memories of Salvation History." In *Women and Theology: The Annual Publication of the College Theology Society, 1994*, ed. Mary Ann Hinsdale and Phyllis H. Kaminski, 109–135. Maryknoll, NY: Orbis, 1995.

Bourg, Florence Caffrey. *Where Two or Three Are Gathered: Christian Families as Domestic Churches*. Notre Dame: University of Notre Dame Press, 2004.

"Breastfeeding: Does it really space babies?" Cincinnati, OH: Couple to Couple League, 1998.

Brock, Rita Nakashima. *Journeys by Heart: A Christology of Erotic Power*. New York: Crossroad, 1989.

Brock, Rita Nakashima, and Rebecca Ann Parker. *Proverbs of Ashes: Violence, Redemptive Suffering, and the Search for What Saves Us*. Boston: Beacon, 2001.

Brock, Rita Nakashima, and Susan Brooks Thistlethwaite. *Casting Stones: Prostitution and Liberation in Asia and the United States*. Minneapolis, MN: Fortress Press, 1996.

Brown, Joanne Carlson, and Carole R. Bohn. *Christianity, Patriarchy, and Abuse: A Feminist Critique*. Cleveland, OH: Pilgrim Press, 1989.

Brown, Raymond E. *An Introduction to the New Testament*. New York: Doubleday, 1997.

Browning, Don, Bonnie Miller-McLemore, Pamela Couture, K. Brynolf Lyon, and Robert Franklin. *From Culture Wars to Common Ground: Religion and the American Family Debate*. Louisville, KY: Westminster John Knox Press, 1997.

Browning, Melissa. *Risky Marriage: HIV and Intimate Relationships in Tanzania*. Lanham, Maryland: Lexington Books, 2014.

Bruckner, Hannan, and Bearman. "After the Promise: The STD Consequences of Adolescent Virginity Pledges," *Journal of Adolescent Health*. May 2005.

Cahill, Lisa Sowle. "The Atonement Paradigm: Does it Still Have Explanatory Value?" *Theo logical Studies* (June 2007): 418–432.

________."AIDS, Justice, and the Common Good" in *Catholic Ethicists on HIV/AIDS Prevention*, ed. James F. Keenan. London: Continuum, 2000.

________. *Family: A Christian Social Perspective*. Minneapolis, MN: Fortress Press, 2000.

________. *Global Justice, Christology and Christian Ethics*. New York: Cambridge University Press, 2013.

________. "Marriage: Developments in Catholic Theology and Ethics." *Theological Studies* 64 (2003): 78–105.

________. "Realigning Catholic Priorities: Bioethics and the Common Good," *America* 191 no. 6 (September 13, 2004):11–13.

________. *Sex, Gender, and Christian Ethics*. Cambridge: Cambridge University Press, 1996.

________. *Theological Bioethics: Participation, Justice, and Change*. Washington, DC: Georgetown University Press, 2005.

Cahill, Lisa Sowle, John Garvey, and T. Frank Kennedy, S. J., eds. *Sexuality and the U.S. Catholic Church: Crisis and Renewal.* New York: Crossroad, 2006.

Campbell, Carole A. *Women, Families, and HIV/AIDS: A Sociological Perspective on the Epidemic in America.* Cambridge, United Kingdom: Cambridge University Press, 1999.

Campbell, Ted A. "The Wesleyan Quadrilateral: A Modern Methodist Myth," In *Doctrine and Theology in the United Methodist Church*, ed. Thomas G. Langford, 127–182. Nashville, TN: Kingswood, 1990.

Cana Conference of Chicago, Family Ministries Office of the Archdiocese of Chicago. *In the Spirit of Cana: Guidelines for Pastoral Outreach to Christian Marriage: Formation, Celebration, and Continuing Education.* Chicago, IL: Archdiocese of Chicago, 2005.

Caravano, Kathryn. "More than Mothers and Whores: Redefining the AIDS Prevention Needs of Women." In *Women's Health, Politics, and Power: Essays on Sex/Gender, Medicine, and Public Health*, ed. Elizabeth Fee and Nancy Krieger, 255–267. Amityville, NY: Baywood Publishing Company, 1994.

Caredy, John J., ed., *The Sexuality Debate in North American Churches, 1988-1995: Controversies, Unresolved Issues, Future Prospects.* Lewiston, NY: Edwin Mellen Press, 1995.

Cassidy, Laurie M., and Alex Mikulich, eds., *Interrupting White Privilege: Catholic Theologians Break the Silence.* Maryknoll, NY: Orbis Books, 2007.

Cekik, Grace [pseud.]. Interviewed by the author. Chicago, IL, October 11, 2006, July 8, 2014.

Centers for Disease Control and Prevention, "Are condoms effective in preventing HIV transmission?" Accessed May 6, 2006.http://www.cdc.gov/nchstp/od/latex.htm.

_______. "Syringe Exchange Programs, United Sates, 2008." *Morbidity and Mortality Weekly Report (MMWR)* 59(45). November 19, 2010.

_______. *Essential Components of a Comprehensive Strategy to Prevent Domestic HIV.* Atlanta: National Center for HIV, STD, and TB Prevention, 2006.

_______. "Fact Sheet: HIV/AIDS among African Americans." Atlanta: United States Department of Health and Human Services, Centers for Disease Control and Prevention, 2014.

_______. "Fact Sheet: HIV/AIDS among Women." Rev. March 6, 2014. Atlanta: United States Department of Health and Human Services, Centers for Disease Control and Prevention, 2014.

_______. "Fact Sheet: The HIV/AIDS Epidemic at a Glance." Rev. November 25, 2014. Atlanta: United States Department of Health and Human Services, Centers for Disease Control and Prevention, 2014.

_______. *HIV/AIDS Surveillance Report, 2012.* Vol. 24. Atlanta: United States Department of Health and Human Services, Centers for Disease Control and Prevention, 2014.

_______. "HIV Related Knowledge and Stigma—United States, 2000," in *Morbidity and Mortality Weekly Report* 49:47. 2000.

_______. "HIV Statistics: Basics." Rev. October 15, 2014. Accessed December 26, 2014. http://www.cdc.gov/hiv/statistics/basics/ .

_______. "Revised Recommendations for HIV Testing of Adults, Adolescents, and Pregnant Women in Health-Care Settings." *Morbidity and Mortality Weekly Report* 55:14 (2006): 1–17.

Champlin, Joseph M. *Together for Life: A Preparation for Marriage and for the Ceremony.* Notre Dame, IN: Ave Maria Press, 2000.

Childress, James F., Eric M. Meslin, and Harold T. Shapiro, eds., *Belmont Revisited: Ethical Principles for Research with Human Subjects.* Washington, DC: Georgetown University Press, 2005.

Christiansen, Demian, and Nanette Benbow. "Chicago HIV/AIDS Brief." Chicago, IL: Office of HIV/AIDS Surveillance, Chicago Department of Public Health, 2005.

Cimperman, Maria. *When God's People Have AIDS: An Approach to Ethics.* Maryknoll, NY: Orbis, 2005.

Confraternity of Christian Doctrine, *Lectionary for Mass for Use in the Dioceses in the United States*, 2nd, NAB. Washington, DC: Confraternity of Christian Doctrine, 2001.

Conn, Joann Wolski, and Walter E. Conn, eds., *Horizons on Catholic Feminist Theology.* Washington, DC: Georgetown University Press, 1992.

Constantine, Norman A. "Converging Evidence Leaves Policy Behind: Sex Education in the United States," *Journal of Adolescent Health* 42:4. April 2008.

Copeland, M. Shawn. "Wading through Many Sorrows: Toward a Theology of Suffering in Womanist Perspective." In *Readings in Moral Theology, No. 9: Feminist Ethics and the Catholic Moral Tradition*, ed. Charles E. Curran, Margaret A. Farley, and Richard A. McCormick, 136–163. New York: Paulist, 1996.

Covino, Paul, ed. *Celebrating Marriage*. Portland, OR: Pastoral Press, 1994.

_______."Marriage Ministry and the Rite of Marriage," *Origins* 37:21. November 2007.

Creswell, John W. *Qualitative Inquiry and Research Design: Choosing Among Five Traditions*. Thousand Oaks, CA: Sage Publications, 1998.

Curran, Charles E. *Catholic Moral Theology in the United States: A History*. Washington, DC: Georgetown University Press, 2008.

_______. *The Catholic Moral Tradition Today: A Synthesis*. Washington, DC: Georgetown University Press, 1999.

_______. *Catholic Social Teaching 1891–Present: A Historical, Theological, and Ethical Analysis*. Washington, DC: Georgetown University Press, 2002.

Curran, Charles E., Margaret A. Farley, and Richard A. McCormick, S. J., eds. *Readings in Moral Theology, No. 9: Feminist Ethics and the Catholic Moral Tradition*. New York: Paulist, 1996.

Daly, Lois K. *Feminist Theological Ethics: A Reader*. Louisville, KY: Westminster John Knox Press, 1994.

Daly, Mary. *The Church and the Second Sex*. New York: Harper & Row, 1968.

Daly, Robert J. *The Origins of the Christian Doctrine of Sacrifice*. Minneapolis, MN: Fortress, 1978.

D'Cruz, Premilla. "Moments of Truth: The Experiences of Wives in HIV/AIDS Affected Nuclear Households in Mumbai." *Journal of Comparative Family Studies* 34:2 (Spring 2003): 255–281.

Deacon, Harriet. "Towards a Sustainable Theory of Health-Related Stigma: Lessons from the HIV/AIDS Literature," *Journal of Community and Applied Social Psychology* 16, 2006.

De La Torre, Miguel A. *A Lily among the Thorns: Imagining a New Christian Sexuality*. San Francisco: Jossey-Bass, 2007.

DeNavas-Walt, Carmen, Bernadette D. Proctor, and Jessica Smith. *Income, Poverty, and Health Insurance in the United States: 2006*. United States Census Bureau Current Population Reports P60-233. Washington, DC: United States Government Printing Office, 2007.

Desilver, Drew. "Who's Poor in America? Fifty Years into the War on Poverty." Pew Research Center Report. January 13, 2014.

DeSnyder, V. Nelly Salgado. "Understanding the Sexuality of Mexican-born Women and Their Risk for HIV/AIDS." *Psychology of Women Quarterly* 24 (2000): 100–109.

Diaz, T. "Socioeconomic Differences among People with AIDS: Results from a Multistate Surveillance Project." *American Journal of Preventive Medicine* 10 (1994): 217–222.

DiSpezio, Michael. *The Science of HIV*, 2nd ed. Arlington, VA: NSTA Press, 2000.

Dixon, Robyn. "With Women Powerless, AIDS Reigns." *Los Angeles Times*, January 23, 2005.

Dorr, Donal. *Option for the Poor: A Hundred Years of Catholic Social Teaching*, Red. Ed. Maryknoll, NY: Orbis, 2001.

Douglas, Kelly Brown. *Sexuality and the Black Church: A Womanist Perspective*. Maryknoll, NY: Orbis, 1999.

Dowling, Kevin. "Let's Not Condemn Condoms in the Fight Against AIDS." *U.S. Catholic*, November 2003, 20–22.

Dube, Musa Wenkosi. "An HIV and AIDS Curriculum for Theological Institutions in Africa." In Musa Wenkosi Dube, ed., *HIV/AIDS and the Curriculum: Methods of Integrating HIV/AIDS in Theological Programmes*. Geneva, Switzerland: World Council of Churches Publications, 2003.

_______. "Theological Challenges: Proclaiming the Fullness of Life in the HIV/AIDS & Global Economic Era." *International Review of Mission* (October 2002): 535–549.

Echegaray, Hugo. *The Practice of Jesus*, trans. Matthew J. O'Connell. Maryknoll, NY: Orbis Books, 1984.

Edlin, Brian et al. "Intersecting Epidemics—Crack Cocaine Use and HIV Infection Among Inner-City Young Adults." *New England Journal of Medicine* 331, no. 21 (1994): 1442.

Farley, Margaret A. "The Church and the Family: An Ethical Task." *Horizons* 10/1. (1983): 50–71.

________. *Just Love: A Framework for Christian Sexual Ethics.* New York: Continuum, 2006.

________. "Partnership in Hope: Gender, Faith, and Responses to HIV/AIDS in Africa." *Journal of Feminist Studies in Religion* 20 (2004): 33–48.

________. *Personal Commitments: Beginning, Keeping, Changing.* San Francisco, CA: Harper & Row, 1986.

________. "Sources of Sexual Inequality in the History of Christian Thought." *Journal of Religion* 56 (April 1976): 163–169.

Farmer, Paul. Editorial. *Lancet* 358 (9279): 404–409, 2001.

________. "Medicine and Social Justice." *America* 173, no. 2. (July 15, 1995): 13–17.

________. *Pathologies of Power: Health, Human Rights, and the New War on the Poor.* Los Angeles, CA: University of California Press, 2003.

Farmer, Paul, Maureen Connors, and Janie Simmons, eds. *Women, Poverty, and AIDS: Sex, Drugs, and Structural Violence.* Monroe, ME: Common Courage Press, 1996.

Feeding America. "Food Insecurity Statistics." Accessed June 23, 2014. http://feedingamerica.org/hunger-in-america/hunger-facts/hunger-and-poverty-statistics.aspx#.

Fife, Wayne. *Doing Fieldwork: Ethnographic Methods for Research in Developing Countries and Beyond.* New York: Palgrave Macmillan, 2005.

Fiorenza, Elisabeth Schussler. *Bread Not Stone: The Challenge of Feminist Biblical Interpretation.* Boston, MA: Beacon Press, 1984.

________. "Feminist Spirituality, Christian Identity, and Catholic Vision. In *Womanspirit Rising,* Carol Christ and Judith Plaskow, eds., 136–148. San Francisco, CA: Harper and Row, 1979.

________. *In Memory of Her: A Feminist Theological Reconstruction of Christian Origins.* New York: Crossroad, 1983.

Flannery, Austin, O.P., ed. *Vatican Council II: Constitutions, Decrees, Declarations.* New York: Costello, 1996.

Flemming, Austin. *Parish Weddings.* Chicago, IL: Archdiocese of Chicago Liturgy Training Publications, 1987.

Fortune, Marie M. "The Conundrum of Sin, Sex, Violence, and Theodicy." In *The Other Side of Sin: Woundedness from the Perspective of the Sinned-Against,* ed. Andrew Sung Park and Susan L. Nelson, 109–142. Albany, NY: State University of New York Press, 2001.

Fuller, Jon. "AIDS Prevention: A Challenge to the Catholic Moral Tradition." *America* 175 (December 28, 1996): 13–20.

________. "Condoms, Catholics, and HIV/AIDS Prevention." *The Furrow* 52, no. 9 (September 2001): 459–467.

Fullilove, Mindy Thompson, M. D. "The Little Handbook." Created for the use of the Qualitative Research Methods 2001 Class, Mailman School of Public Health, Columbia University, 2001.

________."Death and Life in the Great American City," *International Journal of Mental Health* 28:4 (1999–2000).

Fullilove, Robert E., and Mindy Thompson Fullilove. "HIV Prevention and Intervention in the African-American Community: A Public Health Perspective." In *The AIDS Knowledge Base,* ed. P. T. Cohen, M. A. Sande, and P. A. Volberding, 3rd ed. Philadelphia, PA: Lippincott Williams and Wilkins, 1999.

Gaffney, James. *Sin Reconsidered.* New York: Paulist Press, 1983.

Gaillardetz, Richard R. *A Daring Promise: A Spirituality of Christian Marriage.* New York: Crossroad, 2002.

________. "The Ordinary Universal Magisterium: Unresolved Questions." *Theological Studies* 63 (2002): 447–71.

Gallagher, John A. *Time Past, Time Future: A Historical Study of Catholic Moral Theology.* New York: Paulist Press, 1990.

Gallant, Joel, MD, MPH. *100 Questions and Answers about HIV and AIDS*, 2nd ed. Burlington, MA: Jones and Bartlett, 2012.

Garascia, Anthony. *Before "I Do": Preparing for the Sacrament of Marriage*. Notre Dame: Ave Maria Press, 1999.

Genovesi, Vincent J. *In Pursuit of Love: Catholic Morality and Human Sexuality*, 2d ed. Collegeville, MN: Liturgical Press, 1996.

Gilleman, Gerard. *The Primacy of Charity in Moral Theology*. Westminster, MD: Newman Press, 1959.

Gittins, Anthony J. "Sacrifice, Violence, and the Eucharist." *Worship* 65:5 (1991).

_______. *Where There's Hope There's Life: Women's Stories of Homelessness and Survival*. Liguori, MO: Liguori Publications, 2006.

Glynn, J. R., M. Carael, B. Auvert, M. Kahindo, J. Chege, R. Musonda, F. Kaona, A. Buve, and the Study Group on the Heterogeneity of HIV Epidemics in African Cities. "Why do young women have much higher prevalence of HIV than young men? A study in Kisumu, Kenya and Ndola, Zambia." *Journal of Acquired Immunodeficiency Syndromes* 2001: 15 (suppl 4): S51-S60.

Goffman, Erving. *Stigma: Notes on the Management of Spoiled Identity*. Englewood Cliffs, NJ: Prentice Hall, 1963.

Gonzalez, Justo L. *The Story of Christianity, Vol. 1: The Early Church to the Dawn of the Reformation*. San Francisco, CA: Harper, 1984.

Gormally, Luke. *National Catholic Bioethics Quarterly*, January 2005, as reported by John Allen, "The Word from Rome: Vatican in Condom Debate," *National Catholic Reporter*. May 5, 2006.

Grabowski, John S. *Sex and Virtue: An Introduction to Sexual Ethics*. Washington, DC: Catholic University of America Press, 2003.

Grey, Mary. *Redeeming the Dream: Feminism, Redemption, and Christian Tradition*. London: SPCK, 1989.

Gudorf, Christine E. *Body, Sex, and Pleasure: Reconstructing Christian Sexual Ethics*. Cleveland, OH: Pilgrim Press, 1994.

_______. "Contraception and Abortion in Roman Catholicism," in Daniel C. Maguire, ed., *Sacred Rights: The Case for Contraception and Abortion in World Religions*. New York: Oxford University Press, 2003.

_______."Encountering the Other: The Modern Papacy on Women," in *Feminist Ethics and the Catholic Moral Tradition: Readings in Moral Theology, No. 9*, eds., Charles E. Curran, Margaret A. Farley, and Richard A. McCormick, S. J. New York: Paulist Press, 1996.

_______. "To Make A Seamless Garment, Use a Single Piece of Cloth." *Cross Currents* 34 (1984): 473–91.

_______. "The Power to Create: Sacraments and Men's Needs to Birth." *Horizons* 14/2 (1987): 296–309.

_______. "Western Religion and the Patriarchal Family." In *Religion and Sexual Health*, ed. Ronald M. Green, 99–117. Dordrecht: Kluwer, 1992.

_______. "Why Sex is Good For Your Marriage," *U.S. Catholic*. November 1992.

Gula, Richard M., S.S. *The Call to Holiness: Embracing a Fully Christian Life*. New York: Paulist, 2003.

_______. *Moral Discernment*. New York: Paulist, 1997.

_______. "Morality and Spirituality." In *Moral Theology: New Directions and Fundamental Issues*, ed. James Keating. New York: Paulist, 2004.

_______. *Reason Informed by Faith: Foundations of Catholic Morality*. New York: Paulist Press, 1989.

Gunter, W. Stephen, et al. *Wesley and the Quadrilateral: Renewing the Conversation*. Nashville, TN: Abingdon, 1997.

Gutierrez, Gustavo. "Saying and Showing to the Poor: God Loves You," in *In the Company of the Poor: Conversations with Dr. Paul Farmer and Fr. Gustavo Gutierrez*, ed. Michael Griffin and Jennie Weiss Block. Maryknoll: Orbis, 2013.

Haddad, Beverley. "Living It Out: Faith Resources and Sites as Critical to Participatory Learning with Rural South African Women." *Journal of Feminist Studies in Religion* 22:1 (2006): 135–154.

________. "Reflections on the Church and HIV/AIDS." *Theology Today* 62 (2005): 29–37.

Hagan, John, and Ruth D. Peterson, eds. *Crime and Inequality*. Stanford, CA: Stanford University Press, 1995.

Hagedorn, John M., and Paul J. Goldstein, "Murder and Drugs in the Information Age: An Urban Political Economy Approach to Variation in Homicide Rates." *Great Cities Institute*. Chicago, IL: University of Illinois–Chicago, 1999.

Haring, Bernard. *Free and Faithful in Christ: Moral Theology for Clergy and Laity*. New York: Seabury Press, 1981.

Harrington, Daniel J. *Interpreting the New Testament*. Collegeville, MN: Liturgical Press/ Michael Glazier, 1979.

________. *Who Is Jesus? Why Is He Important?: An Invitation to the New Testament*. Franklin, WI: Sheed & Ward, 1999.

Harrington, Daniel J., and James F. Keenan. *Jesus and Virtue Ethics: Building Bridges between New Testament Studies and Moral Theology*. Lanham, MD: Sheed & Ward, 2002.

Hayes, Diana L. *Hagar's Daughters: Womanist Ways of Being in the World*. 1995 Madaleva Lecture in Spirituality. New York: Paulist Press, 1995.

Hayes, Diana L., and Cyprian Davis, eds. *Taking Down Our Harps: Black Catholics in the United States*. Maryknoll, NY: Orbis Books, 1998.

Hays, Richard B. *The Moral Vision of the New Testament: A Contemporary Introduction to New Testament Ethics*. San Francisco, CA: HarperCollins, 1996.

Heise, L., M. Ellsberg, and M. Gottemoeller. "Ending Violence against Women." *Population Reports*. Series L. No. 11. Baltimore, MD: Population Information Program, Johns Hopkins University School of Public Health, 1999.

Hellwig, Monika K. *Jesus: The Compassion of God*. Wilmington, DE: Michael Glazier, 1983.

Hinze, Christine Firer. "Bridge Discourse on Wage Justice: Roman Catholic and Feminist Perspectives on the Family Living Wage," in *Feminist Ethics and the Catholic Moral Tradition*, ed. Charles E. Curran, Margaret Farley, and Richard A. McCormick, S. J. Mahwah, NJ: Paulist, 1996.

Hirsch, Arnold. *Making the Second Ghetto: Race and Housing in Chicago, 1940–1960*. Cambridge: Cambridge University Press, 1983.

Hobgood, Mary E. *Dismantling Privilege: An Ethic of Accountability*. Cleveland: Pilgrim, 2002.

Hogan, Linda. *Confronting the Truth: Conscience and the Catholic Tradition*. New York: Paulist, 2001.

Hollenbach, David. *The Common Good and Christian Ethics*. Cambridge, United Kingdom: Cambridge University Press, 2002.

Holzemer William L., et al. "Validation of the HIV/AIDS Stigma Instrument—PLWA (HASI-P)," *AIDS Care* 19:8. 9/2007.

Horsley, Richard. *Sociology of the Jesus Movement*. New York: Crossroad, 1989.

Howard, Joseph. "The Use of the Condom for Disease Prevention," *Linacre Quarterly* 63. 1996.

Interdicasterial Commission for the Catechism. *Catechism of the Catholic Church*. New York: Doubleday, 1995.

Iozzio, Mary Jo. "Moving beyond the Impasse: Catholics Should Support Use of Federal Funding for Needle Exchange Programs," *Health Progress* 90:2. 2009.

Isasi-Diaz, Ada Maria. *Mujerista Theology*. Maryknoll, NY: Orbis, 2003.

Israel, Barbara A., Amy J. Schulz, Lorena Estrada-Martinez, Shannon N. Zenk, Edna Viruell-Fuentes, Antonia M. Villarruel, and Carmen Stokes. "Engaging Urban Residents in Assessing Neighborhood Environments and Their Implications for Health." *Journal of Urban Health* 83:3 (2006): 523–539.

Jackson, Diva [pseud.]. Interviewed by the author. Chicago, IL, March 16, 2006, July 8, 2014.

John Paul II. *Familiaris consortio*. Washington, DC: United States Catholic Conference, 1981.

________. *Instruction on Certain Questions Regarding the Collaboration of the Non-Ordained Faithful in the Sacred Ministry of Priest.* Vatican City: Libreria Editrice Vaticana, 1997.

________. *Letter to Women.* In *Origins* (25 July 1995): 137–143.

________. *Mulieris dignitatem.* In *Origins* 18/17 (6 October 1988): 261–283.

________. "Pope Addresses Vatican AIDS Conference." *Origins* (November 30, 1989) 19:26, 34–436.

________. *The Theology of the Body: Human Love in the Divine Plan.* Boston: Pauline, 1997.

Johnson, Elizabeth A. *Consider Jesus: Waves of Renewal in Christology.* New York: Crossroad, 1990.

________. *She Who Is: The Mystery of God in Feminist Theological Discourse.* New York: Crossroad, 1992.

Johnson, Luke Timothy. "The Biblical Foundations of Matrimony." In *Readings in Moral Theology, No. 5: Marriage*, eds. Charles E. Curran and Julie Hanlon Rubio. Mahwah, NJ: Paulist Press, 2009.

Jung, Patricia Beattie, Mary E. Hunt, and Radhika Balakrishnan, eds. *Good Sex: Feminist Perspectives from the World's Religions.* New Brunswick, NJ: Rutgers University Press, 2005.

Kaleeba, Noerine. *Open Secret: People Facing Up to HIV and AIDS in Uganda.* Series: Strategies for Hope, no. 15. London: ACTIONAID, 2000.

________. *We Miss You All: AIDS in the Family.* Harare, Zimbabwe: Women and AIDS Support Network, 1991.

Kaufman, Philip S. *Why You Can Disagree and Remain a Faithful Catholic.* New York: Crossroad, 2000.

Keane, Philip S. *Health Care Reform: A Catholic View.* New York: Paulist Press, 1993.

________. *Sexual Morality: A Catholic Perspective.* New York: Paulist Press, 1977.

Keating, James, ed. *Moral Theology: New Directions and Fundamental Issues.* New York: Paulist, 2004.

Keenan, James F., S. J. "Prophylactics, Toleration, and Cooperation: Contemporary Moral Problems and Traditional Principles." *International Philosophical Quarterly* 28 (1988): 201–220.

________. "Proposing Cardinal Virtues." *Theological Studies* 56:4 (1995): 709–729.

________. *Virtues for Ordinary Christians.* Franklin, WI: Sheed and Ward, 1999.

Keenan, James F., S. J., Jon D. Fuller, S .J., M. D., Lisa Sowle Cahill, and Kevin T. Kelly, eds. *Catholic Ethicists and HIV/AIDS Prevention.* New York: Continuum, 2000.

Kelly, David. *Critical Care Ethics* (Kansas City, MO: Sheed & Ward, 1991), 204–209. See also James Drane, "Condoms, AIDS, and Catholic Ethics," *Commonweal* 189. 1991.

Kelly, Kevin T. *New Directions in Sexual Ethics: Moral Theology and the Challenge of AIDS.* London: Geoffrey Chapman, 1998.

Kennedy, C. A. "Gender Differences in HIV-Related Psychological Distress in Heterosexual Couples." *AIDS Care* 7:1 (1995): S33–S38.

Kidder, Tracy. *Mountains Beyond Mountains: The Quest of Dr. Paul Farmer, A Man Who Would Cure the World.* New York: Random House, 2003.

King, Cheryl [pseud.]. Interviewed by the author. Chicago, IL, October 18, 2006, July 15, 2014.

Kippley, John and Sheila. *The Art of Natural Family Planning.*

Kissioki, Seelah, Charlotte Hartwig, and Kari Hartwig. "Church Leaders Confront HIV/AIDS and Stigma: A Case Study from Tanzania," *Journal of Community and Applied Social Psychology* 16. 2006.

Laufer, Franklin N. "Cost Effectiveness of Syringe-Exchange as an HIV Prevention Strategy," *Journal of the Acquired Immune Deficiency Syndrome* 28. 2001.

Lawler, Michael G. *Marriage and the Catholic Church: Disputed Questions.* Collegeville, MN: Liturgical Press, 2002.

Lawler, Michael G., and William P. Roberts, eds. *Christian Marriage and Family: Contemporary, Theological, and Pastoral Perspectives.* Collegeville, MN: Liturgical Press, 1996.

Leo XIII, *Rerun novarum*, no. 9. See also Michael J. Schuck, *That They Be One: The Social Teaching of the Papal Encyclicals 1740–1989*. Washington, DC: Georgetown University Press, 1991.

Levenson, Jacob. *The Secret Epidemic: The Story of AIDS and Black America*. New York: Pantheon Books, 2004.

Lindberg, L. "Changes in Formal Sex Education: 1995-2002," *Contraception* 74:2. August 2006.

Lonergan, Bernard. "The Transition from a Classicist World-View to Historical Mindedness." In *Law for Liberty: The Role of Law in the Church Today*, ed. James E. Biechler, 126–33. Baltimore: Helicon, 1967.

Lorde, Audre. "An Open Letter to Mary Daly." In *Sister Outsider*, 66–71. Trumansburg, NY: The Crossing Press Feminist Series, 1984.

________. *The Cancer Journals*. San Francisco, CA: Aunt Lute Books, 1980.

Machung, Anne, and Arlie Hothschild. *The Second Shift: Working Parents and the Revolution at Home*. New York: Viking, 1989.

Mackin, Theodore. *The Marital Sacrament*. New York: Paulist Press, 1989.

________. *What Is Marriage? Marriage in the Catholic Church*. New York: Paulist Press, 1982.

Mahoney, John. *The Making of Moral Theology: A Study of the Roman Catholic Tradition*. Oxford: Oxford University Press, 1987.

Massachusetts Bishops, "Sex Education: Information or Formation?" *Origins* 17. December 31, 1987.

Massaro, Thomas J. *Catholic Social Teaching and United States Welfare Reform*. Collegeville, MN: Liturgical Press, 2002.

Massingale, Bryan N., Reverend. "Stigma: The Other Virus," Presentation, National Catholic AIDS Network Annual Clergy and Religious HIV/AIDS Roundtable. Chicago, IL: Loyola University Chicago, June 2, 2006.

Martey, Emmanuel. "Church and Marriage in African Society: A Theological Appraisal." *African Theological Journal* 20:2 (1991): 136–147.

Martos, Joseph. *Doors to the Sacred: A Historical Introduction to Sacraments in the Catholic Church*, expanded ed. Liguori, MO: Liguori/Triumph, 1991.

McAreavey, John. *The Canon Law of Marriage and the Family*. Dublin, Ireland: Four Courts Press, 1997.

McCormick, Richard A. S.J., "*Humanae vitae* 25 Years Later," in Odozor, *Sexuality, Marriage*, 478-485.

McIntosh, Peggy. "Unpacking the Invisible Backpack." *Independent School* 49:2 (Winter 1990): 31–36.

Melton, Sue [pseud.]. Interviewed by the author. July 18, 2006, July 3, 2014.

Mendoza, Lettie [pseud.]. Interviewed by the author. July 14, 2006, September 9, 2007. Personal communication with loved ones occurred on November 1, 2007, July 6, 2014, July 8, 2014, and July 9, 2014.

Mertens, Jennifer. "Catholic Sex Ed 101: How Can the Church Empower Teen Girls?" *National Catholic Reporter*. June 20–July 3, 2014.

Messer, Donald E. *Breaking the Conspiracy of Silence: Christian Churches and the Global AIDS Crisis*. Minneapolis, MN: Fortress Press, 2004.

Miller, J. Michael, ed. *The Encyclicals of Pope John Paul II*. Huntington, IN: Our Sunday Visitor, 2001.

Miller-McLemore, Bonnie J. "Family and Work: Can Anyone 'Have It All'?" in Anne Carr and Mary Stewart Van Leeuwen, eds., *Religion, Feminism, and the Family*. Louisville, KY: Westminster John Knox Press, 1996.

Mohrmann, Margaret E., M.D., *Attending Children: A Doctor's Education*. Washington, DC: Georgetown University Press, 2005.

________. *Medicine as Ministry: Reflections on Suffering, Ethics, and Hope*. Cleveland, OH: Pilgrim Press, 1995.

Moller, David Wendell. *Dancing with Broken Bones: Portraits of Death and Dying Among Inner-City Poor*. Oxford: Oxford University Press, 2004.

Morenoff, Jeffrey, and Robert J. Sampson. "Violent Crime and the Spatial Dynamics of Neighborhood Transition: Chicago 1970–1990." *Social Forces* 76 (1997): 31–64.

National Center for Health Statistics. *Health, United States, 2007*. Hyattsville, MD: United States Department of Health and Human Services National Center for Health Statistics, 2007.

National Conference of Catholic Bishops Committee on Pastoral Practices. *Faithful to Each Other Forever: A Catholic Handbook of Pastoral Help for Marriage Preparation*. Washington, DC: United States Conference of Catholic Bishops, 1988.

National Institutes of Allergy and Infectious Diseases (NIAID). "HIV Infection and AIDS: An Overview." October 2007. Accessed March 11, 2008. http://www.niaid.nih.gov/factsheets/hivinf.htm.

Nelms, Bobbie Crew. "Adolescent Sex Education: Making It a Priority," *Journal of Pediatric Health Care* 17:5. Sept/Oct 2003.

Noonan, John T., Jr. *A Church that Can and Cannot Change: The Development of Catholic Moral Teaching*. Notre Dame, IN: University of Notre Dame Press, 2005.

_______. "Contraception: The Doctrine and the Context," in Paulinus Ikechukwu Odozor, C. S. Sp., ed., *Sexuality, Marriage, and Family: Readings in the Catholic Tradition*. Notre Dame, IN: University of Notre Dame Press, 2001.

Nothwehr, Dawn M. *Mutuality: A Formal Norm for Christian Social Ethics*. Eugene, OR: Wipf & Stock, 1998.

Nouwen, Henri J. M. *Life of the Beloved: Spiritual Living in a Secular World*. New York: Crossroad, 1992.

O'Brien, David J., and Thomas A. Shannon, eds. *Catholic Social Thought: The Documentary Heritage*. Maryknoll, NY: Orbis, 1992.

O'Collins, Gerald, S. J. and Edward G. Farrugia, S. J. *A Concise Dictionary of Theology*, Rev. Ed. New York: Paulist, 2000.

O'Donnell, T.J. *Medicine and Christian Morality*, 2nd ed. New York: Alba House, 1991.

Okie, Susie. "Sex, Drugs, Prisons, and HIV." *New England Journal of Medicine*. 365:2 (11 January 2007): 105–108.

O'Neill, Mary Aquinn. "The Mystery of Being Human Together." In *Freeing Theology: The Essentials of Theology in Feminist Perspective*, ed. Catherine Mowry LaCugna. New York: HarperCollins, 1993.

Orsy, Ladislas. *The Church Learning and Teaching: Magisterium, Assent, Dissent, Academic Freedom*. Collegeville, MN: Liturgical, Press, 1991.

________. *Marriage in Canon Law: Texts and Comments, Reflections and Questions*. Wilmington, DE: Michael Glazier, 1986.

Ortega, Mariana. "Being Lovingly, Knowingly Ignorant: White Feminism and Women of Color." *Hypatia* 21:3 (Summer 2006): 56–74.

Outka, Gene. *Agape: An Ethical Analysis*. New Haven, CT: Yale University Press, 1972.

Paterson, Gillian. *Women in the Time of AIDS: Women, Health, and the Challenge of HIV*. Maryknoll, NY: Orbis, 1996.

Patrick, Anne. *Liberating Conscience: Feminist Explorations in Catholic Moral Theology*. New York: Continuum, 1996.

Patton, Michael Quinn. *Qualitative Evaluation and Research Methods*, 2nd ed. Newbury Park, CA: Sage, 1990.

Paul VI. *Humanae vitae*. In *The Papal Encyclicals, 1958-1981*, ed. Claudia Carlen, 223–36. Wilmington, NC: McGrath, 1981.

Peters, Edward N., ed. *The 1917 or Pio-Benedictine Code of Canon Law*. San Francisco, CA: Ignatius Press, 2001.

Pew Research Center. "Breadwinner Moms." May 29, 2013. Accessed June 23, 2014.http://www.pewresearch.org/key-data-points/gay-marriage-key-data-points-from-pew-research/.

Phelps, Jamie T. *Black and Catholic: The Challenge and Gift of Black Folks*. Milwaukee: Marquette University Press, 1997.

Phiri, Isabel Apawo, and Sarojini Nadar, eds. *African Women, Religion, and Health: Essays in Honor of Mercy Amba Ewudziwa Oduyoye*. Maryknoll, NY: Orbis, 2006.

Piux XI, *Casti connubii*, no. 26. Accessed July 9, 2014. http://www.vatican.va/holy_father/pius_xi/encyclicals/documents/hf_p-xi_enc_31121930_casti-connubii_en.html.

Pope Francis. Apostolic Exhortation *Evangelii Gaudium: The Joy of the Gospel*. Washington DC: United States Conference of Catholic Bishops, 2013.

Pope, Stephen. "Expressive Individualism and True Self-Love: A Thomistic Perspective." *Journal of Religion* 71:3 (1991): 384–99.

Procter-Smith, Marjorie. "Images of Women in the Lectionary." In *The Power of Naming: A Concilium Reader in Feminist Liberation Theology*, ed. Elisabeth Schussler Fiorenza, 175–186. Maryknoll, NY: Orbis, 1996.

Purvis, Sally. "A Common Love: Christian Feminist Ethics and the Family," in *Religion, Feminism, and the Family*, ed. Anne Carr and Mary Stewart Van Leeuwen. Louisville, KY: Westminster John Knox Press, 1996.

Ramirez, Carmen [pseud.]. Interviewed by the author. Chicago, IL, August 13, 2006, July 8, 2014.

Reid Jr., Charles J. "The History of the Family," in *Concilium 1995/4: The Family*. Maryknoll, New York: Orbis, 1995.

Richardson, Lynda. "Condoms in School Said Not To Affect Teenage Sex Rate," *New York Times*. September 30, 1997.

Risch, Gail S., and Lisa A. Riley, and Michael G. Lawler. "Problematic Issues in the Early Years of Marriage: Content for Premarital Education," *Journal of Psychology and Theology* 31. 2003.

Risch, Gail S., and Michael G. Lawler. Time, Sex, and Money: The First Five Years of Marriage," *America*. May 14, 2001.

Ross, Susan A. "The Bride of Christ and the Body Politic: Body and Gender in Pre-Vatican II Marriage Theology." *Journal of Religion* 71 (1991): 345–61.

________. *Extravagant Affections: A Feminist Sacramental Theology*. New York: Continuum, 1998.

________. *For the Beauty of the Earth: Women, Sacramentality, and Justice*. 2006 Madaleva Lecture in Spirituality. New York: Paulist Press, 2002.

________. "Liturgy and Ethics: Feminist Perspectives." In *Annual of the Society of Christian Ethics* 20 (2000): 263–74.

Rubio, Julie Hanlon. *A Christian Theology of Marriage and Family*. New York: Paulist, 2003.

Ruether, Rosemary Radford. "Birth Control and the Ideals of Marital Sexuality." In *Contraception and Holiness: The Catholic Predicament*, ed. Thomas D. Roberts, 72–91. New York: Herder and Herder, 1964.

________. *Christianity and the Making of the Modern Family*. Boston: Beacon Press, 2000.

________. *Sexism and God-Talk: Towards a Feminist Theology*. Boston, MA: Beacon Press, 1983.

Ryan, Maura. "Beyond a Western Bioethics?" *Theological Studies* 65 (2004): 158–177.

________. *Ethics and Economics of Assisted Reproduction: The Cost of Longing*. Washington, DC: Georgetown University Press, 2001.

Sacred Congregation of Rites. *Rite of Marriage*. Collegeville. MD: The Liturgical Press, 1970.

Salzman, Todd A., ed. *Method and Catholic Moral Theology: The Ongoing Reconstruction*. Omaha: Creighton University Press, 1999.

________. *What Are They Saying about Catholic Ethical Method?* New York: Paulist, 2003.

Salzman, Todd A, and Michael G. Lawler, *Sexual Ethics: A Theological Introduction*. Washington DC: Georgetown University Press, 2012.

Sampson, Robert J., Jeffrey D. Morenoff, and Stephen Raudenbush, "Social Anatomy of Racial and Ethnic Disparities in Violence." *American Journal of Public Health* 95 (2005): 224–232.

Sanders, E.P. *Jesus and Judaism* (Minneapolis: Fortress, 1985); John Dominic Crossan, *The Historical Jesus: The Life of a Mediterranean Jewish Peasant*. New York: Harper, 1993.

Scharen, Christian, and Aana Marie Vigen. *Ethnography as Christian Theology and Ethics*. New York: Continuum, 2011.

Schneiders, Sandra, IHM. *Beyond Patching: Faith and Feminism in the Catholic Church*. New York: Paulist, 1991.

_______. *The Revelatory Text: Interpreting the New Testament as Sacred Scripture*. San Francisco, CA: Harper, 1991.

_______. *Women and the Word*. New York: Paulist, 1986.

Schott, Robin May. *Discovering Feminist Philosophy: Knowledge, Ethics, Politics*. Lanham, MD: Rowman & Littlefield, 2003.

Schuller, Eileen. "Women in the Lectionary." *National Liturgy Bulletin* (Canada) 27 (1994).

Searle, Mark, ed. *Liturgy and Social Justice*. Collegeville, MN: Liturgical Press, 1980.

Seewald, Peter. *Light of the World*. San Francisco: Ignatius Press, 2010.

Second Vatican Council. *Dogmatic Constitution on Divine Revelation (Dei Verbum)*. November 18, 1965.

_______. *Gaudium et Spes*: Pastoral Constitution on the Church in the Modern World. December 7, 1965.

Selling, Joseph A., ed. *Embracing Sexuality: Authority and Experience in the Catholic Church*. Burlington, VT: Ashgate, 2001.

Sharpe, Ursula, with Noerine Kaleeba. *Witness to Faith: AIDS and Development in Africa*. Series: Pope Paul VI Memorial Lectures. London: CAFOD, 1993.

Shilts, Randy. *And the Band Played On: Politics, People, and the AIDS Epidemic*. New York: St. Martins Press, 1987.

Siplon, Patricia D. *AIDS and the Policy Struggle in the United States*. Washington, DC: Georgetown University Press, 2002.

Smith, Crystal [pseud.]. Interviewed by the author. Chicago, IL, August 3, 2006.

Somfai, Bela. "AIDS, Condoms, and the Church," *Compass*. November 1987.

Sontag, Susan. *AIDS and Its Metaphors*. New York: Farrar, Straus, and Giroux, 1988.

_______. *Illness as Metaphor*. New York: Farrar, Straus, and Giroux, 1977.

Spohn, William C. *Go and Do Likewise: Jesus and Ethics*. New York: Continuum, 1999.

Spradley, James P. *The Ethnographic Interview*. New York: Holt, Rinehart, and Winston, 1979.

Stevenson, Kenneth W. *Nuptial Blessing*. London: Alcuin, 1982.

_______. *To Join Together: The Rite of Marriage*. New York: Pueblo, 1987.

Stillwaggon, Eileen. *Ecology of AIDS*. New York: Oxford, 2006.

_______. *Ecology of Poverty*; Paul Farmer, Margaret Connors, Janie Simmons, Eds, *Women, Poverty, and AIDS: Sex, Drugs, and Structural Violence*. Monroe, ME: Common Courage Press, 1996.

Substance Abuse and Mental Health Services Administration, *Results from the 2009 National Survey on Drug Use and Health, vol. 1: Summary of National Findings* (NSDUH Series H-38A, HHS Publication No. SMA 10-4856). Rockville, MD: Office of Applied Studies, 2010.

Sulmasy, Daniel P., O. F. M. "Catholic Participation in Needle- and Syringe-Exchange Programs for Injection-Drug Users: An Ethical Analysis" *Theological Studies* 73. 2012.

Teaford, Jon C. "Urban Renewal and Its Aftermath." *Housing Policy Debate* 11, no. 2 (2000): 443–465.

"The Deadly After-Effect of Abortion: Breast Cancer," "The Pill," "Tubal Ligation," and "Vasectomy." Cincinnati, OH: The Couple to Couple League.

"The First Three Years: They're Important." Cincinnati, OH: Foundation for the Family, 1999.

Thiel, John E. *Senses of Tradition: Continuity and Development in Catholic Faith*. Oxford: Oxford University Press, 2000.

Thomas, David M. *Christian Marriage: The New Challenge*. Collegeville, MN: Liturgical Press, 2007.

Thorsen, Donald A. D. *The Wesleyan Quadrilateral: Scripture, Tradition, Reason, and Experience as a Model of Evangelical Theology*. Grand Rapids, MI: Zondevan, 1990.

Tillich, Paul. *Love, Power, and Justice*. London: Oxford University Press, 1954.

Tillman, Fritz. *The Master Calls: A Handbook of Christian Living*. Baltimore, MD: Helicon Press, 1960.

Townes, Emilie M., ed. *A Troubling in My Soul*. Maryknoll, NY: Orbis, 1993.

_______. *Breaking the Fine Rain of Death: African American Health Issues and a Womanist Ethic of Care*. New York: Continuum, 2001.

_______. *Womanist Ethics and the Cultural Production of Evil*. New York: Palgrave Macmillan, 2006.
Traina, Cristina L.H. *Feminist Ethics and Natural Law: The End of the Anathemas*. Washington, DC: Georgetown University Press, 1999.
_______. "Papal Ideals, Marital Realities: One View from the Ground." In *Sexual Diversity and Catholicism: Toward the Development of Moral Theology*, ed. Patricia Beattie Jung and Joseph Andrew Coray, 269–88. Collegeville, MN: Liturgical Press, 2001.
Trelstad, Marit A. *Cross Examinations: Readings on the Meaning of the Cross Today*. Minneapolis, MN: Fortress, 2006.
Trible, Phyllis. *Texts of Terror: Literary-Feminist Readings of Biblical Narratives*. Philadelphia, PA: Fortress, 1984.
Trussell, James, and Laurence Grummer-Strawn. "Contraceptive Failure of the Ovulation Method of Periodic Abstinence," *Family Planning Perspectives* 22. March/April 1990.
UNAIDS. "AIDS by the Numbers 2013." Geneva, Switzerland: UNAIDS, 2013.
_______. *AIDS Epidemic Update 2007, with Global Summary*. Geneva, Switzerland: UNAIDS, 2007.
_______."Call for Urgent Action to Improve Coverage of HIV Services for Injecting Drug Users." March 2010. Accessed July 30, 2014. http://www.unaids.org/en/Resources/PressCentre/Featurestories/2010/March/20100310IDU/.
_______. *Women and HIV/AIDS: Confronting the Crisis*. New York: United Nations Publications, 2004.
_______. "World AIDS Day Report." Geneva, Switzerland: UNAIDS, 2012.
United Nations Department of Economic and Social Affairs. *Population, Development, and HIV/AIDS with Particular Emphasis on Poverty: The Concise Report*. New York: United Nations Publications, 2005.
United States Conference of Catholic Bishops. Accessed January 25, 2008.
www.foryourmarriage.org.
United States Conference of Catholic Bishops. *Marriage: Love and Life in the Divine Plan*. Washington, DC: USCCB Publishing, 2009.
United States Census. Current Population Survey (CPS), 2013 Annual Social and Economic Supplement (ASEC). Accessed June 23, 2014. https://www.census.gov/hhes/www/poverty/about/overview/.
UNFPA. *State of the World Population 2004: The Cairo Consensus at Ten-Population, Reproductive Health and the Global Effort to End Poverty*. New York: United Nations Populations Fund, 2004.
UN Millennium Project. *Taking Action: Achieving Gender Equality and Empowering Women. Task Force on Education and Gender Equality*. Sterling, VA: Earthscan, 2005.
United States Catholic Conference Administrative Board. *The Many Faces of AIDS: A Gospel Response*. In *Origins* 17:28 (December 24, 1987): 481–493.
United States Catholic Bishops. *Called to Compassion and Responsibility: A Response to the HIV/AIDS Crisis*. In *Origins* 19:26 (December 5, 1989): 423-436.
_______. *Economic Justice for All*. In *Catholic Social Thought: The Documentary Heritage*, ed. David J. O'Brien and Thomas A. Shannon, 572–680. Maryknoll, NY: Orbis, 1992.
_______. *Ethical and Religious Directives for Catholic Health Care Services*, 4ed. Washington, DC: USCCB Publishing, 2001.
_______. *Faithful Citizenship: A Catholic Call to Political Responsibility*. In *Origins* 33 (2003): 321–330.
_______. "Pastoral Letter on Health and Health Care." In *Medical Ethics: Sources of Catholic Teaching*, ed. Kevin D. O'Rourke and Philip Boyle, 264–67. St. Louis, MO: Catholic Health Association of the United States, 1989.
United States Conference of Catholic Bishops, *When I Call For Help*. Washington, DC: United States Conference of Catholic Bishops, 2002.
Vacek, Edward Collins. *Love, Human and Divine: The Heart of Christian Ethics*. Washington, DC: Georgetown University Press, 1994.

Varvaro, W. A. "Prohibition Against Marriage of AIDS Victims," in *Roman Replies and Canon Law Society of America Advisory Opinions*. Washington, DC: Canon Law Society of America, 1987.

Wallace, Rodrick. "A Synergism of Plagues: 'Planned Shrinkage,' Contagious Housing Destruction, and AIDS in the Bronx." *Environmental Research* 47 (1988).

Walker, Keesha [pseud.]. Interviewed by the author. Chicago, IL, August 4, 2006.

Walker, Sharon E. *Women with AIDS and their Children*. New York: Garland, 1998.

Ward, Darrell E. *The AmFAR AIDS Handbook: The Complete Guide to Understanding HIV and AIDS*. New York: W.W. Norton & Company, 1999.

Weaver, Darlene Fozard. *Self Love and Christian Ethics*. New York: Cambridge University Press, 2002.

________. "Taking Sin Seriously." *Journal of Religious Ethics* 31:1 (March 2003): 45–74.

Weaver, J. Denny. *The Nonviolent Atonement*. Grand Rapids, MI: Eerdmans, 2001.

Weiss, Robert S. *Learning from Strangers: The Art and Method of Qualitative Interview Studies*. New York: Free Press, 1994.

Whitehead, Evelyn Eaton, and James D. Whitehead. "Marriage Becomes a Journey," in *Perspectives on Marriage: A Reader*, 2nd ed., ed. Kieran Scott and Michael Warren. New York: Oxford University Press, 2001.

Whiteside, Alan. *HIV/AIDS: A Very Short Introduction*. New York: Oxford University Press, 2008.

Whitmore, Todd David. "Crossing the Road: The Case for Ethnographic Fieldwork in Christian Ethics." *Journal of the Society of Christian Ethics* 27:2 (2007): 273–294.

Wiley, Tatha. *Original Sin: Origins, Developments, Contemporary Meanings*. Mahwah, NJ: Paulist, 2002.

Williams, Delores. *Sisters in the Wilderness*. Maryknoll, NY: Orbis, 1993.

Williams, Lee M., Lisa A. Riley, Gail S. Risch, and David T. Van Dyke. "An Empirical Approach to Designing Marriage Preparation Programs," *American Journal of Family Therapy* 27. 1999.

Wodak, Alex, and Annie Cooney. "Do Needle Syringe Programs Reduce HIV Infection among Injecting Drug Users? A Comprehensive Review of the International Evidence," *Substance Use and Misuse* 41. 2006.

Wolfe, W.R., et al. "Effects of HIV-related stigma among an early sample of patients receiving antiretroviral therapy in Botswana," *AIDS Care* 18:8. 2006.

World Council of Churches Global Consultation on Ecumenical Responses to the Challenges of HIV/AIDS in Africa, "Plan of Action," Adopted in Nairobi, Kenya, November 28, 2001.

World Health Organization. *Effectiveness of Sterile Needle and Syringe Programming in Reducing HIV/AIDS Among IDUs: Evidence for Action Technical Paper and Policy Brief.* Geneva: World Health Organization, 2004.

_______. *HIV Transmission through Breastfeeding: A Review of Available Evidence*. Geneva, Switzerland: World Health Organization Publications, 2004.

Varvaro, W. A. "Prohibition Against Marriage of AIDS Victims," in *Roman Replies and CLSA Advisory Opinions*. 1987.

Vigen, Aana Marie. *Women, Ethics, and Inequality in U.S. Healthcare: To Count Among the Living*. New York: Palgrave Macmillan, 2006.

Vlahov, D., and B. Junge. "The Role of Needle Exchange Programs in HIV Prevention." *Public Health Reports*. June 1998.

Vogt, Christopher P. "Fostering a Catholic Commitment to the Common Good: An Approach Rooted in Virtue Ethics," *Theological Studies* 68. 2007.

_______. "Locating the Church in the World: Ethnography, Christian Ethics, and the Global Church." *Journal of Moral Theology* 2:2 (2013): 158–172.

Yin, Robert. *Case Study Research: Designs and Methods*. Thousand Oaks, CA: Sage, 1994.

Young, Pamela Dickey. *Feminist Theology/Christian Theology: In Search of Method.* Minneapolis, MN: Fortress, 1990.

Index

About the Author

Emily Reimer-Barry holds a Ph.D. in Christian Ethics from Loyola University Chicago. She is assistant professor in the Department of Theology and Religious Studies at the University of San Diego, where she teaches undergraduate courses in Catholic theology, sexual ethics, and Catholic social thought. Emily is particularly interested in the intersection of social ethics and sexual ethics. Her publications include an article co-authored with Melissa Browning, entitled "Preaching, Sexuality, and Women Religious: Listening to Prophetic Voices at the Margins of Religious Life," in *Theology and Sexuality* (2013), and an article, "HIV Prevention for Incarcerated Populations: A Common Good Approach," in the *Journal of the Society of Christian Ethics* (2011). She has also contributed to edited volumes on ethnography and feminist ethics, and writes for the blog http://www.catholicmoraltheology.com. Emily remains committed to developing and maintaining collaborative relationships with research partners, and has continued to do fieldwork and community-based research in her new home of San Diego, California. For more information about her work, visit her website at http://www.emilyreimerbarry.com.